Population Policies Reconsidered

Health, Empowerment, and Rights

This volume is published under an arrangement with the Swedish International Development-ment Authority (SIDA), as part of the Swedish contribution to the United Nations Conference on Population and Development, Cairo 1994. This contribution also includes four other volumes, listed below:

Understanding Reproductive Change — Kenya, Tamil Nadu, Punjab, Costa Rica. Edited by Bertil Egerö and Mikael Hammarskjöld, Programme on Population and Development. PROP. Published by Lund University Press, Sweden.

The Challenge of Complexity — Third World Perspectives on Population Research. Edited by Tomas Kjellqvist. Published by SAREC, the Swedish Agency for Research Cooperation with Developing Countries, Sweden.

Women, Children, and Work in Sweden 1850–1993, by Ann-Sofie Ohlander. Published by the Ministry for Foreign Affairs, Sweden.

Sex Education and Reproductive Health in Sweden in the 20th Century, by Marc Bygdeman and Katarina Lindahl. Published by the Ministry for Foreign Affairs, Sweden.

Population Policies Reconsidered

Health, Empowerment, and Rights

Gita Sen
Adrienne Germain
Lincoln C. Chen

EDITORS

Harvard Center for Population and Development Studies

Department of Population and International Health
Harvard School of Public Health
Boston, Massachusetts

International Women's Health Coalition
IWHC
New York, New York

March 1994
Distributed by Harvard University Press

HARVARD SERIES ON POPULATION AND INTERNATIONAL HEALTH

Library of Congress Cataloging-In-Publication Data

Population policies reconsidered : health, empowerment, and rights/
    Gita Sen, Adrienne Germain, Lincoln C. Chen, editors.
        p.   cm. – – (Harvard series on population and international
    health)
        "March 1994"
        Includes bibliographical references and index.
        ISBN Number 0-674-69003-6 (pbk.) : $14.95
        1. Population Policy.   I. Sen, Gita.   II. Germain, Adrienne.
    III. Chen, Lincoln C.   IV. Series.
    HB883.5.P65 1994
    363.9– –dc20   94-8443
                                                                          CIP

International Women's Health Coalition (IWHC)
24 East 21 Street
New York, NY 10010
(212) 979-8500

Harvard Center for Population and Development Studies
9 Bow Street
Cambridge, MA 02139
(617) 495-0000

Books in the Harvard Series on Population and International Health

Population Policies Reconsidered: Health, Empowerment and Rights
Edited by Gita Sen, Adrienne Germain and Lincoln C. Chen

Power & Decision: The Social Control of Reproduction
Edited by Gita Sen and Rachel Snow

Health and Social Change in International Perspective
Edited by Lincoln C. Chen, Arthur Kleinman and Norma C. Ware

Assessing Child Survival Programs in Developing Countries
By Joseph J. Valadez

Table of Contents

Tables and Figures iii

Boxes v

Contributors vii

Preface xiii

Overview

1. Reconsidering Population Policies: Ethics, Development, and Strategies for Change 3
   Gita Sen, Adrienne Germain, and Lincoln C. Chen

Section One: Premises Re-Examined

2. Population and Ethics: Expanding the Moral Space 15
   Sissela Bok

3. Setting a New Agenda: Sexual and Reproductive Health and Rights 27
   Adrienne Germain, Sia Nowrojee, and Hnin Hnin Pyne

4. Challenges from the Women's Health Movement: Women's Rights versus Population Control 47
   Claudia García-Moreno and Amparo Claro

5. Development, Population, and the Environment: A Search for Balance 63
   Gita Sen

6. Population, Well-being, and Freedom 75
   Sudhir Anand

Section Two: Human Rights and Reproductive Rights

7. Honoring Human Rights in Population Policies:
    From Declaration to Action 89
    Reed Boland, Sudhakar Rao, and George Zeidenstein

8. Reproductive and Sexual Rights: A Feminist Perspective ... 107
    Sônia Correa and Rosalind Petchesky

Section Three: Gender and Empowerment

9. The Meaning of Women's Empowerment:
    New Concepts from Action 127
    Srilatha Batliwala

10. Women's Burdens: Easing the Structural Constraints 139
    Sonalde Desai

11. Women's Status, Empowerment, and
    Reproductive Outcomes 151
    Simeen Mahmud and Anne M. Johnston

12. Gender Relations and Household Dynamics 161
    Alayne Adams and Sarah Castle

Section Four: Reproductive and Sexual Health

13. Reproductive and Sexual Health Services:
    Expanding Access and Enhancing Quality 177
    Iain Aitken and Laura Reichenbach

14. A Reproductive Health Approach to the Objectives
    and Assessment of Family Planning Programs 193
    Anrudh Jain and Judith Bruce

15. Reaching Young People: Ingredients of
    Effective Programs 211
    Kirstan Hawkins and Bayeligne Meshesha

16. Fertility Control Technology: A Women-Centered
    Approach to Research 223
    Mahmoud F. Fathalla

17. Financing Reproductive and Sexual Health Services 235
    Jennifer Zeitlin, Ramesh Govindaraj, and Lincoln C. Chen

Abbreviations and Acronyms 249
Index 253

Tables and Figures

Chapter 3
Table 1   Interpretations of Quality of Care Concepts 35

Chapter 6
Figure 1   Male and Female Life Expectancy at Birth,
           and GNP Per Capita, 1990 78

Chapter 10
Table 1   Results from Time-Use Studies in Developing Countries 141
Table 2   Proportion of Time Potentially Spent Living
           Apart from Mother or Living with Mother Only
           by Country through Age 15 144
Figure 1   A Model of Child Health and Survival 146

Chapter 12
Table 1   Percent of Children Living Away from
           Their Biological Mother by Age in West Africa 165
Figure 1   Women's Life Cycle in West Africa 167
Figure 2   Women's Roles throughout the Life Cycle
           in West Africa 169

Chapter 13
Table 1   Reproductive and Sexual Health Problems,
           Estimated Impacts, Program Interventions 179
Figure 1   Distribution of Disease Burden in Disability-Adjusted
           Life Years (DALYs) Lost in Demographically Developing
           Countries, 1990 181
Figure 2   Percentage of DALYs Lost Contributed by Reproductive
           Health Problems, Women Aged 15-44, by Region 181
Table 2   Cost-Effectiveness of Reproductive Health Interventions..... 182
Figure 3   Births Attended by Trained Personnel, by Region, 1985 184
Table 3   Reproductive Health Tasks at Different Levels of Care 186

Chapter 14
Figure 1   Classification of Clients According to Success or Failure...... 202
Figure 2   Percentage of Women Using a Specified Method at 30
           Months after the Initiation of an IUD, Compared with
           1967-70 HARI Index, Taiwan 204
Figure 3   HARI Index for Selected Countries...................................... 205

Chapter 16

Table 1   Contraceptive Prevalence in the Developing
          World by Region 225
Table 2   Percentage Distribution of Contraceptive Users by
          Method in Developed and Developing Countries 226
Figure 1   The Annual Number of New Cases of Sexually
          Transmitted Disease Worldwide 229
Figure 2   Steps in Contraceptive Research and Development 233

Chapter 17

Table 1   Projected Resource Requirements for Population
          Programs in the Year 2000 237
Figure 1   Percentage Distribution of Health and Population
          Expenditures, and of World Population, by
          Type of Economy, 1990 240
Table 2   Regional Population and Health Public-Sector
          Expenditures in Developing Countries, 1990
          ($U.S. millions) 240
Table 3   Selected Developing Countries Categorized
          according to Percentage of Contraceptive Users
          Served by the Commercial Private Sector 241
Table 4   Population Aid Disbursements by Major Donors,
          1990 ($U.S. millions) 242
Figure 2   Health and Population Aid Disbursements, 1990
          ($U.S. millions) 243
Figure 3   Percentage Distribution of External Assistance to
          Health and Population Sectors, and to Reproductive
          Health Services, by Program Type, 1990 244
Table 5   External Assistance to Health and Population Sectors,
          by Program Type, 1990 ($U.S. millions) 245

Boxes

Chapter 1
Box 1   Excerpts from the Harare Statement
by Parliamentarians 12

Chapter 2
Box 1   Definitions of Population 16

Chapter 3
Box 1   Women's Declaration on Population Policies
(In Preparation for the 1994 International
Conference on Population and Development) 31
Box 2   Meeting Women's Sexual and Reproductive
Health Needs in Sierra Leone 38
Box 3   Meeting Male Reproductive Health Needs
in Latin America 40

Chapter 4
Box 1   Examples of Women-Centered Government
Health Policies 50

Chapter 7
Box 1   Excerpts from John D. Rockefeller 3rd's Address
at the World Population Conference, 1974 92
Box 2   Population Policies in China 98

Chapter 9
Box 1   Women's Mobilizing: Anti-Liquor Agitation
by Indian Women 133
Box 2   Empowerment: Three Approaches 136

Chapter 10
Box 1   Why Holistic Approaches Are Needed 140
Box 2   Taking Care of Our Children: The Experiences
of SEWA Union 136

Chapter 11
Box 1   The Consequences of Forced Marriage
in a South African Community 155
Box 2   Marriage under Customary Law
in Sub-Saharan Africa 156

Chapter 12
Box 1   Calculating the Value of a Woman 164
Box 2   Conflicting Loyalties: Marital Obligations and
             Natal Affiliations in West Africa 168

Chapter 13
Box 1   Controlling HIV and Sexually Transmitted Diseases 180
Box 2   The Loneliness of a Front-Line Health Worker 187
Box 3   Silent Endurance: Women in Rural Egypt 188
Box 4   Integrating Women's Health into Development: BRAC in
             Bangladesh 189

Chapter 15
Box 1   Reaching Young People in Ethiopia 218

Chapter 16
Box 1   Reproductive Suffering in History 224
Box 2   Excerpts from the Declaration of the International
             Symposium, "Contraceptive Research and
             Development for the Year 2000 and Beyond" 231

Chapter 17
Box 1   Are Reproductive Health Services Affordable? 246

Contributors

Alayne Adams is a David E. Bell/MacArthur Fellow at the Harvard Center for Population and Development Studies, where she is pursuing research in household demography, food security, and nutrition. A graduate of McGill University, she completed her doctorate at the London School of Hygiene and Tropical Medicine on seasonal food insecurity, and nutritional, social, and economic risk among agriculturalists in central Mali.

Iain Aitken is a medical graduate from the University of Cambridge. After specialty training in tropical medicine and pediatrics, he spent fifteen years in the development of health systems and the training of physicians and other health workers in Papua New Guinea, West Africa, and the Middle East. He became interested in reproductive health because he found it to be a neglected area. He joined the faculty of the Harvard School of Public Health in 1989 and continues his work in reproductive health with the World Health Organization and in Africa and Asia.

Sudhir Anand is Fellow in Economics at St. Catherine's College, Oxford, and Visiting Professor at the Harvard Center for Population and Development Studies. His current research interests include inequality, poverty, food, and undernutrition in developing countries. He is the author of *Inequality and Poverty in Malaysia: Measurement and Decomposition*, as well as of numerous articles in development economics. Dr. Anand is a graduate of Oxford University, where he received a B.A. and an M.A. in mathematics, and a B.Phil. and D.Phil. in economics.

Srilatha Batliwala is an activist and researcher. Currently coordinating DAWN (Development Alternatives with Women for a New Era) activities in India, she was formerly director of Mahila Samakhya Karnataka, a government-sponsored project for the education and empowerment of women. She has worked in both rural and urban grass-roots programs, and has focused on women's empowerment issues for the past decade.

Sissela Bok is a Distinguished Fellow at the Harvard Center for Population and Development Studies. Dr. Bok, a former Professor of Philosophy at Brandeis University, has written extensively in the fields of medical ethics, practical ethics more generally, literature, and biography. She is the author of *Lying: Moral Choice in Private and Public Life*; *Secrets: On the Ethics of Concealment and Revelation*; *A Strategy for Peace: Human Values and the Threat of War*; and *Alva Myrdal: A Daughter's Memoir*. A graduate of George Washington University, she received her Ph.D. from Harvard University.

Reed Boland is Editor-in-Chief of the *Annual Review of Population Law*, published jointly by Harvard Law School and the United Nations Population Fund. Dr. Boland is a leading researcher in world-wide reproductive health law and has published articles on such topics as abortion, RU-486, population policy, family planning, and assisted reproduction. Dr. Boland, a graduate of Cornell, received his Ph.D. from Harvard University and his J.D. from Harvard Law School.

Judith Bruce holds a B.A. from Harvard University in biological anthropology. She has worked extensively in Asia, the Middle East, and Africa. As Senior Associate in the Programs Division of the Population Council, she coordinates a program of policy-oriented research and field projects related to women's productive and reproductive roles. In the reproductive health field, Ms. Bruce's primary contribution has been a framework to evaluate quality of care. She coordinates two programs at the Population Council: Women's Roles and Status, and Improving Reproductive Health Care. In both of these programs, numerous articles, case studies, and volumes of readings for use by development scholars and practitioners have been published.

Sarah Castle is a Mellon Fellow at the Population Studies and Training Center at Brown University, where she is pursuing research in the household determinants of children's care and illness management. Formerly a David E. Bell/MacArthur Fellow at the Harvard Center for Population and Development Studies, Dr. Castle completed her Ph.D. at the London School of Hygiene and Tropical Medicine, examining intrahousehold variations in female status and their impact on children's health outcomes among the Malian Fulani.

Lincoln C. Chen is Taro Takemi Professor of International Health at the Harvard School of Public Health and Director of the Harvard Center for Population and Development Studies. Dr. Chen, a public health physician, worked with the Ford Foundation in India and Bangladesh and the International Center for Diarrhoeal Disease Research, Bangladesh, for 14 years before joining

Harvard in 1987. His interests include health, population, and international development policy research. Dr. Chen, a graduate of Princeton, received his M.D. from Harvard Medical School, and his master's degree in Public Health from Johns Hopkins University.

Amparo Claro has been working with Isis International since 1984. She is in charge of the Latin American and Caribbean Women's Health Network (LACWHN), which has a membership of about 2,000 groups and organizations, mostly from Latin America. She is Director of the LACWHN publications, *Revista* (Spanish) and *Women's Health Journal* (English). As a therapist working for social change, she has conducted workshops in diverse communities on sexuality, bodily awareness, and well-being, emphasizing reproductive rights. She has been involved in Chile's feminist movement since its inception, as well as in the creation of the Women's House — "La Morada."

Sônia Correa, DAWN Research Coordinator on Population and Reproductive Rights, is a Brazilian researcher and activist from SOS Corpo, of which she is a founding member. In 1991, Ms. Correa was awarded a grant from the Brazilian Fellowship Program of the John D. and Catherine T. MacArthur Foundation to develop conceptual interlinkages and international networking across the overlapping fields of gender, development, population, and reproductive rights. She is also a member of the Brazilian Commission on Citizenship and Reproduction and of the Brazilian Association of NGO's Collective Boards. She holds degrees in architecture and anthropology.

Sonalde Desai is currently an Associate in the Research Division of the Population Council. She received an M.A. in sociology from Case Western Reserve University and a Ph.D. in sociology from Stanford University. Dr. Desai's research interests include social demography, family sociology, fertility in developing countries, gender stratification in labor markets, and the effect of women's employment on child development.

Mahmoud F. Fathalla, M.D., Ph.D., FACOG (Hon.), FRCOG (Hon.), Dr. Hon. Causa (Uppsala), is Senior Advisor for Biomedical and Reproductive Health Research at the Rockefeller Foundation, and Professor of Obstetrics and Gynecology at Assiut University, Egypt. He is President-Elect of the International Federation of Gynecology and Obstetrics, Chairman of the International Medical Advisory Panel of the International Planned Parenthood Federation, and former director of the WHO Special Program of Research, Development and Research Training in Human Reproduction.

Claudia García-Moreno was until recently the Oxfam Health Unit Coordinator in Oxford, England. She has worked in primary health care in development and refugee settings. From 1984 to 1993 she worked for Oxfam, overseeing health programs, mainly in Africa and Latin America. Her current interests include primary health care, women's health, AIDS, and population and development. She hold a degree in medicine from LaSalle University and an M.Sc. in Community Medicine from the London School of Hygiene and Tropical Medicine.

Adrienne Germain is Vice-President of the International Women's Health Coalition in New York. Ms. Germain served with the Ford Foundation for 14 years and was the Foundation's country representative in Bangladesh from 1981 to 1985. Since 1985, Ms. Germain has worked with IWHC to support women's health advocates, donors, and international agencies to bring the perspectives and voices of women into decision making on population policies and programs. Ms. Germain, a graduate of Wellesley, holds an M.A. in Sociology from the University of California, Berkeley.

Ramesh Govindaraj is a Research Associate at the Harvard Center for Population and Development Studies. He is a physician with an M.S. in Health Policy and Management from the Harvard School of Public Health, where he is currently pursuing a doctorate in International Health Policy and Economics. Before coming to Harvard in 1992, Dr. Govindaraj was International Projects Director for Southeast Asia and the Pacific for Johnson & Johnson International, Inc. His research interests include pharmaceutical policy and the financing of health care — including the economics of reproductive health.

Kirstan Hawkins is a Research Officer with the International Planned Parenthood Federation. She is a social anthropologist by training and is currently carrying out part-time research for a doctoral thesis at the Centre for Development Studies, University of Swansea. Her research interests are developmental anthropology and the cultural contexts of fertility. She is also trained in social work and has practiced as a youth counselor. During her work with IPPF, she has taken a particular interest in the development of sexual and reproductive health programs for young people.

Anrudh Jain, Ph.D., is Senior Associate and Deputy Director, Programs Division, of the Population Council. His current interests include activities designed to broaden the content of population policy and improve the quality of care in family planning programs. He has extensive experience working with professionals and institutions in developing countries; analyzing and evaluating family planning programs; and assessing the fertility impact of development projects. As Deputy Director of the Programs Division, he assists the Director in program development and management of the Council's activities overseas. He has published extensively in international journals and has co-edited *Fertility in Asia: Assessing the Impact of Development Projects* and *Infant Mortality in India: Differentials and Determinants*. He was the editor of *Managing Quality of Care in Population Programs*.

Anne M. Johnston is a David E. Bell/MacArthur Fellow at the Harvard Center for Population and Development Studies. She has served as both Director of Women in Development and Advisor for Women, Health, and Population in the South Pacific for the Australian International Development Assistance Bureau. In these capacities, she represented Australia on the OECD DAC Expert Group for Women in Development. Ms. Johnston has a master's degree in public health from the University of Minnesota. She has lectured in the United States, Australia, and South East Asia and conducted extensive fieldwork throughout the South Pacific, Central America, and the Caribbean in gender and environment, community health, and population development.

Simeen Mahmud was a David E. Bell/MacArthur Fellow at the Harvard Center for Population and Development Studies in 1992–1993. Currently, she is a Research Fellow in the Population Studies Division at the Bangladesh Institute for Development Studies. Ms. Mahmud holds a M.Sc. in Medical Demography from the London School of Hygiene and Tropical Medicine. Her research interests include: the influence of women's work on status and reproduction, women's entrepreneurship in water selling and its impact on productivity, and evaluating the effect of development interventions on women's lives.

Bayeligne Meshesha has been Manager of the Youth Counselling and Family Planning Services Project for the Family Guidance Association of Ethiopia since its inception in 1990. Mr. Meshesha has worked with adolescents for over a decade as both teacher and headmaster, and as program officer in an NGO that dealt with child sponsorship programs. He holds a degree from Addis Ababa University in Educational Administration. He is involved in the development of youth programs for adolescent reproductive health.

Sia Nowrojee is a consultant in sexual and reproductive health. She was formerly Assistant Program Officer for Global Policy at the International Women's Health Coalition, where she coordinated work on sexuality and gender and population issues. Ms. Nowrojee has a master's degree in clinical social work from the Bryn Mawr College Graduate School of Social Work and Social Research. She has worked in Kenya and in the United States in women's health and family planning clinics and adolescent health and sexuality programs.

Rosalind Pollack Petchesky is a Professor of Political Science and Women's Studies at Hunter College of the City University of New York. Her book *Abortion and Woman's Choice: The State, Sexuality and Reproductive Freedom* (1990, revised edition) and many published articles on reproductive rights and feminist theory have been translated into several languages. She has been an activist in feminist movements for reproductive rights and gender equality in New York City, the United States, and worldwide since the 1970s.

Hnin Hnin Pyne is an AIDS specialist in the Asia technical department of the World Bank. She received her master's degree in planning from the Massachusetts Institute of Technology, concentrating on gender and development. Her thesis research focused on AIDS and prostitution of Burmese women in Thailand. As a David E. Bell/ MacArthur Fellow at the Harvard Center for Population and Development Studies in 1992– 1993, she continued to work in the areas of women's reproductive health and rights.

Sudhakar Rao is a member of the Indian Administrative Service, with 20 years of diverse work experience at both the policy-making and implementation levels. He holds a master's degree in economics from the Delhi School of Economics and a master's degree in public administration from Harvard University. He was a Visiting Fellow at the Harvard Center for Population and Development Studies in 1992–1993, where he worked on issues concerning health and population.

Laura Reichenbach completed her master's degree in public administration from the John F. Kennedy School of Government at Harvard and is currently pursuing a doctorate in international health policy and economics at the Harvard School of Public Health. She is interested in the policy and management issues affecting the development of women's reproductive health policy.

Gita Sen is a Professor of Economics at the Indian Institute of Management, Bangalore, and an Adjunct Professor of Development Economics at the Harvard Center for Population and Development Studies. A leading researcher on women-in-development, Dr. Sen is pursuing policy research on women, development, health and population, and the environment. She is a founding member of DAWN, Development Alternatives with Women for a New Era. Dr. Sen received an M.A. from the Delhi School of Economics and a Ph.D. in economics from Stanford University.

George Zeidenstein is a Distinguished Fellow at the Harvard Center for Population and Development Studies. From 1976 until 1993, he was President of the Population Council. He is a graduate of Harvard Law School and has devoted his career to public service since the summer of 1964, when he served in Mississippi and Arkansas as a volunteer lawyer in support of a campaign to register African-American voters. For the next 30 years, Mr. Zeidenstein was a public sector entrepreneur and executive, living with his family for several years in South Asia and traveling widely for work throughout developing countries. He is the author of many articles and speeches concerning population policy and international development. He was decorated in recognition of his work by the presidents of Finland and Senegal.

Jennifer Zeitlin is a doctoral candidate in the Department of Population and International Health at the Harvard School of Public Health, and a David E. Bell/MacArthur Fellow at the Harvard Center for Population and Development Studies. Her current research is on women's labor-force participation and its impact on demand for health services and on maternal and child health. Ms. Zeitlin has worked on public health projects in India, Indonesia, Bangladesh, Mexico, France, and the United States. She holds a graduate degree in International Relations from the Institut d'Études Politiques de Paris.

Preface

Population Policies Reconsidered brings together an unusual combination of scholars, social activists, and policy-makers from diverse backgrounds and many disciplines — ethics and law, demography, and the social and health sciences — to critically re-examine population policies and family planning programs.

Late in 1992, the editors of the volume and staff of the Swedish International Development Authority (SIDA) realized that fresh, dynamic, and forceful critiques of population policies and family planning programs were emerging rapidly, especially from women who have too long been voiceless in policy formulation and implementation. We agreed, therefore, to produce a volume by academics and women's health advocates who would jointly review the underlying premises, field experiences, and the scientific literature, in order to propose directions for the future.

In putting the book together, we invited the authors to freely probe and debate selected topics. While diversity and independence characterize the final contributions, the invitations to authors were based on our sense of the critical issues to be explored and our sense that population policies can and should be defined within a broader human development approach.

Initially we considered the task of articulating new directions for population policies, based upon the universally accepted goals of health, empowerment, and human rights, to be relatively straightforward. The writing of the pa-

pers, however, proved to be far more demanding. A series of weekly seminars during the spring of 1993 and a special authors' workshop that May at the Harvard Center for Population and Development Studies highlighted the complexity and contentiousness of the themes and strategies to be addressed. Terminologies varied, value systems clashed, and scientific methods differed between disciplines. There was also the daunting task of creating a balanced synthesis of science and the voices of diverse groups whose insights come from experience.

A preponderance of the authors are associated with the sponsoring institutions and countries of the editors, and we are keenly aware of the resulting regional imbalances. Furthermore, because we are breaking new ground, we found few national-level population policies or large-scale programs based on a human development approach. Nonetheless, the authors marshall considerable evidence to support such an approach.

The seventeen chapters address the cutting edge of current debates on population policies. Although none of the contributions provides definitive answers, all raise provocative questions, challenge established thinking, and propose specific ways to transform population policies to place central importance on overcoming poor health, lack of reproductive choice, poverty, and oppression. Our aim is to contribute to a new consensus on policy directions for the twenty-first century.

Population Policies Reconsidered represents only one stop in a journey of discovery. With thirty contributors and three editors scattered around the world, the logistics of bringing this volume to fruition within a very short time-frame was indeed complex. For helping us complete this first leg, we are grateful to many people, including Laura Reichenbach, Liz Pelcyger, Sarah Hemphill, Deborah Smullyan, Winifred Fitzgerald, and Charlie Mitchell of the Harvard Center for Population and Development Studies. We appreciate the fine work of Edith Barry, Gail Cooper, and Dore Hollander in copy editing and production. Special thanks go to Carmen Díaz-Olivo of the International Women's Health Coalition (IWHC) for her commitment under pressure; to Jane Ordway, also of IWHC, for her editorial and management expertise; and to David Bell, Sissela Bok, and Ruth Dixon-Mueller, who provided continuing and penetrating advice on the draft manuscripts.

Most of all, we are grateful to SIDA for its generous financial support of the project, and to Göran Dahlgren, Anna Runeborg, Nils Öström, and Eva Wallstam, who initiated and provided continuing moral support for this book.

Gita Sen
Adrienne Germain
Lincoln Chen

Overview

1

Reconsidering Population Policies: Ethics, Development, and Strategies for Change[1]

Gita Sen, Adrienne Germain, Lincoln Chen

The twentieth century has witnessed many human achievements — dazzling technological breakthroughs, unparalleled economic prosperity, remarkable advances in human survival, and the transition of former colonial states to political independence. The fruits of progress, however, have not been equitably shared. Much of humankind still lives in poverty, and many material gains have been achieved through means that ravage the resource base upon which we and future generations depend. Eradicating mass poverty, protecting human rights, stabilizing the environment, empowering people — especially women — and rectifying economic inequities between North and South and rich and poor, are among the major challenges of our times. Attaining equitable and sustainable development between and within nations is thus an unfinished agenda that will carry us well into the next century.

To what extent can population policies, in their current forms, contribute to achieving these objectives? How must population policies be transformed to maximize their contributions to human well-being? How can they be translated into effective program strategies?

In this introduction, we address these ques-

tions: first by reviewing contemporary population policies, and second by providing an overview of the themes of this book. Throughout the volume, three major themes recur that challenge the fundamental premises of current population policies — ethics, human rights, and human development; women's empowerment; and reproductive and sexual health. These themes together present a new approach to population based on a solid ethical foundation and aimed at sustainable human development.

Contemporary Population Policies

Dramatic changes in the demographic characteristics of the world's population are a hallmark of this century. At no earlier time in human history has the number, composition, and distribution of human populations undergone such rapid and profound transitions. Since their beginnings four decades ago, modern population policies have sought to manage some of these demographic changes, principally, rapid population growth in high-fertility countries. The major instrument employed has been family planning programs. About half of all couples in the world now use contraception, but contraceptive services are by no means universally accessible or afford-able. As many as one-third of all pregnancies end in induced abortion, often illegally and with great hazard to women's health and even their lives. To buttress family planning programs, population policies have also supported social and demographic research to identify the determinants and consequences of demographic change, and biomedical research to develop safer and more effective fertility control technologies.

The population field has undergone many changes, as lessons from experience have been incorporated into policy and action. The 1950s and 1960s witnessed the emergence of neo-Malthusian concerns that too many people reproducing too rapidly retards economic growth, destroys the environment, overstretches social services, exacerbates poverty, and fuels conflict. As a consequence, the population field promoted public understanding and support for birth control, the development of better contraceptive technologies, and family planning programs around the world. Northern governments went to the 1974 World Population Conference at Bucharest with the position that family planning programs should be the primary means to achieve population control. Many Southern countries countered that "development is the best contraceptive," arguing that equitable socio-economic development was the answer to perceived demographic threats. This debate was partly reflective of, and strengthened emergent understanding of, the relationships among advances in education, the status of women, and human fertility.

By the 1980s, family planning activities had expanded greatly throughout the developing world. This growth occurred despite the chilling effect of the United States government's position at the 1984 World Population Conference in Mexico City that population growth is a "neutral" phenomenon. At the same time, dissatisfaction with vertical contraceptive delivery systems[2] designed to achieve demographic goals became widespread among diverse groups, including actual and potential clients, the women's health movement, health professionals, social scientists, and some

family planning providers. The United Nations Decade of Women, the Child Survival movement, and the Safe Motherhood Initiative brought new actors into the debate who promoted integration of family planning with broader programs for health and women's advancement. Paradoxically, the 1980s also witnessed shifts in development policies away from the 1970s' interest in poverty alleviation and meeting basic human needs, toward macroeconomic policies that emphasized economic growth, fiscal responsibility, and reduction of state-provided social services.

In the 1990s, alarm in some quarters over impending environmental catastrophe has refocused public and political attention on population, the environment, and development. A crisis mentality has even generated extreme assertions that population control should take precedence over other development investments and can be successful in settings of entrenched poverty and human underdevelopment. Many consider such narrow demographic approaches to be neither ethically sound nor effective. Reconsideration of population policies is urgently needed to resolve these conflicting views and re-establish a strong consensus for public action.

Throughout this recent history, the basic premise of population policy has remained unchanged. Government (public) intervention has been thought to be necessary to influence or control individual (private) action in the interest of the common good. Demographically driven population policies have assumed that individual welfare would be advanced by collective action to assist, persuade, or induce individuals to increase or decrease their fertility to meet socially desirable goals. This premise has come increasingly under fire, and population policies are at a crossroads.

Furthermore, the social context of reproduction and sexual relations is dramatically different in the 1990s than in previous decades. The STD/HIV/AIDS pandemics, international economic crises, deterioration in social services, widespread infringements of human rights, environmental degradation, and a resurgence of conservatism that opposes modern fertility regulation and women's advancement powerfully affect people's lives. At the same time, new voices, earlier dormant or suppressed, have emerged. In particular, women's health activists have joined the debate. They have diverse ideologies and deep roots in the community, and are therefore increasingly accepted as legitimate advocates for those who have been too often the objects, and not the subjects, of population policies.

Population Policies Reconsidered examines the ethical basis, the objectives, and the methods of current population policies. In challenging these specific population policies, we strongly support — in its own right — a human development approach within which reproductive health, empowerment, and rights are central objectives. The enabling environment thus created for women and men to decide if and when they want children is — from a population policy point of view — the focal point. Empirical evidence clearly indicates that this approach, in most societies, is closely related to reduced fertility. Furthermore, a human development approach is essential to ensure adequate planning to accommodate additional people who will be born. Within this approach, demographic facts would be used, along with others, to plan for improved living conditions and sustainable development for all.

Population Policies Reconsidered

Section I of this book, "Premises Reconsidered," offers a wide-ranging exploration of population policies: their ethical implications, linkages with development and the environment, and the perspectives of women's health advocates. Together, the five chapters challenge the fundamental premises of contemporary policies and make powerful arguments for transforming them to be compatible with our growing understanding of how population, development, human rights, and the environment are linked. This opening section is followed by three others that assess how new policies should be designed.

The two chapters of Section II, "Human Rights and Reproductive Rights," find that existing international documents, treaties, and declarations concerned with population, women, and human rights are often ambiguous and mutually contradictory. The authors propose reformulation of population policies based on an unambiguous acceptance of universal human rights, including not only civil and political rights but also social and economic rights.

The two remaining sections review program strategies and methods that are essential to translate this new vision into practice. In Section III, "Gender and Empowerment," four chapters underscore the centrality of women's empowerment as a strategy. The section argues for a shift from passive concepts of women's education and status to promotion of social changes necessary to achieve women's empowerment. Sustained leadership and organization by women, generation of political will, provision of basic infrastructure and social services to reduce women's triple workloads, and fundamental changes in the power dynamics between women and men, as well as among women themselves, are proposed.

Section IV, "Reproductive and Sexual Health Services," describes the challenges to be met if family planning programs are to be improved and made more effective in providing reproductive and sexual health services. The five chapters outline several key actions required, including redefining the objectives of family planning programs; improving their quality and effectiveness; expanding their coverage to reach all those in need, including young people; improving fertility regulation technologies; and enhancing resource allocation. All of these proposals are well within the reach of sound public policy.

Ethics and Human Development

Three major themes echo throughout the book. The first is that population policies should be transformed to reflect a fundamental commitment to ethics and human rights. The second is that population policies, rather than concentrating simply on fertility control, can only be effective and humane as part of broader human development approaches that create an enabling environment within which people can attain their health and rights. The third theme gives priority to two strategies: women's empowerment and reproductive and sexual health services.

Ethical Underpinnings

In the population field, research has been undertaken on specific ethical issues — for example, the rights of human subjects in biomedical research, flagrant abuses of human rights such as compulsory abortion or sterilization, and the ethics of using incentives and disincentives. More fundamental questions need, however, to be systematically considered.

Where an imbalance of power exists between the objects and the formulators of policy, or where class or gender disparities are severe, how much and what kind of intervention by the state is ethical? For instance, in what circumstances, if any, can the state override individual interest in reproduction? What if the pronatalist behavior of an individual is driven by dependence on child labor for survival or old-age security? What if it is driven by women's need to produce sons in a patriarchal society that values boys over girls? Is the state obligated in such cases to provide remedial measures while advocating birth control? Can or should policy-makers be entrusted to define the social interest? Many people in Southern countries do not trust the motives of Northern governments in promulgating population control policies, and many poor women and men in the South do not trust the functionaries of state-operated family planning programs. Can such trust be built? What if a society has few functioning institutional mechanisms for appeal or redress of grievances, especially those of the poor and powerless, against an omnipotent state or international agencies? How can abuses be prevented and redressed? What is the appropriate and ethically acceptable balance between the quantity and the quality of services?

What are an individual's rights and responsibilities vis-à-vis his or her sexual partner and society? What does it mean to decide "freely *and* responsibly"? Should women's biological and social positioning in reproduction give primacy to their choices and also their voices in the definition of rights and responsibilities? What are men's responsibilities regarding reproduction, transmission of disease, and their children's well-being? How can men be encouraged to assume more responsibility for their own behavior without compromising women's autonomy?

Sissela Bok notes that such ethical issues, which lie at the heart of controversies about current population policies and family planning programs, have often been glossed over or ignored altogether. She suggests that it is essential to define clear ethical guidelines, both for the objectives of policies and also for the means employed to implement them. In the rapidly changing and uncertain terrain of population policy, Bok argues that an "expansion of moral space" for dialogue is critical to the development of an ethically sound consensus on the rights and responsibilities of citizens and the nation state.

Sudhir Anand asserts the ethical soundness of viewing "population" as people, not as instruments to serve some impersonal economic objective. He argues that the intrinsic importance of individual well-being and freedom, including the right of reproductive choice and the reduction of inequalities, especially between women and men, far outweighs an instrumental rationale for population control in the alleged interest of the social good.

Reed Boland, Sudhakar Rao, and George Zeidenstein find that lack of clarity in population documents, together with the fact that these documents are not legally binding on states, means that abuses of human rights, when they occur in population programs, have no legal basis for correction. While human rights and women's rights instruments that are legally binding could, the authors suggest, be used to better effect, population policies should themselves be reformulated, based on unqualified respect for individual human rights and gender equity. Such policies would, among other actions, accord primacy to the choices of women, who bear most of the biological and social burden of reproduction.

Sônia Correa and Rosalind Petchesky define

reproductive and sexual rights on the basis of four principles: bodily integrity, personhood, equality, and respect for diversity. These rights include both the power to make informed decisions about one's own fertility, child-bearing, gynecological health, and sexual activity, and access to resources to carry out such decisions safely and effectively. Like other contributors, Correa and Petchesky conclude that states should be obliged to provide the enabling conditions (social welfare, personal security, and political freedom) required for realization of reproductive rights and responsible choices. By grounding rights in their social context and spelling out correlative duties of the state, the authors dissolve the boundaries among human rights, sexuality, reproduction, and development. In so doing, they offer a basis for a feminist social-rights approach to population and development.

These four chapters, together with the women's health movement agendas described by Claudia García-Moreno and Amparo Claro, make a compelling case for giving primacy to individual well-being and rights, and for reconciling these with public concerns in consistently humane and balanced ways.

Sustainable Human Development

Debate over population policies comes at a time of profound and rapid transitions in the world economy and the everyday lives of ordinary people. The "lost decade" of the 1980s brought economic stagnation and crisis to many economies. Mass poverty persists and has probably worsened, in both the South and the North. Economic adjustment programs imposed on many Southern countries have helped only a few. Many now believe that the conditions of life and the livelihoods of large numbers of poor people, especially women and girls, have worsened as a result of development policies favoring macroeconomic stabilization. In contexts where the financial and institutional bases for health and education are being eroded by macroeconomic policies, the priority accorded by some funding agencies to population control as a precondition

for development assistance seems disingenuous, at best. These economic difficulties have been accompanied by massive over-consumption of energy and resources in most Northern countries, which are also promoting a global private market for the free flow of goods and services.

Left unchecked, these economic and market forces can be extremely unfriendly to people's economic and social security. If population stabilization is to be achieved with human dignity, without coercion, and without inordinate burdens imposed on women, then investments must be channeled to poverty alleviation, universal access to health care and education, and the advancement of equity — all as part of sustainable and human development.

How can population policies be made compatible with newer theories of human development? In reviewing the literature on equitable human development and poverty alleviation, Sudhir Anand concludes that population policies should be directly aimed at advancing people's well-being and freedom. They should foster enabling conditions both on their own merit and as a means to achieve human development. Such population policies would introduce critical new dimensions to customary notions of human development. Individuals' control over their reproduction and sexuality, gender equity, and freedom and empowerment would complement and strengthen the narrower focus of human development programs on health, education, and income.

A particularly important aspect of the linkages between population and human development is the interaction between people and the environment. Gita Sen, recognizing that data on population–environment relationships are inconclusive at best, questions environmentalists' rationale for narrow population control strategies. She argues that espousal of top-down population control runs counter to the tactics of mobilizing people's energies that have been so central to the best of the environmental movement. Sen concludes that policies that build on popular participation and directly address human development needs have both moral value and efficacy. Further, they provide a basis on which environmentalists and women's health activists can build alliances for strategies that promote secure livelihoods, basic needs, and gender equity, not just economic development.

Sonalde Desai argues that population and development policies must also recognize and alleviate, rather than exacerbate, women's already-heavy burdens of household maintenance, childbearing and child-rearing, income generation, and community participation. This requires increased investment in, among other things, basic infrastructure for water and sanitation, and access to fuel.

Strategies for Change

How would population policies that are ethically sound and reinforce human development translate into program strategies? We focus on two means: first, empowering women in order to overcome one of the most pernicious inequities in the distribution of resources, as well as in the exercise of human rights; and second, providing reproductive and sexual health services. These two strategies are priorities in their own right. While they are not alone sufficient, they are necessary for the achievement of human development goals and of population stabilization with dignity and without coercion.

Empowering Women

Population policies can play a major role in rectifying the power imbalances between women and men that severely constrain achievement of human development and population goals.

The vital role played by the international women's health movement in shifting the objectives of population policy towards women's empowerment is documented by Claudia García-Moreno and Amparo Claro. They describe how those with the most at stake personally in the population debate have succeeded in making their voices heard at national and international levels. Bringing to bear grassroots experience, communications skills, networking, advocacy,

and astute political positioning, women's health advocates have challenged the ethical as well as practical dimensions of population policies and family planning programs. At the same time, they have argued strongly for increased investment in human development and equity, giving central importance to women's empowerment, including their self-defined needs, their creativity and efficacy, and their right to accountability from policy agents, communities, and men.

But what exactly does "empowerment" mean? Srilatha Batliwala explains that empowerment views women as active subjects and agents, not as passive objects, of social change. Her assessment of the rich program experiences of South Asia demonstrates that changing power relations across many levels of society is a complex process requiring many different actions. Three possible strategies — economic self-sufficiency and security, integrated development, and consciousness-raising — all place primary importance on the power of women in groups, rather than simply as individuals, to challenge existing oppressive gender relations, alter the distribution and control of resources, and address the wider practical and strategic needs of women.

While empowering women requires fundamental changes at many levels of society, arguably the most complex and elusive transformations may be in the relations within the household and family. Alayne Adams and Sarah Castle examine women's reproductive decisionmaking within the dynamics of households in Sub-Saharan West Africa. The authors demonstrate that women's empowerment requires changes not only in the relationships between women and men, but also in power relations among women across generations. They conclude that younger women who bear the main burdens of reproduction and have the least power need more policy and program attention.

The concept of empowerment is relatively new to the population field. Simeen Mahmud and Anne Johnston review the literature on the relationships between fertility, women's status, their education, and employment, and conclude that most of it uses vague concepts of "women's status," or concentrates on the relationship between female education and fertility. The narrow, instrumental focus on female education has had at least three questionable consequences. First, it has masked the multifaceted nature of gender relations as relations of power that subordinate women to the will of others — in households, villages, communities, labor and other markets, and vis-à-vis the state. These relations determine women's access to both material and nonmaterial resources, their ability to control their bodies and their lives, and their decision-making capability. Second, an overemphasis on formal education downplays other aspects of gender relations and disparities that affect women's reproductive health and their health generally. Third, the emphasis on education alone ignores the state's responsibility to provide reproductive health services, clean water, sanitation, and other basic needs that also critically affect reproductive outcomes. While education can certainly help reduce some power imbalances, the millions of highly educated women who have little reproductive control bear testimony to the fact that education ("schooling") is not enough. Furthermore, pious assertions of the value of girls' and women's education have ignored the many changes necessary to make it possible for girls and women to have access to education.

Promotion of women's empowerment — in concept, language, and practice — can help bridge the distance between women's rights language increasingly used in policy statements, and the actual implementation of population policies, which continues to emphasize contraceptive services. As important, because women's empowerment requires changes in male power and dominance, an empowerment approach would increase policy and program attention to male responsibility for their own fertility, disease transmission, and child care.

Exercising reproductive control means making decisions, not only about contraception, but also about other sexual and reproductive health needs, and about sexuality itself. Women's ability to make decisions requires alterations in power relations within the *home* between women and men, and between younger and older women; within the *community*, which generates and enforces a wide range of sanctions and practices affecting health, from son preference to female genital mutilation; vis-à-vis the *state*, whose functionaries and policy-makers ignore or downgrade women's concerns; and in relation to the *scientific community*, whose research and technology development determine the fertility regulation technologies women and men can choose from.

Providing Reproductive and Sexual Health Services

Our proposed transformation of population policies requires redefinition of the objectives, expansion of the scope, and improvements in the quality of sexual and reproductive health services to serve all of those in need. Adrienne Germain, Sia Nowrojee, and Hnin Hnin Pyne offer a new agenda to assure healthful, voluntary reproduction, to prevent and control STDs and HIV/AIDS, to reduce gender-based violence, and to promote mutually caring and responsible sexual relationships. This agenda, espoused by most women's health advocates, includes broader information and services for women, programs to encourage men's responsibility for their own sexual behavior, and research and action to promote healthful and equitable sexuality and gender relations.

As Anrudh Jain and Judith Bruce point out, progress toward achieving such an agenda requires redefinition of family planning program objectives to focus on human well-being, rather than on demographic targets. The measure of success would be an individual's ability to undertake sexual relations and reproduction in a healthful manner, rather than measures such as numbers of contraceptives delivered or births averted, which are currently used to evaluate family planning programs.

Authors differ on the range of services that can be realistically offered. While recognizing the ideal goal of comprehensive reproductive health services and basic health care for all, Jain and Bruce argue for a more limited constellation of reproductive health services in the short run, with emphasis on improving their quality. On the other hand, Iain Aitken and Laura Reichenbach propose a more comprehensive group of sexual and reproductive health services, arguing that this larger cluster of services ranks highly in terms of cost-effectiveness, and that together they reinforce each other's effectiveness. The efficacy of integrated services would therefore justify or even outweigh the costs. Among the many challenges to be met, Aitken and Reichenbach identify three: technical and social support for health workers to ensure strong provider–client relationships; functional linkages among community, health center, and hospital; and integration of services to attain program efficacy.

Kirsten Hawkins and Bayeligne Meshesha assert that the young and unmarried, who often are excluded from family planning services although they are at great risk of STDs, violence, and unwanted pregnancy, must have access to reproductive and sexual health services. Furthermore, they propose significant changes in conventional population education and family-life education programs to ensure that these programs are relevant to the lives of young people today, engage young people as full participants in their design and implementation, enable them to make informed and effective choices about sexuality and reproduction, and foster more equitable gender relations.

Another comparatively neglected clientele is men. It is not sufficient, nor is it equitable, simply to "empower" women to use services or to support their children. Germain, Nowrojee, and Pyne propose increased attention to men, not simply to persuade them to "allow" women to practice birth control, but to encourage their own participation in and responsibility for fertility regulation, disease prevention, and child-rearing.

A necessary component of services is, of course, fertility regulation technologies. Mahmoud Fathalla argues for a women-centered approach to contraceptive research based on collaboration among women's health activists, scientists, and policy makers. This research agenda gives priority to the development and introduction of women-controlled methods that protect against STDs (with and without concomitant protection against unwanted conception), post-ovulatory methods such as menses inducers, and safe male methods. Fathalla points out that achievement of this agenda will require reinvigorated science that is gender-sensitive, and also greatly enhanced resources from both the public sector and private industry.

The final chapter in the book, by Jennifer Zeitlin, Ramesh Govindaraj, and Lincoln Chen, examines current levels of and approaches to financing reproductive and sexual health services. The authors demonstrate that existing projections of resource requirements, especially in the population field, are both methodologically flawed and based on restrictive assumptions about the services to be provided (generally contraceptives only). Better estimates of the likely costs of the various components of reproductive and sexual health services are essential, along with sharper assessment of the sources and flows of financing, especially by developing countries themselves. In most Southern countries, population and health investments are currently at levels far below those required to achieve reproductive health and rights. Even the lowest-income countries, however, have scope to accelerate health expenditures by (for example) reducing military expenditures and corruption. International development assistance can play a critically important role in promoting increased allocation of resources to reproductive and sexual health and rights.

Population Policies: A New Vision

Although the terms "health," "empowerment," and "human rights" are being increasingly used in population discourse, the words have not yet been sufficiently translated into action. Several arguments have repeatedly been raised for retaining narrow population policies. Some point to the estimated 100 million married women of reproductive age at risk of unwanted pregnancy who do not yet have access to contraceptive services.

Others assert that improving the quality and extending the scope of services would require resources far beyond those currently or foreseeably available. Still others argue that this new approach should not be labelled "population," because the scope has been so broadened that it encompasses all of human and sustainable development.

We argue that investing in people's health, empowerment, and human rights is not only worthy in its own right, but would probably be more conducive to population stabilization than narrowly conceived policies of population control. Nearly all Northern countries that have achieved population stabilization have done so through promoting better quality of life rather than explicitly trying to reduce population growth. Policies that are supportive of human development would also offer a sound ethical basis for resolving some of the most vexing contradictions in the field. Although most population policies affirm that people have the right "freely and responsibly" to decide on the number and spacing of children, many family planning programs exclude youth, the unmarried, and even men from information and services; fail to provide safe and legal abortions; emphasize quantity rather than quality of services; and in too many circumstances use compulsion or coercion. Policies founded on health, empowerment, and rights would reduce such contradictions, promote fresh program approaches, and foster close collaboration with other development sectors.

This new population approach would be distinct from, as well as complement, current approaches to both sustainable and human development, for several reasons. First, beyond the customary focus of human development on education, infant mortality, and income, transformed population policies would add human reproduction and

sexuality as inalienable components of sustainable and human development. Second, the proposed empowerment and reproductive health service strategies would complement current human development programs. Finally, the approach would be inclusive and participatory, giving voice and decision-making power to those with the most at stake in human reproduction and sexuality.

This new vision of population policies does not call for a retreat from government intervention in population affairs. Rather, it seeks a qualitative shift in state actions to promote the quality of life and the services that could advance human well-being and freedom into the next century. As documented throughout this book, and as reflected in recent statements by parliamentarians (see Box 1 on next page), powerful momentum for such a transformation of population policies already exists.

As worldwide debate intensifies over the distribution and use of resources, opportunities for employment and livelihoods, and peace and security, so also are pressures generated to advance the alleged public good over individuals' well-being and liberties. If we are to promote human rights and grapple humanely and successfully with demographic change, we must accord primacy to the quality of life and equity for everyone. Through such an approach, population policies would reinforce social and economic advances that not only could encourage smaller family sizes but also would provide decent living standards for all.

Notes

1 The editors are solely responsible for this chapter's contents.

2 International agencies and governments have tended to segment related health services — such as contraception, child health, and "safe motherhood" — into separate, or "vertical," budget categories and delivery systems.

Excerpts from the Harare Statement by Parliamentarians

The population concept has to be reconsidered. We must find constructive views, well founded and relevant to the men and women who are the final executors of every population policy. Population policies can seldom be treated as such; you have to find out how they are related to other issues. We note that countries which have reached a balanced development make no effort to limit their population, but rather stress improving living qualities. It is important to develop population related issues as education, housing, water facilities and health services.

Why an ethical dimension?

Sexuality and reproduction constitute the very heart of human life. It is a fundamental human right that men as well as women should be met with dignity and concern for their individual problems. Population issues must respect the integrity of the individual and comprehend the deeply personal interests involved in these private matters.

Why a gender approach?

We believe that it is important to find a gender balanced approach to population issues. Thus we are concerned about the empowerment of women as well as men - women being disregarded in many places in their roles outside the family, while men have been neglected in their important roles within the family as fathers and husbands.

Teenagers and their perspectives

The future of any society lies in the integration of social and cultural norms with individual perspectives and expectations in the transitory and formative stage of life called teenage. In Africa, teenagers are not only omitted in most family planning programmes, they are increasingly left without traditional guidance.

Quality of reproductive health services

Quality of care implies a continuity of supply of contraceptive commodities in a broad mix of choice, training of personnel, and maintenance of services. Reproductive health facilities should be expanded to more easily accessible also to the rural population. The services should be integrated in the Mother and Child Health concept. Where demanded and possible special facilities for men should be provided.

Programme for action

On Family Planning and Contraception

To amend any law that limits the access to family planning services to adolescents and adult women, by requiring the consent of parents or spouses; to introduce sexual education courses for boys and girls since the early years of schooling; to make family planning counseling as well as post-delivery and post-abortion services available on demand.

On abortion

To provide timely and adequate treatment for complications related to spontaneous or induced abortions; to amend national laws in order to decriminalize abortion, bearing in mind the large number of clandestine abortions as well as the high mortality rate resulting from them.

On Women's Equal Rights and Opportunities

To recognize the value of women's domestic work in the National Accounts; to guarantee women's access to land ownership, credit and education; to legislate women's maternity leave, making sure that no woman is dismissed during pregnancy as a result of it; to promote the sharing of responsibilities for child-rearing and domestic activities among spouses; to promote massive information and sensitization campaigns on women's rights.

On Violence against Women

To streamline and expedite procedures to control and sanction sexual harassment in the work place as well as domestic violence, especially that among spouses and partners, establishing mandatory programmes to reeducate perpetrators; to promote a nationwide debate on the issue of violence against women, seeking to raise the public consciousness on its status as a criminal act; to ban circumcision of girls as a violation of human rights.

Lastly, it is highly recommended that parliamentarians take upon themselves to periodically prepare National Reports on "legislative, judicial, administrative and other measures" adopted by Member Countries, to be submitted to the UN Secretary General every four years on the Elimination of All Forms of Discrimination Against Women (Art. 19).

Excerpted from: Statement of Parliamentarians attending the Conference "Population Reconsidered: Empowerment, Health and Human Rights," Harare, Zimbabwe, December 10, 1993.

Premises Re-Examined

2

Population and Ethics: Expanding the Moral Space

Sissela Bok

The primary focus of postwar population policy has been on aggregate numbers of human beings. In recent years, this focus has been increasingly challenged. Population experts have been criticized for conducting their research and debating policies at a level so abstract as to leave out of account the felt experience of the *people* whose procreative activities are at issue. To be sure, it will never be possible to formulate population policy without a degree of abstraction. Populations are by definition multitudes, or people in the aggregate, and must be viewed as such for purposes of policy making. But when experts do so too single-mindedly, they risk ignoring the impact of their policies on the lives of individual human beings — of women, men, and children in villages and cities the world over, whose activities go to make up the population statistics.

The result of such a narrow emphasis has often been that fundamental ethical issues at stake in policy debates about matters as central to human lives as sexuality, procreation, and family life have been given short shrift. This is not to say that participants in policy debates do not have frequent recourse to the language of ethics — as when they argue that a particular policy is just or unjust, admirable or reprehensible, respectful of autonomy or coercive, conducive to greater well-being or likely to increase suffering. The use of moral terms is inescapable as soon as a course of action is evaluated or advocated on normative grounds.[1] But moral language is used as often to shield against inquiry as to pursue it. In debates over population policy, uncritical cost-benefit analyses and vacuous moral rhetoric alike have been employed to deflect attention from the concerns of those whose lives are directly and intimately affected by different population policies.

The word *population* can also be taken in the sense of an action or process of peopling a place or region, or the increase, over time, in the number of people in a place or region (see Box 1 on next page).

In this temporal sense of the word, too, policy experts in the population field have often given short shrift to crucial ethical considerations by focusing exclusively on the needs either of future or (more rarely) of present populations.

As the controversies over population policy have intensified over the past decade, it has become clear that ethical concerns are at their heart. Previously neglected ethical issues, moreover, have come to the forefront, in large part because many of those with most at stake personally in the population debate have succeeded in making their voices heard as never before. Women's groups, including members of the growing women's health movement; human rights advocates; environmentalists; supporters of labor, business, and farming interests; representatives of nongovernmental organizations; and grassroots activists in every region — all have insisted on making their different, at times clashing, positions heard.

The resulting debates have brought searing moral conflicts into the open and, while hardly resolving them, at least have succeeded in delineating them more sharply than in the past. And although abstract moral rhetoric still resounds on every side of such debates, it no longer drowns out the voices of those most affected by the outcomes. In consequence, it has become more difficult for policy analysts, agency representatives, religious leaders, and public officials simply to ignore or to downplay the impact of their policies on human lives.

Contexts of Moral Choice Regarding Population Issues

Ethical conflicts over population policies concern not only the aims that we should pursue, singly and collectively, but also the means that we can legitimately employ and that are most desirable in the course of this pursuit. The choices about ends and means when it comes to sexuality, family planning, and childbearing take place at every level, from the individual all the way to the international. Because these choices arise in contexts of great diversity, involving gender, class, ethnicity, and religion, there are wide variations in what individuals are able to do, depending on the power relationships in which they stand. But no matter how varied the contexts in which such choices are made, it is important to recognize that the resultant policies often place the largest burden on women, and it is they who have been most often at risk from errors in, or abuses of, policies, customs, and rules.

Works of literature have conveyed women's experiences in this regard magnificently: from Homer's *Iliad* to Thomas Hardy's *Tess of the D'Urbervilles;* from the seventeenth-century *The True Relation of My Birth, Breeding, and Life,* by Margaret Cavendish, to Tolstoy's *Anna Karenina;*

BOX 1

Definitions of Population

Population (1)
   Devastation, laying waste (obsolete).
Population (2)
   1. A peopled or inhabited place (obsolete).
   2. The state of a country with respect to numbers of people: the degree in which a place is populated or inhabited; hence, the total number of persons inhabiting a country, town, or other area; the body of inhabitants.
   3. The action or process of peopling a place or region; increase of people.

Source: Oxford English Dictionary, Second Ed.

---

from *The Confessions of Lady Nijo,* written in fourteenth-century Japan, across the world to Sigrid Undset's account, in *Kristin Lavransdatter,* of a woman's life in medieval Norway; and from the Indian villagers described in Kamala Markandaya's *Nectar in a Sieve* to the women of Zimbabwe in Tsitsi Dangarembga's *Nervous Conditions.*

No matter how diverse the conditions of the women's lives depicted in these works, their responses to pregnancy and childbirth are strikingly similar: the intense exhilaration, longing, fear, or dejection associated with thoughts of becoming pregnant, depending on the circumstances; the desperate furtiveness often associated with extramarital pregnancies; the bonding with a newborn baby or, at times, its rejection; the anguish about one born too early or in poor health; and the blending of love and suffering when the birth of a child is welcomed by one parent but not the other.

Our century has seen the advent of remarkable technological innovations in the areas of contraception, sterilization, safe abortion, in vitro fertilization, surrogate motherhood, fetal monitoring and therapy, and safe premature deliveries. These new technologies have greatly increased procreative choice for many, while also generating new ethical dilemmas. For instance, in societies where son preference is strong, the availability of amniocentesis or other forms of prenatal screening places new pressures on women to abort fetuses found to be female, as reported in China and India. The fundamentals of the experiences of pregnancy and childbirth have nevertheless not shifted for the vast majority of women. Since early times, the personal and social pressures associated with these events have resulted not only from community and interpersonal attitudes toward sexuality, courtship, marriage, and family life, but also from population policies of a sort, whether pronatalist or antinatalist, often rooted in particular religious doctrines or aiming at the welfare of particular societies.

While such policies are still common today, the major issues driving the population debate since the early 1950s have been global. Opinions have differed sharply regarding the long-range economic, environmental, and social consequences to societies of this century's unprecedented population growth, but few experts have doubted that they will be felt worldwide. Already, more people live at or near starvation levels than were even alive in 1900. The growing pressures for access to water, energy, and food transcend all cultural and national boundaries.

Among the many analysts who have viewed the escalating population figures with alarm, further differences have arisen respecting the policies to be undertaken in response. Should the focus be on economic and social reforms, or more directly on population growth in its own right? And what role should the richer nations, where population growth has on the whole stabilized, play with respect to population policy in poorer societies? Over the years and in shifting coalitions, Marxists, Catholics, Western liberals, Reagan conservatives, and many others have locked horns over the answers to these questions. But whoever has prevailed at any one time and in any one place, the resultant policies have too often continued to leave women without any say, even about matters that affect their lives as intimately and powerfully as sexuality and procreation.

By now, individuals traditionally left out of the population debate are increasingly insisting on being heard. As a result, a widening split can be perceived in the population field that throws into new relief long-standing conflicts regarding goals and means. It is a split between those who give priority to population control and those who stress, in the first place, individual choice and human rights — a division of opinion that culminated in the sharp disagreements before and at the 1992 United Nations Conference on Environment and Development, in Rio de Janeiro, Brazil. Advocates of the first position include many population and environmental experts. They claim that without more forceful efforts to control the world's population, individual choice and human rights will come to be increasingly violated as resources are depleted and poverty, disease, and social unrest place an ever greater burden on peoples worldwide.

Those who uphold the second position stress the lack of respect for the individuals whose procreative practices are affected, sometimes coercively, by pronatalist or antinatalist policies in many nations, or by members of some one community or culture or power sphere — more generally, by haves for have-nots. They point out that most resource depletion and environmental damage stems less from population increases in the poorer nations than from overconsumption in the richer societies; and they argue that policies that run roughshod over individual autonomy often also turn out to be to be counterproductive from the point of view of achieving population control.

Advocates on both sides of this split often appeal to moral principles, rights, responsibilities, and obligations in support of their views. They inevitably bring to bear, implicitly or explicitly, one or more moral principles, such as liberty, equality, or justice. But unless the parties to debates about such moral claims explore the different meanings they attach to these terms, they cannot go far in considering the underlying moral issues at stake. Liberty, most would agree, is a central value; but at what individual or societal cost should it be supported or imposed? And what constraints should operate in cases where the liberties of some injure others directly or thwart their freedom? The same conflicts arise with respect to equality and justice.

Each of these moral principles, moreover, is at stake in two central controversies in political philosophy, both of which must take population into account: how to allocate scarce resources and costs across space, and how to allocate them across time (Shue 1980). Differences concerning allocation across space are regional ones, within nations as between them. Among the most disputed differences concerning allocation across space are those between the interests of richer and poorer nations, often encapsulated as North-South differences. How should the costs of alleviating the present glaring inequities between rich and poor societies be distributed? Do equality and justice call for rich societies to shift resources away from the needs of their own poor as long as others are in greater need elsewhere? And how do justice and expected utility balance out in deciding whether to give priority to cutting back on consumption by richer nations or on population growth in poorer nations? Is it indeed necessary to conceive of a trade-off in this regard, rather than of the necessity for rich and poor societies to cooperate in furthering both goals?

Whereas questions concerning different approaches to allocating costs and resources over space within and between societies have been debated since the beginnings of human history, discussions about allocations over time are of more recent vintage. To be sure, much has been said and written about what the living owe to their successors, and the concept of trusteeship has long been stressed in both religious and secular contexts (Feinberg 1980; Weiss 1989). But not until this century has it come to seem possible that human choices — not least with respect to population policy — might substantially reduce or even exhaust the resources needed by coming generations; and not until the philosopher John Rawls took up the issue of intergenerational justice did thinkers begin to address the vexing problem of what claims the unborn might have upon the living (Rawls 1971).

Can one speak of the rights of the unborn? Many balk at granting to beings who do not exist and who might never come into existence rights comparable to those owed to persons who are alive today. But most find it equally difficult to deny the responsibility on the part of present generations to take the interests of future generations into account, when it comes, for instance, to nonrenewable resources (Bayles 1980). As soon as we accept such responsibility on the part of the living, however, the question arises as to what obligations it entails and, in turn, once again the question of how to allocate among existing societies and groups the burdens of attempting to fulfill those obligations.

The debates about these and other only partially explored ethical issues in population policy are further hampered by inadequate empirical data on which to base policy choices. Contemporary demographic data, while imperfect and subject to inaccurate interpretations, are less of a scientific problem in this respect than are the much more subjective and widely diverging projections about the future. Still more unsettled from a scientific point of view are questions of whether, and if so how, population causally relates to some of the central concerns of our time: environment, poverty, gender, and quality of life. The fact that the linkages between population and these issues, as well as the proposals for what to do about them, are scientifically contentious adds to the difficulty of reaching consensus about the moral issues involved.

Such consensus can be achieved, if at all, only by degrees. An important contribution that a focus on ethics can make to this process is to challenge the self-serving rigidity and premature closure inherent in much moral rhetoric, and instead to create the "moral space" needed for reflection, debate, and joint exploration (Walker 1993). The many new voices now taking part in the debates over population policy can help greatly in opening up this moral space and keeping it open.

The approach to ethics that generates and guards moral space is especially needed for complex and intertwining moral issues, such as those concerning population policy, where the choices arrived at affect numerous groups. It allows for thorough exploration of diverse perspectives; for efforts to perceive and understand the experiences on the basis of which moral claims are made; for helping to sort out and analyze conflicting claims; and for delineating areas, however narrow at first, of general agreement. In this process, greater attention to clarifying definitions, the structure of arguments, and the empirical claims on which they rest will help remove needless causes of disagreement. In turn, this will make it possible to set forth with greater care the moral aspects of the debates regarding population policy.

Ends and Means

Centrally at issue in contemporary debates about population policy are conflicts regarding the ends to be pursued and the means employed in such pursuit. Of necessity, these conflicts raise ethical questions about the justification advanced for particular ends and particular means, as well as the ancient question of whether the ends justify the means or whether the recourse to unethical means inevitably corrupts and at times destroys the pursuit of the ends.

These questions are the more difficult to unravel as both means and ends come together and interact at many levels. We live with interlocking hierarchies of ends, from the most minute aims of everyday life to vast, overriding, ambitious goals for ourselves, our communities, and the world. The narrower ends can also be seen as means or stepping-stones to the larger ones. In this way, recovery from an illness can be seen either as an end in its own right or as a means enabling someone to work toward larger ends, such as family survival, social reform, or artistic creation. As a result, what some view as means — say, literacy, food security, or access to health care and family planning — others can with equal reason see as ends in their own right.

Ends

In theory, the ends, or aims, of population policy could encompass any factor or set of factors that would count as improvements for any group of human beings. In practice, however, population policy has increasingly come to serve two general and often conflicting aims, related to the two sides of the split over population priorities noted above. The first aim pertains to population in the temporal sense of *peopling:* it is to stem the growth of the world's population before it depletes available resources and poses possibly irreversible threats to the earth's environment and thus to all living beings. The second aim has more to do with population in the sense of existing human beings, seen both in the aggregate and individually. It places priority on overcoming the poor health, lack of reproductive choice, subjugation, and poverty of so many members of the world's present population.

For those who see the first aim as primary, the most direct methods of inhibiting population growth have long been celibacy, contraception, sterilization, and abortion. Family planning programs the world over have employed these methods in various mixtures. More recently, it has become clear that socioeconomic factors, especially women's access to health care and education, and a concern for human rights, including reproductive rights, play an important indirect role in fertility regulation as well. Advocates of the second aim, however, stress these factors not merely as indirect means to population control, but instead as ends that must be achieved for their own sake.

High on the agenda in current discussions of family planning is the question of whether there can be agreement among the proponents of the two aims to pursue both, at least where they overlap. Is it possible, in view of the urgency of the problems now so clearly facing individuals and societies, to work together for greater access to education, health care, and means of voluntary family planning, even in the absence of any consensus regarding the underlying question as to which of the two aims is primary and which secondary (Sinding 1992)?

The answers to this question vary, on both sides of the divide. On each side, those most disposed to collaboration accept both aims as worth pursuing as long as the one they see as most urgent receives priority. In a second group on each side are activists who agree with members of the first group in principle, but are unwilling to go along with them in practice. They find it important from a strategic point of view not to budge with respect to furthering the aim they take to be secondary unless priority is granted the one they advocate. In a third group, finally, are persons who take their own preferred aim as not merely the one that should be granted priority but the only one worth striving for, and see danger in accommodation of any competing aim. Among these are individuals of more intense, sometimes more limited vision, as well as battle-weary stragglers from the second group who have concluded that nothing will ever be gained through collaboration.

Each of the two aims carries a different and characteristic danger of what might be a collapse of moral perception for persons in this third group. The work of the biologist Garrett Hardin exemplifies the first aim carried thus to excess. In an influential article, "The Tragedy of the Commons," Hardin maintains that when a large enough number of people make individually justified and reasonable decisions to avail themselves of collective resources, such as a commons for cattle or a body of drinking water, they end by depleting the resource, to the great detriment of all (Hardin 1968). He asserts that population growth threatens humanity with such a tragedy on a large scale, and that only drastic methods can avert it. "Freedom to breed will bring ruin to all." Better to allow starvation and disease to take their course in societies unable to limit their population by other means than to provide food aid that merely makes it possible for their populations to continue to grow.

In later writings, Hardin has elaborated a "lifeboat ethics," according to which rich nations should think of themselves as in a lifeboat, surrounded by the poor of the world swimming in the sea, hoping to be taken in or to be aided in some other way (Hardin 1974, 1993). If we are in such a lifeboat, we may be tempted by the ideal of being our brother's keeper, Hardin suggests, but if we take in more needy people than we can cope with, "the boat is swamped and everybody drowns. Complete justice, complete catastrophe" (Hardin 1974).

Since Hardin first advanced his draconian thesis of coercive population control on a vast scale, with rich nations hoarding their resources in the face of mass Third World starvation, those who dreamed of some lifeboat in which nations could insulate themselves from poverty, disease, environmental damage, wars, and economic dislocations have had a rude awakening. As the Union of Concerned Scientists has put it, "we all have but one lifeboat" (Union of Concerned Scientists 1993). Unless nations collectively respond to threats to the global environment, manage resources more effectively, and stabilize population, no nation will be able to escape injury in conflicts over increasingly scarce resources. It is not altruism, therefore, but enlightened self-interest, for developed nations both to reduce their overconsumption and to provide aid and support to developing nations in order to further collective goals.

It is important to see, too, just how corrupting it would be for societies to act according to Hardin's prescriptions and how destructive, even at home. Communities would be rent asunder by discord about refusing humanitarian aid and closing doors to immigration. And there could be no guarantee that the brutal disregard for human dignity that he advocates would be practiced only toward foreigners.

Meanwhile, the risk of excess, on the part of those who give exclusive priority to the aim of stressing the rights and needs of existing human beings, arises when groups are convinced that their cause is just and that any cooperation with those who disagree will prove destructive to it. Advancing their own goals, no matter what the consequences, then becomes a necessity, and all compromise is ruled out. "Do what is right though the heavens may fall" is a motto with long antecedents (Bok 1988, 1989). Depending, thus, on what is thought to be "right," the motto has great appeal, not only to fanatics but to unscrupulous militants of every persuasion. It is, after all, in the name of liberty, justice, and group rights to survival that the warring factions in Bosnia resort to "ethnic cleansing" and every other breach of the most basic human rights.

Even for those many advocates of both aims who are able to come to agreement on policies to pursue in practice, however, conflicts remain where the overlap between the two aims is less clear-cut, or nonexistent. At what individual or societal cost should either aim then be pursued more vigorously than the other? Should the reproductive freedom stressed by proponents of the second aim be limited for persons with AIDS, for instance, or for those addicted to drugs? Are there demographic projections for a society that are so threatening as to warrant methods of family planning ordinarily rejected as too coercive? And how wise is it to pursue vigorous efforts, through oral rehydration and vaccinations, to ensure the survival of young children in the poorest nations, which are most threatened by population growth and environmental deterioration? Would it be preferable to give priority to family planning efforts over child survival programs, or can both be adequately pursued together (King et al. 1991)?

Means

Conflicts over the various means employed to attain the aims of population policy, such as different methods of contraception, sterilization, and abortion, concern both their efficacy in achieving the intended aims and their moral legitimacy. Judgments about the efficacy of the methods have to rely on evaluations of the degree to which they have achieved the stated goals under different circumstances. Thus, comparisons are made between the levels of success or failure of family planning programs in different communities, and between approaches that focus primarily on family planning and others that also stress economic development and the access of women to education and health care.

Debates about the moral legitimacy of different means of achieving the aims of population policy center, first of all, on whether the means in question are morally illegitimate in their own right, regardless of how voluntarily they may be employed. Contraceptives, sterilization, and abortion are prohibited by the Catholic church, for example, as being contrary to natural law and thus morally illegitimate, yet they are accepted as legitimate by a great many practicing Catholics. Many groups, women's groups foremost among them, argue that the morality of using these methods ought to be evaluated by individuals in the context of their own lives, rather than decided for them by religious or political authorities.

A second and related distinction with respect to the moral legitimacy of methods employed for purposes of population policy is that between voluntary and coerced procreative practices. Coercion — the exertion of force by pressure or threat — need not be morally illegitimate. Every government relies on some measure of coercion — in crime control, for example, or in the collection of taxes (Wertheimer 1987). Such forms of coercion, like all others, are much more widely condemned on moral grounds when they subject individuals to what the United Nations Declaration of Human Rights characterizes as "cruel, inhuman, or degrading treatment" (article 5). Advocates of voluntarism in the use of family planning methods reject the coercion involved in imposing or prohibiting such methods as precisely cruel, inhuman, and degrading.

In our time, perhaps the most publicized state efforts to coerce procreative practices have been those in pre-1989 Romania and present-day China. In Romania, the pronatalist regime of Nicolae Ceausescu prohibited sterilization and abortion, as well as the sale of contraceptives, with disastrous results both for families and for the babies left in foundling homes, many of whom were found to suffer from AIDS. The Chinese government has, on the contrary, enforced the use of these same methods in its pursuit of antinatalist goals. Both approaches have caused bitter anguish on the part of many of the families whose childbearing practices were coerced in these ways; both were held indispensable by government officials for achieving national goals.

The distinction between voluntary and coerced methods is never more fraught with moral significance than when it comes to bodily intrusions against a person's will, as in forced abortions or sterilizations. On the scale of methods regarded by most persons as morally illegitimate, such intrusions rank high; so do threats and other so-called negative incentives, and various forms of deceit and manipulation designed to mislead individuals into adopting or refusing one or another form of family planning.

In evaluating the degree to which different means are coercively or manipulatively imposed, moreover, an individual's socioeconomic status and access to information play an important role. Middle-class women in industrialized democracies who have access to, and are adequately informed about, a number of reproductive technologies are clearly less likely to find themselves coerced or manipulated than poorer women without such access or knowledge. For that reason, legal, religious, and commercial barriers to access, as well as reproductive technologies, must be evaluated from a moral point of view, with sensitivity to their potential for abuse under different circumstances. The same is true of the incentives and disincentives employed by governments, agencies, and community groups to achieve family planning goals (Callahan 1971).

A third set of moral issues relating to means concerns the funding of family planning and other population programs (Callahan, Callahan, and Clark 1981). What moral compromises are funding agencies at times led to make in order to provide aid of a nature they regard as appropriate, and how carefully do they sort out the pros and cons of such compromises? What are the responsibilities of agencies to ensure that the funds provided to pay for the various means are properly used by public officials on the receiving end, rather than siphoned off for per-

sonal gain or used for unrelated expenditures, such as armaments purchases? If funding agencies make the aid they offer conditional, then what conditions are legitimately and illegitimately imposed? And by what means do these agencies seek to induce acceptance of contraceptive methods, abortion, or sterilization?

Opinions divide as to whether morally problematic means are legitimate if they prevent great damage to persons or societies. In philosophical debates, the argument for such legitimacy is often called the "dirty hands" argument (Walzer 1973). It holds that actions violating ordinary moral principles can be excused if they are undertaken in the reasonable expectation that a greater good will thereby be served. In politics, this argument is often invoked by public officials who reject accusations of wrongdoing by claiming to be acting strictly in the public's best interest. Such claims are central to the controversy over human rights in the population field. Thus, at the United Nations World Conference on Human Rights, in Vienna in June 1993, the Chinese government was vehement in defending its coercive population control policies, arguing that its approach was indispensable to achieving the goals necessary to the well-being of Chinese society as a whole and, given the size of China's population, of the world.

Opponents argue that, on the contrary, such policies trample on human rights, destroy the trust without which societies cannot function well, and are not, in fact, uniquely capable of bringing about the necessary limitation of population growth. At the very least, these critics maintain, the burden of proof is on governments wishing to impose coercive methods to show that alternative, voluntary methods have failed; and this they cannot do until they have tried these methods on a large scale with well-financed programs. Until such programs have been shown to be ineffective, the violations of human rights inherent in coercive methods are unacceptable — and never more than when it comes to violations of the integrity of the human body, as in forced sterilization or abortion.

Rights, Obligations, and Responsibilities

The 1993 United Nations World Conference on Human Rights in Vienna carried important implications for the discussion of the role of rights in controversies cutting across national boundaries, including, most prominently, controversies about population, environment, and development. The conference brought to light, as never before, the range of long-standing, profound disagreements often concealed beneath routine invocations of universal human rights, even by governments having not the slightest intention to respect them in practice. The disagreements primarily were as to whether there could be said to be any rights at all that were universal, that is, due all human beings regardless of race, religion, nationality, gender, or other distinctions. (Such universal rights are to be distinguished from rights that people have by virtue of a nation's laws and of private interactions, such as contracts. See Shue 1980; Thompson 1990).

Many delegates to the conference were prepared to agree in principle that the right not to be subjected to torture or assault should count among universal rights (however much their governments might be denying citizens such rights in practice); others stressed the fundamental economic right to subsistence. Many were also prepared to place greater stress on the long-neglected issues of women's rights, including those concerned with sexual life and procreation. But far fewer saw all the political and economic rights mentioned in the final document as being comparably universal. And a group of delegates headed by China, Indonesia, and Malaysia insisted that the idea of human rights was a Western invention that should in no way govern international relations. If the language of rights is to be used at all, these delegates added, the rights to development and economic growth should receive priority over political rights, such as that of free speech.

Still further debates arose as to exactly what having any such set of rights entitled people to, against whom it might claimed, and who might have corresponding obligations toward them on account of it. For example, it is easy enough to see how a universal human right not to be tortured or wrongfully imprisoned can be claimed against all comers, and that this claim asserts that all have the corresponding obligation not to engage in such actions. But what about the right to education, to adequate health care, or to a minimum wage? Is each a right only with respect to one's own state, or should others acknowledge an obligation to see to it that the right is upheld? And at what cost? The questions are even more open-ended when it comes to the right to development: Against whom or what groups can such a right be claimed, and what does having it demand of them? What, in other words, ought to be the obligation of those toward whom claims of such rights are directed?

Onora O'Neill points out that it is surprising that rights should be so much more prominent than obligations in contemporary debate; for whereas "discussions of obligation and justice have been a staple of the most abstract and the most daily ethical discussions since antiquity . . . discussion of rights was an eighteenth-century innovation" (O'Neill 1986). Even though rights are generally thought to entail correlative obligations, "we have no Universal Declaration of Human Duties, and no International Human Obligations Movement."

Any discussion of what such declarations might contain would have to consider not only the extent of, and the justifications for, different sorts of obligations, but also how they relate to responsibilities on the part of the possessors of rights, and what the status of such responsibilities might be. Further questions of responsibility arise whenever there is a conflict between rights, such that stressing a given set of rights makes it difficult, even impossible, to do justice to others. To what extent, for instance, can one advocate both the right to development and full procreative rights?

It would be wrong to conclude, however, from the disparity of views voiced and the complexity of the problems associated with conflicting rights, that the Vienna Conference exposed the vacuity and practical uselessness of the concept of universal human rights. On the contrary, this concept and concern for its application have assumed extraordinary practical importance in recent decades (Jones 1989). And the very fact that governments have argued their case so vehemently bears testimony to all they have seen as riding on which interpretation of universal human rights might prevail.

Debating the Ethics of Population Policies

The call is sometimes made for a new ethics, whereby societies might better make a concerted stand against threats, such as those posed by war, poverty, oppression, environmental degradation, and epidemics that recognize no linguistic, cultural, or other boundaries. But there is no reason to believe that such a new ethics will soon be discovered, much less that it will somehow gain general acceptance in time to serve as the basis for the collective action that is now so urgent. What is needed, rather, is an effort to find common ground, drawing on existing ethical traditions, and to proceed, from such a basis, to undertake dialogue, debate, and critique, within and between otherwise disparate traditions and standpoints (Bok 1992).

Without such a basis for communication, it is unrealistic to imagine that societies will agree upon an adequate set of collective responses to the problems envisaged in the debate over population policy, tied in as it is with development and environmental concerns. Time and again during the past decades, concerted action with respect to the world has been stalled because of ideological gridlock. In the process, many ethical issues have been neglected; those that have been debated often have been taken up from parochial or short-sighted points of view.

By now, the forceful new voices making themselves heard on all points of the political spectrum are calling attention to moral concerns that ought to have been part of the debate from the beginning. There is, in this sense, a new approach to ethics and population policy; but unless long-standing ethical questions are addressed with greater care and willingness to listen to differing views than in the past, there is every risk that ideological barriers will once again obstruct the

collective responses that are now so clearly called for to the interlocking problems peoples confront.

Two approaches to setting forth and analyzing the ethical issues of population policy may make it harder for such barriers to arise. Both are indispensable, but neither of them can suffice on its own. The first approach is the one discussed above — one that seeks common ground, some baseline consensus from which to undertake and facilitate further debate. There is much greater consensus, for example, about the acceptability of voluntary forms of contraception and about the rejection of infanticide than about the role of positive and negative incentives to promote particular population policies. Likewise, there is greater consensus regarding at least the most basic human rights than conflicting government pronouncements might indicate. There is little doubt that if one asked the citizens in states practicing the greatest violations of human rights, and did so in ways that guaranteed their safety from reprisals, they would begin by stressing the right not to be tortured, assaulted, or killed. This means that, at the very least, certain means of population control would have to be ruled out as constituting such assaults.

The second approach begins, in contrast, by setting forth a more complete position regarding, for example, reproductive rights or duties, agendas for national or international family planning programs, or religious guidelines regarding sexuality and reproduction. Rather than starting out from some ground generally shared, those who employ this approach present, for purposes of persuasion, advocacy, and practical application, what might be called an ideal position that they take to be the correct one, whether or not it is generally shared.

Both approaches are familiar in political, as in philosophical and religious, debates. Proponents of each can, in their own way, seek to inspire as well as to persuade. Each approach, moreover, can help overcome ways in which the other might be inadequate by itself, from the point of view of moving the population debate forward: especially the risk, for the first approach, that whatever consensus it achieves will be too limited to allow much progress to be made, and for the second, that its advocates will be tempted to refuse all compromise and adhere to their developed position, come what may. The danger, in each case, is one of ideological balkanization, of topics' being set aside as taboo, and of practical action's languishing because of factional disputes that seem impossible to overcome.

Efforts to coordinate the two approaches and to move back and forth between them are essential at such times. The debate about ends and means, as about rights, obligations, and responsibilities, can then proceed both from the top down, on the basis of fully delineated positions, and from the bottom up, on the basis of shared premises. Such a debate will inevitably, like all debates about population policy, be fundamentally about ethics: about individual and collective choice concerning how we should live and how we should treat one another. As experts, advocates, and others come together to discuss population policies for the coming century, they have a special obligation to consider the impact of their choices on great numbers of individuals. They must take more seriously than ever, therefore, the moral issues raised by different policy choices. It will matter, in this regard, that they strive not to forget the impact of what they do and fail to do on the individual human fates of those who make up the populations targeted by population policies, both immediately and for generations to come.

Note

1 The word *moral*, used in this sense, notes the presence of normative aspects of the value claims being made, however much one may disagree with the claims; it should be distinguished from *moral* in the sense of morally right, or praiseworthy.

References

Bayles, M. D. 1980. *Morality and population policy.* Tuscaloosa: University of Alabama Press.

Bok, S. 1992. The search for a shared ethics. *Common Knowledge* 1(3):12–25.

———. 1988. Kant's arguments in support of the maxim "Do what is right though the world should perish." *Argumentation* 2:7–25.

———. 1989. *A strategy for peace: Human values and the threat of war.* New York: Pantheon Books.

Callahan, D. 1971. *Ethics and population limitation.* New York: The Population Council.

Callahan, D., C. Callahan, and P. G. Clark. 1981. *Ethical issues of population aid.* New York: Irvington Publishers.

Cavendish, M., Duchess of Newcastle. 1656. The true relation of my birth, breeding, and life. In *The Life of William Cavendish, Duke of Newcastle.* London: J.C. Nimmo Publisher, 1886.

Dangarembga, T. 1989. *Nervous conditions.* Seattle: Seal Press.

Feinberg, J. 1980. *Rights, justice, and the bounds of liberty.* Princeton, N.J.: Princeton University Press.

Hardin, G. 1968. The tragedy of the commons. *Science* 162(3859):1243–1248.

———. 1974. Living on a lifeboat. *BioScience* 24:561–568.

———. 1993. *Living within limits: Ecology, economics, and population taboos.* New York: Oxford University Press.

Hardy, T. 1891. *Tess of the D'Urbervilles.* New York: Norton.

Homer. *The Iliad.* Trans. R. Fitzgerald. 1974. Garden City, N.Y.: Anchor Press.

Jones, D.V. 1989. *Code of peace: Ethics and security in the world of warlord states.* Chicago: University of Chicago Press.

King, M., et al. 1991. Debate: Population growth and child mortality. *NU* 5(1):3–43.

Nijo, Lady. ca. 1307. *The Confessions of Lady Nijo.* Trans. K. Brazell. 1973. Garden City, N.Y.: Anchor Press.

Markandaya, K. 1954. *Nectar in a sieve.* New York: John Day Company.

O'Neill, O. 1986. *Faces of hunger.* London: Allen & Unwin.

Rawls, J. 1971. *A theory of justice.* Cambridge, Mass.: Harvard University Press.

Shue, H. 1980. *Basic rights: Subsistence, affluence, and U.S. foreign policy.* Princeton, N.J.: Princeton University Press.

Sinding, S. W. 1992. *Getting to replacement: Bridging the gap between individual rights and demographic goals.* New York: The Rockefeller Foundation.

Thompson, J. 1990. *The realm of rights.* Cambridge, Mass.: Harvard University Press.

Tolstoy, L. 1877. *Anna Karenina.* Trans. C. Garnett. 1965. New York: Modern Library.

Undset, S. 1928. *Kristin Lavransdatter*. Trans. C. Archer and J. S. Scott. New York: Knopf.

Union of Concerned Scientists. 1993. *World scientists' warning to humanity*. Cambridge, Mass.

Walker, M. U. 1993. Keeping moral space open: New images of ethics consulting. *Hastings Center Report* 23(2):33–40.

Walzer, M. 1973. Political action: The problem of dirty hands. *Philosophy and Public Affairs* 2:160–180.

Weiss, E. B. 1989. *In fairness to future generations: International law, common patrimony, and intergenerational equity*. Dobbs Ferry, N.Y.: Transnational Publishers.

Wertheimer, A. 1987. *Coercion*. Princeton, N.J.: Princeton University Press.

3

Setting a New Agenda: Sexual and Reproductive Health and Rights

Adrienne Germain, Sia Nowrojee, and Hnin Hnin Pyne

As preparations for the 1994 International Conference on Population and Development (ICPD) gather momentum, debate is intensifying over the validity, objectives, scope, and accomplishments of population policies in Southern countries with high rates of population growth. A variety of groups with starkly different ideological positions have become involved in defining the problems to be addressed and appropriate solutions.

At one end of the spectrum are those who perceive rapid population growth in Southern countries as the most overwhelming threat to the future of the planet, economic growth, and national security.[1] At the other end of the spectrum are those who for religious or other reasons are opposed to induced abortion and to most or all contraceptives, sex education, and women's rights. Between the extremes are various other groups, including family planning "revisionists," who would improve current programs on the margins; feminist activists, human rights advocates, and progressive health and development professionals who seek to transform population policies and programs into reproductive and sexual health programs; and some population professionals who

recognize the necessity both to improve the quality of services and to broaden population policies to encompass women's status and education, their access to material resources, and child health (see Bongaarts 1994; Bruce 1993; see Jain and Bruce; and Sen, in this volume).

These positions derive from four decades of experience with population policies and programs, and debates about them are fueled by varying concerns, perspectives, and interests. In regard to past experience, family planning programs have certainly made services available and have contributed to fertility decline (Mauldin and Ross 1991; Ross and Frankenberg 1993), but not yet sufficiently either to ensure that all who wish to regulate their fertility can do so safely and effectively or to achieve population stabilization. In addition, recent developments in the world pose severe obstacles to universal reproductive health and rights and to population stabilization. Since the early 1980s, the world community has faced severe economic crisis, which is translated into declining real wages, increasing unemployment, and deepening poverty in much of the South (see Anand in this volume). Structural adjustment policies, national government actions such as disproportionate investments in the military and corruption, undermine fragile health, education, and other social services even as the populations in need are ever larger (Antrobus 1993; Due 1991; Elson 1990; Lele 1991; Sen 1991; Weil et al. 1990). The pandemics of Human Immunodeficiency Virus (HIV), AIDS and other sexually transmitted diseases (STDs) are devastating families and communities, as well as placing overwhelming demands upon health systems. While poverty pushes more and more people onto fragile lands and into megacities without adequate shelter, clean water, sanitation, and jobs, some businesses and governments are promoting environmentally damaging approaches to development, and consumption in many Northern societies is placing unsustainable demands on natural resources around the globe. At the same time that Southern governments' social-sector budgets are under severe pressure, many industrialized countries are reducing their foreign assistance budgets, shifting allocations to the former USSR and Eastern Europe, and increasing disaster and emergency aid.

These trends require reassessment of both population and development policies to ensure that they create conditions in which it makes sense for people to have fewer children, the so-called demand side of the population equation. Policies should also ensure that all persons have the means to do so safely and effectively, the "supply" side. To accomplish both, it is necessary to transform population policy, until now narrowly equated with family planning services, to address development and human rights concerns and to transform "family planning" into reproductive and sexual health services that advance health and rights, not simply the achievement of demographic objectives.

In this chapter, we briefly address this need to transform population and development policies. We propose three interrelated investment strategies: women's reproductive and sexual health services, including but not limited to birth control; policies and programs to encourage men to take more responsibility for their *own* fertility, for

prevention of STDs, and for the health and well-being of their sexual partners and the children they father; and policies and programs to address underlying issues of sexuality and gender relations, especially for children and young people.

Creating the Necessary Socioeconomic Conditions

Although the importance of the demand side of population growth has long been recognized (Davis 1967; Davis and Blake 1956; Dixon-Mueller 1993b), and many national population policies have been appropriately adjusted (see, for example, Ethiopia 1993), population resources have been invested primarily in family planning programs, rather than in creating the conditions that facilitate people's use of those programs. Substantially changed definitions of the problem to be addressed, along with new approaches to the solutions, are required. The well-being of *both* current and future generations must be at the center of such policies, which would emphasize investments in people of all ages — their health, education, livelihoods, living conditions, and human rights — *and* would prioritize gender equity and women's empowerment. Despite considerable lip service, the political will to bring about more equitable and sustainable development, especially gender equity, has been sorely lacking (see Anand in this volume).

Investments in human development, including the empowerment of women, and assurance of human rights are essential in their own right. They are also the most effective and humane ways to reduce the continuing demand for many children in most Southern countries. Together, they provide the "enabling conditions" essential for people to exercise their reproductive rights and choose "freely and responsibly" the number of children they have (see Correa and Petchesky in this volume). They may also go a long way to slowing down population momentum[2] by creating conditions that foster later marriage; delay of the first birth, longer intervals between births, and demand for smaller families; more equitable relationships and decisionmaking between women and men; and more equitable parental responsibility for children.

It is increasingly clear that the narrow approach adopted to date, which emphasizes quantity of contraceptive methods provided, is inadequate both to meet people's needs and to achieve fertility change. What is required is systematic and persistent interaction between population professionals and agencies on the one hand, and finance, planning, and development agencies on the other. Over the years, population agencies have mounted various attempts to insert "population" and "women" into the development planning process. Little success has been documented, in part because only demographic objectives have been expressed. As Dahlgren (1993) has pointed out, those concerned with population need to work more actively to integrate their objectives and strategies into mainstream agencies. They can do the following:

■ Persuade ministries of finance to increase investments in *human development*, broadly defined (health, education, water, sanitation, housing, social services).

■ Promote investment in *primary health care* to develop a stronger infrastructure for all health ministry activities.

■ Work for legislation and implementing mechanisms to *empower women* in all spheres of social and political life (marriage, inheritance, and so forth) and require men's responsibility for their own sexual behavior and its consequences.

■ Persuade education ministries to adopt policies that not only eliminate the *gender gap* in education, but also include *sexuality and gender education* in the curricula, foster equitable gender relationships, prevent violence against girls, and eliminate sex role stereotypes from textbooks.

■ Support concerned ministries and agencies to provide credit, training, and other essential inputs for women to earn *decent livelihoods*.

■ *Involve women's advocates* in all levels of decisionmaking.

Such efforts are, of course, important in their own right. If they are adopted at the ICPD in 1994, and carried forward into the Summit on Social Development and the UN International Conference on Women and Development in 1995, the population community will indeed have made a significant contribution toward human security and development for current and future generations. Not only these demand-promoting actions, but also the supply side—namely, the provision of reproductive and sexual health services, rather than contraception alone—should receive priority.

Providing Services

To date, family planning programs have assisted millions of women (and couples) to prevent unwanted fertility. Nonetheless, an estimated 100 million married women of reproductive age still have no access to services and about 170 million married women will be added to the potential user pool in the 1990s (Merrick 1994). Uncounted millions more are excluded from services because they are "too young" or unmarried, or they are poorly served (Dixon-Mueller and Germain 1992); most men are not included in family planning services. As many as 38 million abortions occur annually in Southern countries, an estimated 20 million of them clandestine, a stark testament to the lengths to which women go to prevent an unwanted birth (Germain 1989). In too many cases, subtle or explicit coercion of one sort or another has been used to "persuade" or force individuals to use contraceptives, be sterilized or have abortions (see Boland, Rao, and Zeidenstein in this volume). Despite national and international outcry, such practices persist, and may even increase as growing populations challenge governments to provide social services, jobs, and security.

If we are to achieve truly voluntary fertility control that respects human rights and advances health, our agenda must include not only improved quality of family planning services, but also expanded approaches that encompass the multiple dimensions of sexual and reproductive health for both women and men — sexuality and gender education, STD prevention and treatment, safe abortion, pregnancy and delivery services, postpartum and gynecologic care, and child health. We must enable men to take responsibility for their own behavior, and we must provide services and information to children and young people *before* they are sexually active, as well as in the crucial teenage years of sexual exploration and development. The primary objectives of services should be to assure a healthy and satisfying sexual and reproductive life. This agenda is described in the Women's Declaration on Population Policies (see Box 1; also Correa and Petchesky in this volume).

Policies and programs must, among other precautions, tailor interventions to suit particular situations (for example, not all health infrastructures are strong enough to ensure safe, nonabusive provision of long-acting hormonal contraceptives). While encouraging men to take responsibility for their *own* behavior, they must also assure women's control over their bodies (see Boland, Rao, and Zeidenstein; and Correa and Petchesky, in this volume). Given that women bear the primary burdens of reproduction and STDs,[3] that resources and political will to provide reproductive and sexual health services are limited, and that policy development, institution building, and attitudinal changes cannot be immediately achieved, it is essential that representatives of the women to be served are included in all levels and aspects of decisionmaking. Three priority areas for program investment and development are described below: women's health services, programs for men, and education on sexuality and gender.

Women's Sexual and Reproductive Health Services

The objectives should extend beyond simply fertility control and include the following:

■ Enabling women to manage their own fertility safely and effectively by conceiving when they desire to, terminating unwanted pregnancies, and carrying wanted pregnancies to term.

■ Promoting a healthy, satisfying sexual life, free of disease, violence, disability, fear, unnecessary pain, or death associated with reproduction and sexuality.

■ Enabling women to bear and raise healthy children as and when they desire to do so.

To achieve these objectives, changes are needed in the definition of who is to be served; in how services are to be provided, especially the balance between quantity and quality of care; in what services are provided; and in measures to monitor and evaluate programs. Basically, we need to improve the quality and extend the reach of birth control services, as well as provide other, closely related reproductive and sexual health services to all who need them.

Contraceptive Services

In regard to family planning, debate persists on whether unmarried persons should be included in the population to be served, whether the primary focus should continue to be women, whether persons younger and older than reproductive age should be included, and whether persons who are sterile (whether voluntarily or not) should be considered clients (Dixon-Mueller and Germain 1992). Constraints on financial and human resources, along with religious or other beliefs, are often cited as absolute barriers to broadening program scope. A reordering of program and budgetary priorities, however, would contribute substantially to ensuring that all persons, regardless of gender, age, or fertility status, are reached with a wider range of services.

We would give much higher priority than has heretofore been given to improving the quality of services. As regards family planning, Bruce (1990) conceptualized the primary elements of quality of care to include choice among methods, information on technical competence, client-provider relations, continuity of use, and constellation of services. More recently, the International Planned Parenthood Federation (Huezo and Briggs 1992) has formulated a document, "Rights of the Client," to be posted in all of its clinics. Systematic

Women's Declaration on Population Policies
(In Preparation for the 1994 International Conference on Population and Development)

Introduction

In September 1992, women's health advocates representing women's networks in Asia, Africa, Latin America, the Caribbean, the U.S. and Western Europe met to discuss how women's voices might best be heard during preparations for the 1994 Conference on Population and Development and in the conference itself. The group suggested that a strong positive statement from women around the world would make a unique contribution to reshaping the population agenda to better ensure reproductive health and rights.

The group drafted a "Women's Declaration on Population Policies," which was reviewed, modified and finalized by over 100 women's organizations across the globe.

The Declaration is now being circulated by the initiators to women's health advocates, other women's groups and women health professionals, outside and inside government, for their signatures. In addition, the initiators invite other networks, organizations, governments, and individuals, including men, to endorse the Declaration.

(continued on next page)

Initiators of the Women's Declaration on Population Policies

Peggy Antrobus
DAWN
and Women and Development Unit,
University of the West Indies, Barbados

Marge Berer
Reproductive Health Matters
London, United Kingdom

Amparo Claro
Latin American and Caribbean
Women's Health Network
Santiago, Chile

Sônia Correa
National Feminist Health and
Reproductive Rights Network
Recife, Pernambuco, Brazil

Joan Dunlop
International Women's Health Coalition
New York, United States

Claudia Garcia-Moreno
OXFAM Health Unit Coordinator*
Oxford, United Kingdom

Adrienne Germain
International Women's Health Coalition
New York, United States

Marie Aimee Hélie-Lucas
Women Living Under Muslim Laws
International Solidarity Network
Grabels, France

Noeleen Heyzer
Gender and Development Programme
Asian and Pacific Development Centre
Kuala Lumpur, Malaysia

Sandra Kabir
Bangladesh Women's Health Coalition
Dhaka, Bangladesh

Josephine Kasolo
Safe Motherhood Office, World Bank
Kampala, Uganda

Loes Keysers
Coordination Office, Women's Global
Network for Reproductive Rights
(WGNRR)
Amsterdam, The Netherlands

Frances Kissling
Catholics for a Free Choice
Washington, D.C., United States

Bene E. Madunagu
Women in Nigeria (WIN)
Calabar, Nigeria

Florence W. Manguyu
Medical Women's International
Association
Nairobi, Kenya

Alexandrina Marcelo
Institute for Social Studies & Action
and WomenHealth Philippines
Quezon City, The Philippines

Fatima Mernissi

Florence Nekyon
Uganda National Council of Women
and Organizing Committee for 7th
International Women's Health Meeting
Kampala, Uganda

Eva Njenga
Kenya Medical Women's Association
Nairobi, Kenya

Rosalind Petchesky
Reproductive Rights Education Project
and International Reproductive Rights
Research Action Group (IRRRAG)
New York, United States

Jacqueline Pitanguy
Citizenship, Studies, Research,
Information, Action (CEPIA)
Rio de Janeiro, Brazil

T. K. Sundari Ravindran
Rural Women's Social Education Centre
Tamil Nadu, India

Julia Scott
National Black Women's Health Project
Washington, D.C., United States

Kanwaljit Soin
Association of Women for Action and
Research, Singapore

* for identification purposes only

The initiators asked the International Women's Health Coalition (IWHC) to serve as Secretariat for this effort.

Women's Declaration on Population Policies

(continued)

Preamble

Just, humane and effective development policies based on principles of social justice promote the well-being of all people. Population policies designed and implemented under this objective need to address a wide range of conditions that affect the reproductive health and rights of women and men. These include unequal distribution of material and social resources among individuals and groups, based on gender, age, race, religion, social class, rural-urban residence, nationality and other social criteria; changing patterns of sexual and family relationships; political and economic policies that restrict girls' and women's access to health services and methods of fertility regulation; and ideologies, laws and practices that deny women's basic rights.

While there is considerable regional and national diversity, each of these conditions reflects not only biological differences between males and females, but also discrimination against girls and women, and power imbalances between women and men. Each of these conditions affects, and is affected by, the ability and willingness of governments to ensure health and education, to generate employment, and to protect basic human rights for all. Governments' ability and willingness are currently jeopardized by the global economic crisis, structural adjustment programs, and trends toward privatization, among other factors.

To assure the well-being of all people, and especially of women, population policies and programs must be framed within and implemented as a part of broader development strategies that will redress the unequal distribution of resources and power between and within countries, between racial and ethnic groups, and between women and men.

Population policies and programs of most countries and international agencies have been driven more by demographic goals than by quality of life goals. Population size and growth have often been blamed inappropriately as the exclusive or primary causes of problems such as global environmental degradation and poverty. Fertility control programs have prevailed as solutions when poverty and inequity are root causes that need to be addressed. Population policies and programs have typically targeted low income countries and groups, often reflecting racial and class biases.

Women's fertility has been the primary object of both pro-natalist and anti-natalist population policies. Women's behavior rather than men's has been the focus of attention. Women have been expected to carry most of the responsibility and risks of birth control, but have been largely excluded from decision-making in personal relationships as well as in public policy. Sexuality and gender-based power inequities have been largely ignored, and sometimes even strengthened, by population and family planning programs.

As women involved directly in the organization of services, research and advocacy, we focus this declaration on women's reproductive health and rights. We call for a fundamental revision in the design, structure and implementation of population policies, to foster the empowerment and well-being of all women. Women's empowerment is legitimate and critically important in its own right, not merely as a means to address population issues. Population policies that are responsive to women's needs and rights must be grounded in the following internationally accepted, but too often ignored, ethical principles.

Fundamental Ethical Principles

1. Women can and do make responsible decisions for themselves, their families, their communities, and, increasingly, for the state of the world. Women must be subjects, not objects, of any development policy, and especially of population policies.

2. Women have the right to determine when, whether, why, with whom, and how to express their sexuality. Population policies must be based on the principle of respect for the sexual and bodily integrity of girls and women.

3. Women have the individual right and the social responsibility to decide whether, how, and when to have children and how many to have; no woman can be compelled to bear a child or be prevented from doing so against her will. All women, regardless of age, marital status, or other social conditions have a right to information and services necessary to exercise their reproductive rights and responsibilities.

(continued on next page)

Women's Declaration on Population Policies

(continued)

4. Men also have a personal and social responsibility for their own sexual behavior and fertility and for the effects of that behavior on their partners and their children's health and well-being.

5. Sexual and social relationships between women and men must be governed by principles of equity, non-coercion, and mutual respect and responsibility. Violence against girls and women, their subjugation or exploitation, and other harmful practices such as genital mutilation or unnecessary medical procedures, violate basic human rights. Such practices also impede effective, health- and rights-oriented population programs.

6. The fundamental sexual and reproductive rights of women cannot be subordinated, against a woman's will, to the interests of partners, family members, ethnic groups, religious institutions, health providers, researchers, policy makers, the state or any other actors.

7. Women committed to promoting women's reproductive health and rights, and linked to the women to be served, must be included as policy makers and program implementors in all aspects of decision-making including definition of ethical standards, technology development and distribution, services, and information dissemination.

To assure the centrality of women's well-being, population policies and programs need to honor these principles at national and international levels.

Minimum Program Requirements

In the design and implementation of population policies and programs, policy makers in international and national agencies should:

1. Seek to reduce and eliminate pervasive inequalities in all aspects of sexual, social and economic life by:

- providing universal access to information, education and discussion on sexuality, gender roles, reproduction and birth control, in school and outside;
- changing sex-role and gender stereotypes in mass media and other public communications to support more egalitarian and respectful relationships;
- enacting and enforcing laws that protect women from sexual and gender-based violence, abuse, or coercion;

- implementing policies that encourage and support parenting and household maintenance by men;
- prioritizing women's education, job training, paid employment, access to credit, and the right to own land and other property in social and economic policies, and through equal rights legislation;
- prioritizing investment in basic health services, sanitation, and clean water.

2. Support women's organizations that are committed to women's reproductive health and rights and linked to the women to be served, especially women disadvantaged by class, race, ethnicity or other factors, to:

- participate in designing, implementing and monitoring policies and programs for comprehensive reproductive health and rights;
- work with communities on service delivery, education and advocacy.

3. Assure personally and locally appropriate, affordable, good quality, comprehensive reproductive and sexual health services for women of all ages, provided on a voluntary basis without incentives or disincentives, including but not limited to:

- legislation to allow safe access to all appropriate means of birth control;
- balanced attention to all aspects of sexual and reproductive health, including pregnancy, delivery and postpartum care; safe and legal abortion services; safe choices among contraceptive methods including barrier methods; information, prevention and treatment of STDs, AIDS, infertility, and other gynecological problems; child care services; and policies to support men's parenting and household responsibilities;
- nondirective counselling to enable women to make free, fully informed choices among birth control methods as well as other health services;
- discussion and information on sexuality, gender roles and power relationships, reproductive health and rights;
- management information systems that follow the woman or man, not simply the contraceptive method or service;

(continued on next page)

Women's Declaration on Population Policies
(continued)

- training to enable all staff to be gender sensitive, respectful service providers, along with procedures to evaluate and reward performance on the basis of the quality of care provided, not simply the quantity of services;
- program evaluation and funding criteria that utilize the standards defined here to eliminate unsafe or coercive practices, as well as sexist, classist or racist bias;
- inclusion of reproductive health as a central component of all public health programs, including population programs, recognizing that women require information and services not just in the reproductive ages but before and after;
- research into what services women want, how to maintain women's integrity, and how to promote their overall health and well-being.

4. Develop and provide the widest possible range of appropriate contraceptives to meet women's multiple needs throughout their lives:

- give priority to the development of women-controlled methods that protect against sexually transmitted infections, as well as pregnancy, in order to redress the current imbalances in contraceptive technology research, development and delivery;
- ensure availability and promote universal use of good quality condoms;
- ensure that technology research is respectful of women's right to full information and free choice, and is not concentrated among low income or otherwise disadvantaged women, or particular racial groups.

5. Ensure sufficient financial resources to meet the goals outlined above. Expand public funding for health, clean water and sanitation, and maternity care, as well as birth control. Establish better collaboration and coordination among UN, donors, governments and other agencies in order to use resources most effectively for women's health.

6. Design and promote policies for wider social, political and economic transformation that will allow women to negotiate and manage their own sexuality and health, make their own life choices, and participate fully in all levels of government and society.

Necessary Conditions

In order for women to control their sexuality and reproductive health, and to exercise their reproductive rights, the following actions are priorities:

1. Women Decision Makers

Using participatory processes, fill at least 50 percent of decision-making positions in all relevant agencies with women who agree with the principles described here, who have demonstrated commitment to advancing women's rights, and who are linked to the women to be served, taking into account income, ethnicity and race.

2. Financial Resources

As present expenditure levels are totally inadequate, multiply at least four-fold the money available to implement the program requirements listed in this Declaration.

3. Women's Health Movement

Allocate a minimum of 20 percent of available resources for women's health and reproductive rights organizations to strengthen their activities and work toward the goals specified in this declaration.

4. Accountability Mechanisms

Support women's rights and health advocacy groups, and other nongovernmental mechanisms, mandated by and accountable to women, at national and international levels, to:

- investigate and seek redress for abuses or infringements of women's and men's reproductive rights;
- analyze the allocation of resources to reproductive health and rights, and pursue revisions where necessary;
- identify inadequacies or gaps in policies, programs, information and services and recommend improvements;
- document and publicize progress.

Meeting these priority conditions will ensure women's reproductive health and their fundamental right to decide whether, when and how many children to have. Such commitment will also ensure just, humane and effective development and population policies that will attract a broad base of political support.

implementation of these guidelines has not yet been achieved. In fact, clinics are still struggling to define specific standards of care, and to establish measures to monitor and evaluate the quality of services. While the terminology of quality of care has gained currency, the concepts often have significantly different meanings for women's health advocates and for family planning policy makers (see Table 1).

In debates about quality of care in family planning services, it is commonly argued that "the best is the enemy of the good." Some say that the pursuit of quality for a few would jeopardize access for the many and, in extreme cases, would set up "medical barriers" to access (see, most recently, Shelton, Angle, and Jacobstein 1992). In fact, good-quality care need not be expensive (see box on page 246; also Kay and Kabir 1988). The motivation of staff and revisions in the allocations of human, not only financial, resources can improve basic program management and logistics systems and, more importantly, the technical quality and interpersonal quality of services (see Aitken and Reichenbach in this volume). It is not acceptable, nor is it effective, for services to be of such poor quality that women "accept" methods for which they have clear contraindications (Hardy et al. 1991); are exposed to high risk of infection or injury, such as uterine perforation during IUD insertion; are given no or insufficient information to use the method effectively, or are sterilized without consent (Khattab 1992); are not counseled adequately regarding side effects and not enabled to switch methods freely; or are persuaded to use a particular method because of the provider's incompetence or preferences (Dixon-Mueller and Germain 1992 and 1993). Clients should be treated with dignity, not disrespect, and with caring about the social and emotional consequences that may result from a decision to practice birth control.

Such shortcomings, which all too commonly occur, can be solved with commitment to improved training and supervision of staff. Critical

---

TABLE 1

Interpretations of Quality of Care Concepts

Concept	Women's health advocates	Family planning policy makers
Information	Education Advantages and disadvantages of methods	Motivation Advantages of methods methods
Scope of services	Sexual and reproductive health	Contraception; sometimes abortion
Counseling	Client-provider dialogue	Persuasion
Choices	All methods Provide safe abortion	"Modern" methods Prevent abortion
Outcome measures	Contraceptive continuation Client satisfaction	Method continuation Long-acting methods
Follow-up	Provide information, routine care, support for switching methods	Manage complications

Source: Marcelo and Germain 1994.

to this effort are new program statistics and evaluation measures that follow each client to assure proper treatment and positive outcomes; skilled staff to assist clients with emotional or social, not just physical, consequences of birth control; program managers who are alert to quality control problems; and reward systems for staff and programs based on how well they serve people, not on how many contraceptives they dispense (see Jain and Bruce in this volume).

Three other *essential* elements of good-quality birth control services are often resisted, but are of equal priority: safe abortion services; STD prevention, diagnosis, and treatment; and improved technologies.

Safe Abortion Services

Women are demonstrating with their lives and their health that abortion is, for them, a method of family planning (Dixon-Mueller 1993a). It is impractical, as well as unethical, not to provide safe abortion services. The ideal is, of course, to both remove legal restrictions and assure provision of safe services to all who need them. Even where abortion is illegal, however, or where political and social factors are serious obstacles, governments and other agencies in a number of countries have found means to provide this critical service for women's health.

STD Prevention, Diagnosis, and Treatment

In the face of the STD and HIV pandemics, it is mandatory that all programs that serve sexually active people offer information and services for the prevention and control of STDs, including HIV, to all clients. In fact, many family planning services have often given low priority to condom introduction and distribution, although condoms are currently the only means, other than abstinence, to reduce exposure to disease (Liskin, Wharton, and Blackburn 1990). Few, if any, family planning programs in Southern countries, as far as we are aware, systematically screen and treat clients for STD infection. Yet, contraceptive safety is compromised by these diseases; STDs are the major cause of infertility; and the presumed

clients of family planning services, married women of reproductive age, have virtually no access to specialized STD services (Dixon-Mueller and Wasserheit 1991; Elias 1991; Elias, Leonard, and Thompson 1993; Germain et al. 1992).

Improved Technologies

The third necessary change in the birth control dimension of reproductive and sexual health has to do with technology and the ways in which research and development priorities are determined. As described by Fathalla (in this volume), a major reorientation of research priorities and process is needed to pursue critical technological gaps: woman-controlled methods that will protect against infection, with or without protection against pregnancy; abortifacients; and male methods. Simpler, less-expensive diagnostic techniques and treatments for conventional STDs are urgently needed (Wasserheit and Holmes 1992). Substantial changes are also needed in the research process to ensure that the women to be served are fully represented at all stages, and that introductory trials are conducted in such a way as to ensure that service delivery systems are strong enough to protect and follow up on clients' safety and well-being (see García-Moreno and Claro in this volume; Spicehandler and Simmons 1993; WHO/HRP and IWHC 1991).

Other Reproductive Health Services

In addition to these essential investments to transform family planning services into truly voluntary and safe birth control services, investments must be made in *broader reproductive and sexual health services for women* (see Aitken and Reichenbach in this volume). In 1987, the International Women's Health Coalition defined and promoted a reproductive health approach to meet women's needs by encouraging enhanced collaboration among disparate vertical programs for family planning, maternal and child health, and STD control (Germain and Ordway 1989). Since then, many in population and related health fields have adopted the language and the concept of reproductive health. But until now, "reproductive health" has been at best understood and implemented as a combination of conventional contraceptive services, child survival interventions, and pregnancy care (see box on page 246; also Sí Mujer 1992). Recently, some agencies — notably, the Ford Foundation, the John D. and Catherine T. MacArthur Foundation, IPPF, the Population Council, and the World Bank — have begun to incorporate "sexuality," "sexual health," or STDs into their agendas (Ford Foundation 1991; IPPF 1993; Population Council 1989; Senanayake 1992). Such programs represent a significant advance over narrower approaches and serve well those whom they recognize as their clients.

Most programs, however, have approached women as means to the ends of fertility control and child health. They have concentrated on married, fertile women in their reproductive years, and have left many girls and women seriously underserved or unserved. Although family planning has been combined with maternal and child health (for example, Coeytaux 1989; Otsea 1992), such programs have had very little interaction with AIDS and STD programs until quite recently (see, for example, Berer and Ray 1993; World Health Organization 1993). Debates over integrated vs. vertical approaches continue unresolved, leaving most women with no option but to travel to and wait at multiple clinics on multiple days (see Aitken and Reichenbach in this volume).

By the time girls and young women reach family planning and maternal and child health services, they are, in many countries, severely anemic, malnourished and stunted, pregnant, or infected with STDs. Child health programs have as yet invested little in ending discriminatory and abusive treatment of girls by families, communities, and health services. Unmarried, but sexually active young people who do not have children are generally excluded from services; when served, they may be treated punitively (see Hawkins and Meshesha in this volume). Services for childbearing women remain woefully inadequate in preventing death and treating morbidity (see, for

example, Brady and Winikoff 1992). At the other end of the age spectrum, preventive health services have generally had no interest in women who are sterile or beyond reproductive age even though they remain sexually active. At the same time, tertiary health services see increasing numbers of older women with preventable cancers; STDs, including HIV and AIDS; and the effects of menopause, some of which may be inappropriately treated as illness.

Thus, we propose that policies and programs seek to meet the *sexual* and reproductive health needs of girls and women of all ages throughout their life cycles, regardless of whether their sexual relations have a reproductive purpose. Services would include the following:

- Fully voluntary birth control for individuals (a full range of contraceptive methods and safe abortion).

- Services related to pregnancy (prenatal and postnatal care, safe delivery, nutrition, child health).

- STD prevention, screening, diagnosis, and treatment.

- Gynecologic care (screening for breast and cervical cancer).

- Sexuality and gender information, education, counseling.

- Health counseling and education in all services.

- Referral systems for other health problems.

How this agenda is accomplished, short- and longer-range priorities, and specific investments will, of course, need to be adjusted for particular settings (see Box 2 on next page). What is important is an overall strategic vision against which specific plans can be made, implemented, and monitored (see box on page 50). Certainly, these services, and the agencies that fund and administer them, should no longer be driven solely or primarily by demographic concerns.

Meeting Women's Sexual and Reproductive Health Needs in Sierra Leone

My friend said, [The clinic] is so good, I cannot explain. Go ahead and you will see for yourself. As soon as I enter, the place feels like a clinic. It is tidy, neat and clean...There is no waste of time, you are constantly cared for.
—*Primary school teacher, age 31, on her first visit to the Marie Stopes clinic*

For the average Sierra Leonean, life is a constant struggle for survival. The public sector is able to provide only minimal social services. The majority of women learn about womanhood and reproduction only through initiation ceremonies for traditional secret societies. As a result, Sierra Leone has one of the world's highest child mortality rates (150–200 per 1000 births), and one of Africa's highest maternal mortality rates (estimated at 2,500 per 100,000 births). The average woman bears 6–7 children during her lifetime.

Since 1988, the Marie Stopes Society of Sierra Leone (MSSL) has overcome social and economic barriers to provide high-quality reproductive and sexual health services, including contraception, diagnosis and treatment of STDs, Pap smears, prenatal care, services for women with unwanted pregnancies, simple operative procedures, and counseling for menopausal women. General health and nutrition services are also provided, especially for children under age five and malnourished pregnant women. Special care is given to counseling and follow-up to reassure clients and ensure their concerns are met, even by the pharmacist:

I make sure I explain the use of all medications I dispense and confirm that the client absorbed [the information]. It does not take that much time, really.
—*Nurse/pharmacist at the Aberdeen clinic*

Staff training includes, not only technical skills, but also continuing orientation to the goals and ethics of MSSL, to ensure high quality client care and staff harmony despite escalating hardships. Every day, new solutions have to be found to endlessly vexing problems, such as assuring adequate supplies and maintaining accounting procedures in the face of fluctuating exchange rates, inflation, and lack of computerization.

Nonetheless, the rewards are worth the hardships. By the end of 1991, MSSL boasted two main clinics that provide a full range of services (including operating theaters for menstrual regulation and minor gynecologic procedures), and eight satellite clinics. By August 1991, MSSL clinics were seeing about 4,000 clients per month. Most are low-income, petty traders in their middle or late twenties.

Donor contributions are still required, primarily to purchase supplies and spare parts from abroad. Local currency, raised chiefly from clinic charges, is used to pay for staff salaries, other operating costs, and local supplies. The fees MSSL charges clients are minimal, within a range most clients are able to afford. In some cases, fees are waived for clients unable to pay.

MSSL's goal is to fulfill the reproductive and sexual health needs of women throughout their life cycles. Currently, MSSL youth programs include awareness campaigns through radio; talks and videos in schools; a network of youth clubs; and workshops, plays, and singing groups. MSSL advises young people to postpone sexual activity until they feel they are ready. If they are already sexually active, MSSL encourages them to use their clinic's contraceptive and STD information and service.

Although MSSL's primary purpose is to create a space for women, it is very aware that women's lives are closely tied to both their children and their male partners. Thus, it has welcomed men and encouraged them to be involved in the welfare of their partners and children. Employment-based clinics provide regular seminars for male workers on family planning and responsible parenthood. Staff explain to the men all the services that are offered to women and children, and what they are for. As a result, men's interest and participation has increased significantly, and a clinic providing STD and contraceptive services for men opened in 1994.

Source: Adapted from Toubia 1994, with permission.

Men's Responsibility and Behavior

Generally, population policies in Southern countries, concerned international agencies, and demographers have focused on women, since it is they who bear children.[4] While it is essential that women have access to services with which to control their health and fertility, it is entirely inappropriate for policy to allow, even enable, men to abdicate their responsibility for their own fertility, prevention of STDs, and the well-being of their sexual partners and the children they father. Men remain fertile longer than women and continue sexual activity into their older years, often with multiple partners. As a result, evidence from some countries shows that many men actually have higher fertility than their wives, and much of this excess occurs after age 45 (Bruce 1993).

Although vasectomy is significantly cheaper and safer than female sterilization procedures, tubal ligation is nearly three times as frequent as vasectomy in Southern countries. The only other male contraceptive method, the condom, has more often than not been offered as a last choice for women who cannot or will not use modern, more "effective" contraceptives. In any case, many men refuse to use condoms at all, or consistently, or with their regular partners, leaving their partners at risk of STDs (Rosenberg and Gollub 1992; Stein 1993). In general, men have not been welcomed or encouraged to participate in family planning services designed for women. Separate programs for men have generally been of much smaller scale and focused on vasectomy.

It is thus not surprising that contraceptive use data show that in "less-developed" regions of the world, methods that require men's initiative and cooperation (vasectomy, condom, rhythm, and withdrawal) account for only 26 percent of contraceptive use. (In "more-developed" regions, these methods account for 57 percent of use.) Even taking into account the likelihood of underestimation, the great discrepancy between the female and male burdens of responsibility for contraception is stark (see Table 2 on page 226; Mauldin and Segal 1988; Ross and Frankenberg 1993).

Refusing to use contraceptives themselves, many men also resist their partners' desire to use a method (Liskin, Wharton, and Blackburn 1990; Ruminjo et al. 1991). At the same time, in many cases they abdicate responsibility for their children to the woman or women who bore them (Bruce 1989; Bruce and Lloyd 1992). In Costa Rica, where over 80 percent of first births are to adolescent women, a 16-year-old girl described how her boyfriend reacted when she told him she was pregnant: "He told me he didn't want to hear anything about babies because he wasn't interested. He said it probably wasn't his baby anyway. And then he left." (Castillo 1993)

Because their objective has been fertility control, vasectomy services have missed an extremely important opportunity to work with men on other aspects of sexual health (see, for example, Lynan et al. 1993). Programs could provide information, screening, and treatment for STDs; promote continued condom use beyond the initial period following vasectomy; and provide counseling and educational activities to promote healthy sexuality and equitable gender relations (Liskin, Benoit, and Blackburn 1992). Box 3 (on the next page) describes two projects that demonstrate not only how to move from a simple vasectomy clinic to a men's reproductive health program, but also that men can become interested in such services (Rogow 1990; see also Mtsogolo 1992).

Overall, substantially greater investments are needed in vasectomy services and condom promotion, as well as STD control and broader reproductive health services for men. Across regions, men have sometimes shown more interest in family planning than is usually assumed by service providers and policy makers (Hawkins 1992; Liskin, Benoit, and Blackburn 1992; Liskin, Wharton, and Blackburn 1990). It seems that men often prefer separate service facilities from women and, sometimes, male providers (Rogow 1990; Mtsogolo 1992), but experimentation is needed to determine suitable approaches in each country.

More profound changes will also be needed, however, to increase use of vasectomy and condoms, to ensure men's respect for their partners' contraceptive choices, and to motivate men to take responsibility for sexual health and the children they father (see, for example, Savara and Sridhar 1992). Socialization practices and other social institutions that condone or promote severe imbalances of power and other inequities between women and men, along with exploit-

---

B O X 3

Meeting Male Reproductive Health Needs in Latin America

Not much is known about how men view their reproductive and sexual lives. Limited available evidence suggests that they are highly concerned with achieving effective and satisfying sexual function and treating STDs. But what moves men to be concerned about unwanted pregnancy?

A combination of male attitudes and provider bias has meant that men are both a neglected and a poorly prepared constituency for family planning and reproductive health care. Frequently, pride makes men reluctant to ask about reproduction, sexuality, and contraception. Men seldom learn about contraception from health professionals, who themselves have little information.

The experiences of PRO-PATER in Brazil and Profamilia's Clínica para el Hombre in Colombia may help answer the question "How can men's interests be better understood and addressed by reproductive health programs?" The former is a reproductive health service for men only; the latter, a clinic created as an adjunct to a long-standing program for women.

Pro-Pater

This clinic was conceived in 1981 as a "space for men to participate more fully in family planning" through vasectomy, which is almost unknown in Brazil (even though 27 percent of all women aged 15–49 in union have been sterilized). The clinic now also provides counseling, screening and treatment for sexual dysfunction and infertility. It does not provide condoms, nor is it willing to sell them — an important shortcoming given the prevalence of STDs, including HIV, in São Paulo. Clinic staff do treat clients with STDs (except AIDS), but do not publicly promote this service, as STD clinics generally have a poor reputation. In the future, PRO-PATER may form adolescent groups focusing on birth control and sexuality.

PRO-PATER's technical competence is measured by its low complication and failure rates.

The adequacy of the program's counseling is evident from client satisfaction at the initial visit and during follow-up visits, and the virtual absence of requests for vasectomy reversal.

Clínica para el Hombre

To meet the needs of a wide range of clients, this clinic in Colombia combines vasectomy services with testing and treatment of urological problems, sexual problems, infertility, and STDs; general physical examinations; condom distribution; and family planning education. Initially, the clinic faced substantial cultural resistance, staffing problems, and a small case load; but after three years, it was 92 percent financially self-sufficient, had expanded to five cities, and was serving 750 new clients each month. By 1990, the clinic was seeing more than 500 men for follow-up and selling well over 2,000 condoms. Clinic staff also provide care for the female partners of STD and infertility clients.

The clinic is a training resource for other institutions in Colombia and elsewhere in Latin America. The key to its success: careful determination of what is most important to clients, a very attractive facility, individualized care, a wide range of services, low-cost vasectomy, and Saturday hours.

The Future

For the time being, to increase male contraceptive, use we must make the best of the two available methods. This can be done by increasing general acceptance of these methods, improving access to them, and putting greater emphasis on the quality of care provided. Over the longer term, it is essential that new choices for men be developed, whether better condoms or entirely new approaches. Increasingly, the issue is, not lack of demand, but appropriate supply and technology.

Source: Adapted from Rogow 1990, with permission.

---

ative, abusive, and unhealthful sexuality, need to be changed (Aral, Mosher, and Cates 1992; see also Correa and Petchesky in this volume). The greatest hope for such changes lies with young people, who, with support, can challenge gender role stereotypes as they participate in social life, explore their sexuality, and build relationships with each other (S. Nowrojee 1993b).

Sexuality and Gender Relations

Until the advent of HIV and AIDS, and even since then, the family planning field, especially government programs, has generally ignored the fact that reproduction takes place through sexual relations, which are conditioned by broader gender relations. A review of the conventional demographic and family planning literature illustrates that the population field has neglected sexuality, gender roles, and relationships, focusing instead largely on outcomes, such as contraceptive efficacy, unwanted pregnancy, and, more recently, infection (Dixon-Mueller 1993c). Similarly, health and education policies and programs in most countries have rarely dealt with sexuality and have understood very little about how gender relations affect achievement of their goals. Overall, population and health policies and programs continue to be rooted in and reinforce existing gender relations and traditional constructions of sexuality, rather than transforming them. Examples include public campaigns on child health that feature only mothers, family planning education materials or condom packaging that use aggressive images, and STD or HIV campaigns that portray women as vectors of infection.

Socialization into sexuality and gender roles begins early in the family and community, and is reinforced by basic social institutions, the mass media, and other factors (Miedzian 1993; Obura 1991). Political, economic, legal, and cultural subordination of women generally means they are easily subject to violence and unable to protect themselves from risk beginning at a very young age (Fullilove et al. 1990; Handwerker 1994; Heise with Pitanguy and Germain 1994; Worth 1989). Confusing double standards exist for male

and female sexual behavior, under which boys are expected to be sexually aggressive and girls to be both chaste and sexually appealing (Ekwempu 1991; ECOS 1992; S. Nowrojee 1993a; Winn 1992). While women are expected to be submissive, they are also held responsible for sexual interaction. They are the ones expelled from school for pregnancy, or publicly shamed for "loose" behavior. This is well illustrated by boys in India, who identified "good" girls as those who ignored boys when they whistled at them, and "bad" girls as those who "turned and smiled" (Bhende 1992; Savara and Sridhar 1992). Even extreme behavior by boys is rarely questioned — and is sometimes condoned. From Kenya to the United States, boys who rape have been publicly exonerated by parents who say "boys will be boys" (Gross 1993; Perlez 1991), or school officials who say "they meant no harm" (V. Nowrojee 1993).

Women's reproductive and sexual well-being, self-perceptions, and self-esteem are directly and indirectly affected by rape, battery, homicide, incest, psychological abuse, genital mutilation, trafficking of women and children, dowry related murder, and forced sterilization and forced abortion (Adekunle and Ladipo 1992; Dawit 1994; Edemikpong 1990; Ghadially 1991; Maggwa and Ngugi 1992; Pyne 1992; Toubia 1993). The 1993 *World Development Report* indicates that "women ages 15 to 44 lose more Discounted Healthy Years of Life (DHYLs) to rape and domestic violence than they do to breast cancer, cervical cancer, obstructed labor, heart disease, AIDS, respiratory infections, motor vehicle accidents, or war" (World Bank 1993).

Other beliefs and practices regarding women's bodies and sexuality also have important health consequences. Beliefs that women should not know about sexuality can result in high risk of STDs, unwanted pregnancy, and inability or reluctance to seek health care. For example, STD symptoms are often believed by women to be normal, not problems to be treated. A rural Indian woman said, "Like every tree has flowers, every woman has white discharge" (Bang and Bang 1992; Dixon-Mueller and Wasserheit 1991; Pyne 1992; Ramasubban 1994). Widespread beliefs that menstrual blood and normal vaginal discharge are dirty, shameful, or distasteful to the sexual partner lead to poor menstrual hygiene or vaginal cleansing, which increase the risk of vaginal infection and reduce women's sexual pleasure (Dixon-Mueller and Wasserheit 1991; International Center for Research on Women 1994; Ramasubban 1990; Sabatier 1993; Wambua 1992).

Finally, gender differentials in access to health care put girls and women in unnecessary jeopardy. Women, more than men, have to overcome economic and cultural barriers to seeking and receiving information and care. Social constructions of "proper" female behavior and sexuality deter women from using STD clinics for fear of being regarded as promiscuous or defiled (Dixon-Mueller and Germain 1993; Elias and Heise 1993). Single women and adolescents may not approach family planning services, for fear of being seen as sexually active or being refused service. Even medical research has been discriminatory, giving little attention to breast and cervical cancer; using only male subjects for research on heart disease; and, until recently, excluding female-specific symptoms such as cervical cancer or vaginal candidiasis from the case definition of AIDS (Corea 1992; Hamblin and Reid 1991; Reid 1992).

Clearly, social constructions of sexuality and gender relations are major deterrents to sexual and reproductive health and rights. They are generally considered "politically sensitive," which has prevented necessary policy and program development in most countries, although the World Health Organization developed guidelines as early as 1975 (WHO 1975). When the state does intervene, mechanisms must be carefully designed to protect basic rights, including privacy and bodily integrity. Perhaps the most urgent investment needed is in young people, who are being severely injured, and even dying, as a result of societies' unwillingness to invest in sexuality and gender education and services for both unmarried and married young people.

A narrow message of abstinence and dire warnings about the consequences of poorly managed sexuality is not the answer. Sexuality is a basic dimension of human life, and young people, especially under contemporary conditions, experiment in many societies. The message needs to be one of mutual caring and respect, with full knowledge of negative consequences and how to prevent them. A number of innovative efforts have been launched to engage young people in dialogue with each other and with adults on their perceived needs, and to provide them necessary information and services (Francis and O'Neill 1992; see also Hawkins and Meshesha in this volume). Sweden is one country that has adopted a transforming approach to sex education that recognizes sexuality as good and lovemaking as something people should know how to do well. Many other cultures have, or used to have, social institutions to support young people in sexual initiation. Much could be done simply by recovering, re-creating, or building on those traditions.

As experimentation proceeds with programs to support young people in their exploration of their sexuality and their gender roles, we must provide the opportunities for education and work that will encourage and enable them to delay marriage and childbearing. We must also work with other major social institutions, especially the mass media, to promote more equitable and positive images of gender relations and sexuality.

Conclusion

Our proposed approach is twofold. *First*, transform population policies to help achieve human development equity and human rights. *Second*, put sexuality and gender relations at the center of reproductive and sexual health and rights policies and programs to empower women, to ensure their health, and to motivate men to take responsibility for their own behavior. The outcome should be mutually caring, respectful, and pleasurable sexual relationships, and a solid foundation for reproductive and sexual health and rights, as well as for human development and rights overall.

This is a sweeping agenda, which reflects especially women's perceived needs and experiences and recognizes that fundamental social and policy changes are needed. Significant changes are already occurring on a small scale in many countries and even at the level of international diplomatic debate. Women's empowerment, reproductive health, sexuality and many of the other issues are being actively and broadly discussed. What is still needed is the political will to reallocate resources to this agenda, imaginative strategies to use those resources well in the particular circumstances of each country, and the inclusion of representatives of women, who have most at stake, in all levels of decisionmaking.

Notes

1 Some of these also acknowledge that Northern overconsumption is an equal, if not greater, threat, but believe that interventions to restrict consumption are more difficult than population control and therefore urge pursuit of the latter (see, for example, McNamara 1991).

2 Despite falling fertility rates, the number of couples in the reproductive ages has doubled since 1960, and the number of births continues to rise, a phenomenon referred to as "population momentum." Because of the young age structure of Southern populations, the momentum factor will be pronounced in the next 20 years (Merrick 1994).

3 For example, the rate of transmission of STDs from men to women is higher than from women to men. Women suffer much worse consequences than men, including increased risk of ectopic pregnancy and pregnancy wastage, and pelvic inflammatory disease (Dixon-Mueller and Wasserheit 1991; Germain et al. (eds.) 1992).

4 An important exception was India, which put very strong emphasis on vasectomy in the national population program until the early 1970s.

References

Adekunle, A. O., and O. A. Ladipo. 1992. Reproductive tract infections in Nigeria: Challenges for a fragile health infrastructure. In A. Germain et al. (eds.), *Reproductive tract infections: Global impact and priorities for women's reproductive health*. Plenum Press: New York and London.

Antrobus, P. 1993. The impact of structural adjustment policies on women's health. Paper presented at the Medical Women's International Association, Africa and Near East First Regional Congress on Safe Motherhood and the Health of Women, November 29 – December 3, in Nairobi.

Aral, S. O., W. Mosher, and W. Cates, Jr. 1992. Vaginal douching among women of reproductive age in the United States: 1988. *American Journal of Public Health* 82(2):210–214.

Bang, R., and A. Bang. 1992. Why women hide them: Rural women's viewpoints on reproductive tract infections. *Manushi — A Journal about Women and Society* 69:27–30.

Berer, M., and S. Ray. 1993. *Women and HIV/AIDS: An international resource book*. London: Pandora Press.

Bhende, A. 1992. Socialization into sex roles: Program implications. Presentation made at Meeting the Sexual Health Needs of Women and Men: Exploring Integration of Family Planning, AIDS and STD Programs, June 18–19, in Arlington, Va.

Bongaarts, J. 1994 (forthcoming). Population policy options in the developing world. *Science*.

Brady, M., and B. Winikoff. 1992. Rethinking postpartum health care. Proceedings of a seminar presented under the Population Council's Robert H. Ebert Program on Critical Issues in Reproductive Heath and Population. New York: Population Council.

Bruce, J. 1989. Homes divided. *World Development* 17(7):979–991.

———. 1990. Fundamental elements of the quality of care: A simple framework. *Studies in Family Planning* 21(2):61–91.

———. 1993. Testimony presented to the House Foreign Affairs Committee, September 22, in Washington, D.C.

Bruce, J., and C. Lloyd. 1992. *Finding the ties that bind: Beyond leadership and household*. Working paper No. 41. New York: Population Council.

Castillo, S. 1993. Tools for teens. *POPULI* 20(2):8.

Coeytaux, F. 1989. Celebrating mother and child on the fortieth day: The Sfax, Tunisia postpartum program. *Quality/Calidad/ Qualité*. New York: Population Council.

Corea, G. 1992. *The invisible epidemic*. New York: Harper Collins.

Dahlgren, G. 1993. Population policies reconsidered. Introduction to SIDA/SAREC Conference, December 7, in Harare, Zimbabwe.

Davis, K. 1967. Population policy: Will current programs succeed? *Science* 158:7304–7739.

Davis, K. and J. Blake. 1956. Social structure and fertility: an analytic framework. *Economic Development and Cultural Change* 4(3):211–235.

Dawit, S. 1994 (forthcoming). *The international human rights dimensions of female genital mutilation*. London: Zed.

Dixon-Mueller, R. 1993a. Abortion *is* a method of family planning. In R. Dixon-Mueller and A. Germain (eds.), *Four Essays on Birth Control Needs and Risks.* New York: International Women's Health Coalition.

————. 1993b. *Population policy and women's rights: Transforming reproductive choice.* Westport, Conn.: Praeger.

————. 1993c. The sexuality connection in reproductive health. *Studies in Family Planning* 24(5):269–282.

Dixon-Mueller, R., and A. Germain. 1992. Stalking the elusive "unmet need" for family planning. *Studies in Family Planning* 23(5):330–335.

————. 1993. Whose life is it, anyway? Assessing the relative risks of contraception and pregnancy. In In R. Dixon-Mueller and A. Germain (eds.), *Four essays on birth control needs and risks.* New York: International Women's Health Coalition.

Dixon-Mueller, R., and J. Wasserheit. 1991. *The culture of silence: Reproductive tract infections among women in the Third World.* New York: International Women's Health Coalition.

Due, J. M. 1991. Policies to overcome the negative effects of structural adjustment programs on African female-headed households. In C. H. Gladwin (ed.), *Structural adjustment and African women farmers.* Gainesville: University of Florida Press.

ECOS (Estudos e Comunicaçã em Sexualidade e Reprodução Humana). 1992. Um abraço ("A hug"). São Paulo.

Edemikpong, N. B. 1990. Women and AIDS. In E. D. Rothblum and E. Cole (eds.), *Women's mental health in Africa.* Binghampton, England: Harrington Park Press.

Ekwempu, F. 1991. The influence of socio-cultural behavioral patterns on the knowledge and practice of contraception and abortion among the Hauda-Fulani adolescents of Northern Nigeria. Research supported by the International Women's Health Coalition, New York.

Elias, C. 1991. *Sexually transmitted diseases and the reproductive health of women in developing countries.* Working Paper No. 5. Programs Division, Population Council.

Elias, C., and L. Heise. 1993. *The development of microbicides: A new method of HIV prevention for women.* Working Paper No. 6. Programs Division, Population Council.

Elias, C., A. Leonard, and J. Thompson. 1993. A puzzle of will: Responding to reproductive tract infections in the context of family planning programs. Paper presented at the Africa Operations Research/Technical Assistance End-of-Project Conference, October, in Nairobi.

Elson, D. 1990. Male bias in macroeconomics: The case of structural adjustment. In *Male bias in the development process.* Manchester, England: University Press.

Ethiopia: Transitional Government, Office of the Prime Minister. 1993. National population policy of Ethiopia. Addis Ababa, April.

Ford Foundation. 1991. Reproductive health: A strategy for the 1990s. New York.

Francis, C., and C. O'Neill. 1992. A strategy for supporting the use of condoms by sexually active youth: The Eastern Caribbean experience. In L. Bond (ed.), *A portfolio of AIDS/STD behavioral interventions and research.* Washington, D.C.: Pan American Health Organization.

Fullilove, M. T., et al. 1990. Black women and AIDS prevention: A view towards understanding the gender rules. *Journal of Sex Research* 27(1):47-64.

Germain, A. 1989. The Christopher Tietze International Symposium: An overview. In *International Journal of Gynecology and Obstetrics*, Special Suppl. Limerick, Ireland: International Federation of Gynecology and Obstetrics.

Germain, A., and J. Ordway. 1989. *Population and women's health: Balancing the scales.* New York: International Women's Health Coalition.

Germain, A., et al. (eds.). 1992. *Reproductive tract infections: Global impact and priorities for women's reproductive health.* New York: Plenum Press.

Ghadially, R. 1991. All for Izzat. *Manushi — A Journal About Women and Society* (September/October).

Gross, J. 1993. Boys will be boys and adults are befuddled. *New York Times,* March 29.

Hamblin, J., and E. Reid. 1991. Women, the HIV epidemic and human rights: A tragic imperative. Paper presented at the International Workshop on AIDS: A Question of Rights and Humanity, at the International Court of Justice, The Hague.

Handwerker, W. P. 1993 (forthcoming). Gender power differences between parents and high risk sexual behavior by their children: AIDS/STD risk factors extend to prior generation. *Journal of Women's Health.*

Hardy, E. E., et al. 1991. Adequaçã do uso de pílula anticoncepcional entre mulheres unidas ("Contraceptive pill: Adequacy of use among women in union"). *Revista Saúde Pública.* São Paulo, 25(2):96–102.

Hawkins, K. 1992. *Male participation in family planning: A review of program approaches in the Africa region.* London: IPPF.

Heise, L., with J. Pitanguy and A. Germain. 1994 (forthcoming). *Violence against women as a health issue.* Washington, D.C.: World Bank (Population, Health, and Nutrition Division).

Huezo, C. M., and C. Briggs. 1992. Rights of the client. *Medical and Service Guidelines for Family Planning*. International Planned Parenthood Federation.

International Center for Research on Women (ICRW). 1994 (forthcoming). Final report of the ICRW Women and AIDS Research program. Washington, D.C.

International Planned Parenthood Federation. 1993. *Strategic plan. Vision 2000*. London.

John D. and Catherine T. MacArthur Foundation. 1993. 1992 Report on activities. Chicago: The John D. and Catherine T. MacArthur Foundation.

Kay, B. J., and S. M. Kabir. 1988. A study of costs and behavioral outcomes of menstrual regulation services in Bangladesh. *Social Science Medicine* 26(6):597–604.

Khattab, H. 1992. *The silent endurance: Social conditions of women's reproductive health in rural Egypt*. Cairo: Nour Arab Publishing House.

Lele, U. 1991. Women, structural adjustment, and transformation: Some lessons and questions from the African experience. In C. H. Gladwin (ed.), *Structural adjustment and African women farmers*. Gainesville: University of Florida Press.

Liskin, L., E. Benoit, and R. Blackburn. 1992. Male sterilization. *Population Reports*, Series D, No. 5.

Liskin, L., C. Wharton, and R. Blackburn. 1990. Condoms — now more than ever. *Population Reports*, Series H, No. 8.

Lynam, P. J., et al. 1993. Vasectomy in Kenya: The first steps. Working Paper No. 4. Association for Voluntary Surgical Contraception.

Maggwa, A. B. N., and E. N. Ngugi. 1992. Reproductive tract infections in Kenya: Insights for action from research. In Germain, et al. (eds.), *Reproductive tract infections*. Plenum Press: New York and London.

Marcelo, A. B., and A. Germain. 1994 (forthcoming). Women's perspectives on fertility regulation methods and services. In P.F.A. Van Look and G. Perez-Palacios (eds.), *Contraceptive research and development 1984– 1994: The road from Mexico City to Cairo and beyond*. New Delhi: Oxford University Press.

Mauldin, W. P., and J. A. Ross. 1991. Family planning programs: Efforts and results, 1982–89. *Studies in Family Planning* 22(6): 350–367.

Mauldin, W. P., and S. Segal. 1988. Prevalence of contraceptive use: Trends and issues. *Studies in Family Planning* 19(6):335–353.

McNamara, R. S. 1991. A global population policy to advance human development in the 21st century. Speech presented at the United Nations, December 10, in New York.

Merrick, T. 1994 (forthcoming). Population dynamics in developing countries. In R. Case (ed.), *Fiction, factions and facts: The population and development debate*. Washington, D.C.: Overseas Development Council.

Miedzian, M. 1993. How rape is encouraged in American boys and what we can do to stop it. In E. Buchwood, P. Fletcher, and M. Roth (eds.), *Transforming a Rape Culture*. Minneapolis: Milkweed Edition.

Mtsogolo, B. 1992. A male oriented child spacing/social responsibility education and services programme — Malawi. In *ODA Annual Progress Report*. London: Marie Stopes International.

Nowrojee, S. 1993a. Sexuality and gender: Impact on women's health. Paper presented at the Medical Women's International Association, Near East & Africa First Regional Congress: The Health of Women and Safe Motherhood, November 29–December 3, in Nairobi.

———. 1993b. Speaking out for sexual and reproductive health. *DIVA: A Quarterly Journal of South Asian Women* 4(1):17–22.

Nowrojee, V. 1993. Kenyan adopting rape culture. *The Nairobi Law Monthly* 50:29–31.

Obura, A. 1991. *Changing images*. Nairobi: English Press Limited.

Otsea, K. 1992. Progress and prospects: The safe motherhood initiative. World Bank Background Document for the Meeting of Partners for Safe Motherhood, March, in Washington, D.C.

Perlez, J. 1991. Kenyans do some soul searching after the rape of 71 school girls. *New York Times*, July 29.

Population Council. 1989. Annual Report 1988. New York: The Population Council.

Pyne, H. H. 1992. AIDS and prostitution in Thailand: Case study of Burmese prostitutes in Ranong. Master's thesis. MIT.

Ramasubban, R. 1990. Sexual behaviour and conditions of health care: Potential risks for HIV transmission in India. Paper presented at the International Union for the Scientific Study of Population Seminar on Anthropological Studies Relevant to HIV Transmission, November 19–22, in Copenhagen.

———. 1994 (forthcoming). Patriarchy and the risks of HIV transmission to women in India. In M. Jasgupta, T. N. Krishnan, and L. Chen, (eds.), *Health and development in India*. Bombay: Oxford University Press.

Reid, E. 1992. Women, the HIV epidemic and human rights: A tragic imperative. Paper presented at the International Workshop on AIDS: A Question of Rights and Humanity, May, in The Hague.

Rogow, D. 1990. Man/hombre/homme: Meeting male reproductive health care needs in Latin America. *Quality/Calidad/Qualité*. New York: Population Council.

Rosenberg, M. J., and E. L. Gollub. 1992. Commentary: Methods women can use that may prevent sexually transmitted disease, including HIV. *American Journal of Public Health* 82(11):1473–1478.

Ross, J., and E. Frankenberg. 1993. *Findings from two decades of family planning research*. New York: Population Council.

Ruminjo, J., et al. 1991. *Consumer preference and functionality study of the Reality female condom in a low risk population in Kenya*. Research Triangle Park, N.C.: Family Health International.

Sabatier, R. (Southern African AIDS Program, Harare, Zimbabwe). 1993. Personal communication.

Savara, M., and C. R. Sridhar. 1992. Sexual behaviour of urban, educated Indian men: Results of a survey. *Shakti — Journal of Family Welfare*. 30–43.

Sen, G. 1991. Macroeconomic policies and the informal sector: A gender sensitive approach. Paper presented at the UN INSTRAW meeting on Macroeconomic Polices towards Women in the Informal Sector, 1991, in Rome.

Senanayake, P. 1992. Positive approaches to education for sexual health with examples from Asia and Africa. *Journal of Adolescent Health* 13(5):351–354.

Shelton, J.D., M. A. Angle, and R. A. Jacobstein. 1992. Medical barriers to access to family planning. *The Lancet* 340:1334–1335.

Sí Mujer. 1992. *Servicios integrales para la mujer*. Cali, Colombia: The Foundation.

Spicehandler, J., and R. Simmons. 1993. Contraceptive introduction reconsidered: A review and conceptual framework. Prepared on behalf of the Task Force on Research on the Introduction and Transfer of Technologies for Fertility Regulation, and presented at the meeting of the Policy and Coordination Committee, World Health Organization Special Programme of Research, Development and Research Training in Human Reproduction, June 23–25, in Geneva.

Stein, Z. A. 1993. HIV prevention: An update on the status of methods women can use. *American Journal of Public Health* 83:1379–1382.

Toubia, N. 1993. *Female genital mutilation: A call for global action*. New York: Women, Ink.

———. 1994 (forthcoming). The Marie Stopes Clinics in Sierra Leone. *Quality/Calidad/Qualité*. New York: Population Council.

Wambua, L. 1992. RTIs in Cameroon. Women's Health Journal 2:45-50.

Wasserheit, J., and K. Holmes. 1992. Reproductive tract infections: Challenges for international health policy, programs, and research. In A. Germain et al. (eds.), *Reproductive tract infections: Global impact and priorities for women's reproductive health*. New York: Plenum Press.

Weil, D. E. C., et al. 1990. *The impact of development policies on health — A review of the literature*. Geneva: World Health Organization.

Winn, M. 1992. Taboo talk: Reproductive health videos by Pacific Island women. *Quality/Calidad/Qualité* 4. New York: Population Council.

World Bank. 1993. *World development report*. New York: Oxford University Press.

World Health Organization (WHO). 1975. Education and treatment in human sexuality: The training of health professionals. Report of a WHO meeting. Geneva.

———. 1993. New approach to fighting AIDS. Press release, Geneva.

World Health Organization/Special Programme of Research, Development and Research Training in Human Reproduction (WHO/HRP) and International Women's Health Coalition (IWHC). 1991. Creating common ground: Women's perspectives on the selection and introduction of fertility regulation technologies. Report of a meeting between women's health advocates and scientists, February 20–22, Geneva: World Health Organization.

Worth, D. 1989. Sexual decision-making and AIDS: Why condom promotion among vulnerable women is likely to fail. *Studies in Family Planning* 20(6):297–397.

4

Challenges from the Women's Health Movement: Women's Rights versus Population Control

Claudia García-Moreno and Amparo Claro

The international women's health movement, which started in the late 1970s and early 1980s, has challenged the rationale on which population policies have been based — namely, that population control in the social interest has precedence over individual well-being and individual rights.[1] The women's health movement has strongly criticized the prevailing emphasis on narrowly construed "family planning programs" (generally equated with delivery of modern contraceptives and sterilization to married women) as the main way to achieve fertility reduction. It has also questioned the safety of modern contraceptive technologies both intrinsically and as actually delivered, the poor quality of services, the failure of governments to address women's health and empowerment more broadly, and the economic policies that jeopardize social services and promote growth over human welfare.

While millions of women have benefited from contraceptive services, some policies and programs to limit (or increase) population growth have had negative effects, especially on poor women. In many countries, abuses such as pressure to use specific types of contraceptives or sterilization, inadequate attention to contracep-

tive safety, poor-quality services that ignore women's multiple reproductive health needs, and barriers to access to contraceptives and safe abortion services have jeopardized women's rights and health. As other contributors to this volume illustrate, women have borne the brunt of the consequences when governments or other agencies have not provided the information, services, and broad social conditions necessary to assure their reproductive health and rights.

A central tenet of the international women's health movement is that women's health and rights, not macrodemographic objectives, are of paramount concern. In general, the movement argues that policies and programs should ensure better quality and provide more holistic approaches to women's health services, particularly in the area of reproductive health. The movement also places great importance on the issues of sexuality and gender relations. Policies and programs should include women's representatives at all levels of decisionmaking; promote increased responsibility among men for their own reproductive behavior, for the prevention of sexually transmitted diseases (STDs), and for the health and well-being of their partners and the children they father; provide equal opportunity for women in all aspects of social, economic, and political life, for its own sake, not simply as a means to reduce fertility; and pursue sustainable approaches to development that invest directly in people's well-being.

The women's health movement has developed differently in different regions, with varying levels of political awareness and involvement. Overall, the movement has grown substantially in both numbers and political strength during the last decade. In many places, women have moved from being a critical voice on the margin to being influential participants in program and policy debates and decisions at both the national and international levels (see, for example, Dixon-Mueller and Germain 1993; Pitanguy 1994).

In this chapter we describe the history and nature of the views and actions of the international women's health movement regarding sexual and reproductive health. Recognizing that great diversity exists among organized women on these issues and that we cannot do justice to all of them, we focus primarily on the discourse at the global level, where women have come together to share their diverse experiences and search for common ground. We consider strategies and accomplishments of women's health advocates at the local, national, and international levels, and show how the various organizations and movements have been effective agents on behalf of women's sexual and reproductive health and rights. Finally, we reflect on the challenges and dilemmas the movement faces in the years ahead.

The Women's Health Movement in Southern Countries

Like all social movements, the women's health movement is shaped by many political, cultural, and socioeconomic factors, and by its interactions with other social movements. Most countries now have at least some individuals and organizations that consider themselves women's health advocates. In a few Asian countries, in Latin America, and in the United States and Western Europe, advocacy groups have coalesced into "movements". Together, these individuals, groups, and movements constitute an international women's health movement. They share similar concerns, communicate through journals and regional and international networks, and meet on a regular basis to discuss and plan strategies.

The movement includes a wide range of organizations, from clearly articulated feminist non-governmental organizations (NGOs) and networks to grassroots women's groups of various sizes and mandates. The exact number of groups in Southern countries is unknown, but some examples will illustrate the size and dynamism of the movement. The Women's Global Network for Reproductive Rights doubled from 800 members and newsletter subscribers in 1988 to 1,655 in 1992. Its membership spans 113 countries, and more than half of its members are in Southern countries (WGNRR 1992a). The Latin American and Caribbean Women's Health Network, created in 1984 by approximately 30 groups and individuals, now has a contact list of 2,000, mostly groups. The International Women's Health Coalition, working with about 30 groups in 1984, now has contact with over 2,000 individuals and groups in Southern countries. About 150 organizations in Asia include women's health on their agendas (Asian and Pacific Women's Resource Collection Network 1990; Isis International 1992).

Critics often assert that the women's health movement, and feminism more generally, are "Western" phenomena imported to Southern countries by elite Northern and Southern women. While Western ideas have played a role, women in Southern countries have generated their own analyses, organizations, and movements, with and without exposure to the West, and there has been considerable cross-fertilization of ideas across many countries and continents. Critics also assert that Southern women's health advocates are elite women isolated from the realities of the mass of women. While elite women are certainly involved, in countries as diverse as Nigeria, India, the Philippines, and Brazil, disadvantaged women have raised their voices along with health professionals, social workers, psychologists, lawyers, and academics of various disciplines.

Women's health groups in Southern countries have grown out of a variety of circumstances. Many drew on women's involvement in broader nationalist, anti-imperialist, and democratization struggles — for example, in Latin America (Jaquette 1989), China and India (Rowbotham 1992), the Middle East (Jayawardena 1986), and the Philippines (Dixon-Mueller and Germain 1993). Others were initiated in direct response to inappropriate government population policies or poorly designed and implemented family planning services — for example, in Brazil (Pitanguy 1994) and India (Chatterjee 1993). Some, but not all, were influenced by the women's health movement that originated in Europe and North America in the 1970s.[2]

Latin America

The movement is highly developed in Latin America. In 1981, the First Latin American Feminist Meeting made visible a women's movement that was autonomous from political parties and other movements. Sexuality, reproductive rights, and violence were important elements of the agenda (Jaquette 1989). The meeting also established that the Latin American women's movement, while sharing certain concerns, was different from that of Europe or the United States. In 1984, the Latin American and Caribbean Women's Health Network was founded to provide information to feminist and other women's organizations, and to health groups and health service providers at local and regional levels, through a documentation center and a journal published in Spanish and English. The Network hosts meetings and coordinates public information campaigns across the region. It has also established links with international health organizations and participated in dialogues with scientists and policy makers working on issues related to women's reproductive health.[3]

Recognizing the political power of alliances, women in several Latin American countries — for example, Brazil, Chile, and Colombia — are now forming national networks. In Brazil, the National Feminist Network for Reproductive Health and Rights, founded in August 1991, has 65 organizational members from all over the country. In Chile, the Open Forum for Reproductive Rights and Reproductive Health, founded in 1989, is an informal coalition of 45 women's groups and NGOs concerned with reproductive health (Matamala 1993). In Colombia, the Women's Network for Sexual and Reproductive Rights, formed in November 1992 by 20 women's organizations, has been working on proposals for the new constitution that will provide for decriminalization of abortion, sex education in schools, and a national women's health program that it helped formulate (see Box 1 on next page). Networks are also developing in Argentina, Mexico, and Uruguay.

In Brazil, the highly organized women's health movement also has campaigned for decriminalization of abortion. In 1988, it succeeded in preventing insertion of a clause to protect the life of the unborn into the new constitution. It has publicized shortcomings in sterilization services, challenged inadequate protection of women's health and rights in contraceptive research (the preintroduction trials of Norplant®, for example), and campaigned for policy changes in these areas. The movement was also instrumental in the development and approval of PAISM, a national policy and program for comprehensive women's health care (see Box 1 on next page). Feminists inside the government have spearheaded implementation of the Comprehensive Women's Health Program in the municipality of São Paulo. This initiative is one of the few examples anywhere of a government program with a feminist perspective. The program has provided access to legal abortion; set up committees to monitor maternal mortality with equal representation from the health department and civil society; trained health center staff on issues of gender, sexuality, women's needs and their relationships with health care providers, and maternal mortality; and it has offered a range of contraceptive methods in almost all health centers (Araujo 1993).

In Peru, feminist organizations have worked with national and international researchers and

health care providers on the introduction of new contraceptive methods, such as Norplant® and Cyclofem, by producing educational materials and ensuring that service providers are respectful

Examples of Women-Centered Government Health Policies

Brazil: The Comprehensive Program for Women's Health Care (PAISM)

The Comprehensive Program for Women's Health Care (PAISM) in Brazil was created in 1983 to provide services for women beyond the existing maternal and child health services. The program includes prenatal care, delivery and post-partum care, family planning, breast and cervical cancer screening, diagnosis and treatment of sexually transmitted diseases, and infertility services, as well as occupational and mental health services. It also expands coverage to include adolescents and post-menopausal women rather than only women of reproductive age. PAISM emphasizes that women need access to preventive as well as curative care, and to information about their bodies and their health. It notes that this knowledge should be empowering to women.

PAISM was the result of an alliance between the Ministry of Health and the women's movement. Feminists were involved in the development of technical guidelines and educational materials, and continue to promote PAISM and to lobby for its implementation. They have also been involved, at national, state, and municipal levels in attempts to implement the policy (Costa 1992). The Newsletter of Brazil's National Network for Reproductive Rights (1992) suggests that three elements made PAISM possible: health care reform which was moving towards decentralization of health care and addressing health needs; the presence of feminists in government; and the action of the women's movement, which pressed for comprehensive services and for a wider choice in contraceptives. Implementation of PAISM has faltered, but examples in the state of Goias and the municipality of Sao Paulo show that where there is political will and pressure from women, much can be achieved.

Colombia: Health for Women, Women for Health

Willingness on the part of the government, support from the Pan American Health Organization, and the action of feminists have led to a

national women's health policy. The policy lays out five programs: promotion of self–help; reproductive health and sexuality; prevention and care for victims of violence; mental health; and occupational health (Posada 1993).

"Health for Women, Women for Health" explicitly aims to reduce inequalities between women and men and sees women as "subjects of the decisions over their lives, their body, their sexuality and their health" (Colombia Ministry of Health 1992:24). Women, it contends, should be participants in planning and implementing health programs. The policy stresses the importance of a gender perspective in understanding health and illness, as well as poverty and other forms of inequity. It emphasizes the need for a comprehensive approach to women's health, but also recognizes the individuality of women. "The woman has the right to treatment and care from the health services as a whole being, with specific needs — according to her age, activity, social class, race, and place of origin, and not to be treated exclusively as a biological reproducer. She has the right to respectful and dignified treatment by health workers of her body, her fears, and her needs for intimacy and privacy" (Colombia Ministry of Health 1992:25).

The policy recognizes the problem of violence against women, which it notes is the main cause of death among women 15-44 years of age. It also recognizes the need for special attention to adolescents. Regarding sexual and reproductive health it goes beyond the Constitution, which gives couples the right to decide on the number of children they will bear. The policy states that the decision is the right of individuals. It stresses that family planning should be available to all, regardless of age or civil status, with information and counseling provided. It supports a national strategy for education on sexuality "to promote a healthy, pleasurable and responsible sexuality," independent of its link to reproduction (Colombia Ministry of Health 1992:31).

of women's concerns, of their right to informed choice, and of their rights as research subjects (Cambria 1993). In Brazil, Chile, and Mexico, among other countries, women are promoting decriminalization of abortion through public education campaigns and legislative lobbying. In several Latin American countries, feminist organizations provide comprehensive reproductive and sexual health services, including safe abortions, to women. Although these services reach only a few of the thousands of women in need, they provide examples of what can be done.

Asia

In Asia, women's health activism has taken shape largely in response to strong antinatalist (and in a few cases pronatalist) government programs. About 150 women's groups are involved in women's health, in such areas as service delivery, advocacy, education, counseling, and prevention of violence against women (Isis International 1992). Roughly 40 percent of these groups were established during the 1980s. Most of the groups that responded to a survey by Isis International in Asia identified a need to establish a East and Southeast Asia–Pacific Regional Women and Health Network, and an initial meeting was held in December 1993, where the Woman and Health Network for East and Southeast Asia was established.

Women's groups working on health in India and the Philippines are perhaps the most advanced in Asia, but have emerged from rather different circumstances. In India, they have reacted to authoritarian population control efforts by the government; in the Philippines, they have reacted to government policies and pressure from the Roman Catholic hierarchy to restrict access to safe abortion and contraceptive choice. Women's groups in both countries have lobbied on a wide range of issues, including provision of a broad range of health services, not just family planning; elimination of prostitution and violence against women; and the need for broader socioeconomic policies to improve human well-being. Groups in the Philippines have worked to prevent constitutional

restrictions on abortion and to ensure contraceptive access (see Dixon-Mueller and Germain 1993). Some Indian women's groups have campaigned against specific contraceptives and against the use of amniocentesis for sex-selective abortion (Shah 1993). The groups in India span a wide range of perspectives and ideologies, and generally act independently except during focused campaigns. The groups in the Philippines, which also span a range of perspectives, have coalesced into an alliance called WomanHealth. WomanHealth brings together over 50 networks and groups working nationally in health, media, law, academia, and other professions (Fabros 1994). In other countries of the region, such as Indonesia, Bangladesh, and Malaysia, very few individuals and groups are involved in health.[4]

Africa

In Africa, an organized women's health movement is slowly beginning to develop.[5] Women are increasingly involved in a wide range of groups concerned with health and other socioeconomic and political issues. Government agencies — such as the Ministries of Women's Affairs or of Women and Development — and women's organizations linked to political parties are often important actors. NGOs active in the health field address women's need for basic health services, especially those which prevent maternal mortality and infertility. Some women's groups have organized around specific health concerns, such as female genital mutilation in countries of the Horn and West Africa; vesicovaginal fistula, abortion, and infertility in Nigeria; violence against women in Cameroon; and annual campaigns to prevent maternal mortality in many countries. The need to address Human Immunodeficiency Virus (HIV) and AIDS has raised awareness about sexuality and women's lack of power in sexual relations, leading to the creation of organizations like the Society for Women and AIDS in Africa, a regional network with chapters in many French- and English-speaking African countries.

Meetings sponsored by the United Nations and African population groups in preparation for the 1994 International Conference on Population and Development (ICPD) have included women's representatives more systematically than in the past. These meetings, and others, like the Seventh International Women and Health Meeting, held in Uganda in September 1993, and the Medical Women's International Association First Regional Congress on "The Health of Women and Safe Motherhood," held in Nairobi in November and December of 1993, have provided opportunities for African women to meet at the national and regional levels and to build action agendas for their communities.

The Global Women's Health Movement

The First International Women and Health Meeting was convened in the late 1970s by European and North American women; growing numbers of Southern women have attended the six subsequent meetings. These meetings have been particularly important in fostering debate on a wide variety of issues and in uniting the movement into a political force.

In 1984, the Fourth International Women and Health Meeting, the "International Tribunal on Reproductive Rights," was organized by the International Contraception, Abortion and Sterilization Campaign (ICASC). The meeting was attended by women from many Southern and Northern countries, who testified about reproductive rights abuses. "Reproductive rights" emerged as a major issue, and ICASC became the Women's Global Network for Reproductive Rights (WGNRR) with headquarters in Amsterdam.[6] WGNRR publishes a newsletter, and coordinates with other national and international networks and organizations to plan international action campaigns to promote safe abortion, reduce maternal mortality, and, most recently, oppose research on contraceptive vaccines.

Also in 1984, the International Women's Health Coalition (based in New York) and Catholics for a Free Choice (based in Washington, D.C.), which share many of the concerns of the WGNRR, expanded their networks and activities. These international organizations and oth-

ers, like the older Boston Women's Health Book Collective[7] and Isis International, seek to enable women's health groups and networks worldwide to learn from each other and to build solidarity in their search for solutions to the problems women define.

At about the same time, Southern women researchers and activists created an international South–South network, Development Alternatives with Women for a New Era (DAWN), which promotes development from a feminist perspective (Sen and Grown 1987). Initially, DAWN devoted little attention to population issues except to assert women's right to control their own bodies and reproduction. In 1990, DAWN decided that its new five-year agenda should specifically address population and reproductive rights, along with economic structures and the environment, as priority concerns (Correa 1993). Other international networks concerned with women's rights and development also give women's health high priority and serve as important channels for communication and action. For example, the Women Living under Muslim Laws Network, which exists in over 40 countries, has included reproductive rights as a significant component of its research on women and the law (Hélie–Lucas 1993). The Network is drafting a statement to be used in connection with the ICPD that will give voice to both the common threads and the diverse conditions that shape the reproductive lives of women in Muslim countries and communities.

Women's Health Agendas

Despite substantial differences in women's life experiences and views, there is widespread agreement that women around the world generally lack control over their sexual lives, their health, and their bodies, and that external control takes many forms. One can cite as examples the forced sterilization of women in Puerto Rico; lack of access to sterilization for women in France; authoritarian and narrowly conceived family planning programs in Bangladesh, China, India, and Indonesia; pronatalist policies in Malaysia, Romania, and Singapore; restrictions on abortion funding in the United States; forced marriages in Islamic and other societies; and harmful practices such as genital mutilation or unnecessary caesarean sections.

The basic message of the women's health agenda is clear: access to quality health services — particularly reproductive health services that include safe and effective contraception and abortion — and respect for reproductive rights are fundamental demands from women worldwide. Most women in the movement agree that the design, implementation, and evaluation of these services should be shaped by a concern for reproductive health and rights, not by demographic objectives, and that policies and programs must treat women as their subjects, not their objects. Thus reproductive health service programs should, at a minimum, ensure the broadest possible choice of fertility regulation methods — not only modern methods generally asserted to be most effective, but also barrier methods and male methods — and safe abortion. These programs should also provide screening and treatment for sexually transmitted diseases, including HIV, and other reproductive health services. Additionally, women have highlighted the need to address sexuality.[8]

Another fundamental premise of the movement is that women's health and empowerment are goals in their own right, not means to reduce fertility. The Women's Declaration on Population Policies (see box on page 31), as well as DAWN's Population Policies and Reproductive Rights Project, emphasize not only the empowerment of women, but also gender equity, including men's responsibility for their own sexual behavior and fertility (Correa 1993). Calls to reconsider debt repayment, international trade agreements, and structural adjustment programs, and to provide adequate funds and support in government budgets for health and other basic needs, are among the strongest demands made by Southern women in international forums. They believe that changes in these policies are essential for the lasting achievement of health and rights (Correa 1993; Sen and Grown 1987; see also

Anand; Correa and Petchesky; and Desai, in this volume). These demands were central to the lobbying of government delegations by the Women's Caucus at the May 1993 ICPD Preparatory Committee meeting (Women's Caucus 1993).

Despite solidarity on these fundamental points, substantial diversity has emerged in the movement on matters of substance as well as political strategy, both across and within countries. A fundamental dilemma for feminists continues to be how to campaign for access to birth control and reproductive health services without being seen as colluding with proponents of population control. The need to be sensitive to the individual needs and differences of Third World countries and to refine the meaning of "choice" in relation to reproductive technologies have been recurrent themes. More recently, debate has developed over the universal applicability of the concept of reproductive rights (see Correa and Petchesky in this volume; WGNRR 1993b).

Diversity also exists on which issues should be given priority, and on how to devise strategies and implement actions that are both suitable and feasible in various contexts and situations. This diversity is reflected in debates over population policies and programs. At one end of the spectrum are feminists who work inside family planning and population agencies as service providers, researchers, and managers. Although they are few and often isolated in their agencies, they attempt, frequently in alliance with feminists outside the population establishment, to improve the quality of family planning services, to expand services to encompass other aspects of reproductive health, and to provide information and services to young people and others excluded from programs. They also work to transform policies to meet women's needs, to secure financial support for women's health groups, and to include women's health advocates in the work of their agencies (Claro 1993).

At the other end of the spectrum are those who strongly oppose population policies and programs of any kind and, in some cases, most or all modern reproductive technologies.[9] As described by Barroso (1993), other women's health advocates, while not agreeing entirely with this position, consider current population policies to be against women's interests and argue that population policies can never be feminist (see Comilla Declaration 1993;[10] WGNRR 1993a). These groups believe that action should be directed toward dismantling population policies, rather than toward modifying them to meet women's needs. Collaboration with the establishment is thought to lead inevitably to co-optation and is therefore rejected (Comilla Declaration 1993). These groups have participated in such international conferences as the 1992 UN Conference on Environment and Development (UNCED) and the International Women and Health meetings. They also convene meetings on issues such as contraceptive safety, and document and publicize the shortcomings of current policies and programs.

Between the two ends of the spectrum are a wide range of women's health advocates who recognize that population policies will continue in the foreseeable future. They therefore work with each other and in collaboration with feminists and other sympathetic people in the establishment to transform population policies, contraceptive research, and family planning programs to ensure women's reproductive health and rights. The rest of this chapter will describe some of their efforts.

Activities of the Women's Health Movement

At both the national and international levels, women's health advocates and organizations undertake a variety of activities that provide a strong and credible base for their involvement in policy change.

Alternative Service Provision[11]

Service provision at the grassroots level gives women the experience and insight necessary not only to critique policies and programs, but also to make informed recommendations for change.

The experiences of these organizations are important examples for governments seeking to improve public services. Work at the grassroots level has also contributed to international efforts to develop and refine the concept of "quality of care," first codified by Bruce (1989), and to examine and redefine the services needed for women's reproductive health, first described by Germain and Ordway (1989).[12]

Research

In this as in other fields, feminist research "asks new questions and seeks new answers" (Oakley and Mitchell 1976) about women's perceptions and experiences. As a contribution to wider discussions on health policy, for example, the Women's Health Project in South Africa conducted research on how women feel about contraception and contraceptive services (Women's Health Project Newsletter 1992). To inform efforts by the medical community to develop more effective public policies to control STDs in Nigeria, the Women's Health Research Network has focused on infertility, which is widely feared by women in Nigeria and experienced by many (Kisekka 1989). The International Women's Health Coalition has commissioned experts to conduct literature reviews — for example, on reproductive tract infections in women — that are based on a gender perspective and are specifically directed to policy change (Dixon-Mueller and Wasserheit 1991; Germain et al. 1992). At the conceptual level, the International Reproductive Rights Action Group was formed in 1992 to conduct research on the meaning of "reproductive rights" to women in Brazil, Egypt, Mexico, Malaysia, Nigeria, the Philippines, and the United States.

Public Education Campaigns and Publications

Public education campaigns are another important strategy of the global movement pursued primarily through national level efforts. These include annual campaigns on September 28 to decriminalize abortion in Latin America, and global campaigns on May 28, the International

Day of Action for Women's Health, to raise public consciousness and to advocate changes in policies and services.[13]

The women's movement has given considerable importance to disseminating what is learned from their experience of service provision, other community-level work, and research. A number of country-based feminist journals publish articles on women's health. Regional and international feminist journals addressing women's health issues include the Women's Global Network for Reproductive Rights *Newsletter*; *The Women's Health Journal/La Revista,* published by the Latin American and Caribbean Women's Health Network; *Women in Action,* published by Isis; and *Mujer/Fempress*, published by Alternative Communication Network in Santiago, Chile. *Reproductive Health Matters*, based in London with an international editorial board, is a new journal that brings a women-centered perspective to bear on laws, policies, research and services. The journal seeks to encourage cooperation between the women's health movements and professionals and policy makers.

Women's Strategies for Policy Change

Both within countries and internationally, the activities described above are the building blocks of broader strategies to promote change. Women's health advocates differ significantly among themselves on these strategies while, for the most part, adhering to a common reproductive health and rights agenda. This section focuses on strategies at the global level, although we recognize that much of the groundwork takes place at the national level.

Overall, major segments of the movement are concluding that critiques of shortcomings in policies, programs, and technologies are insufficient on their own. Rather, multidimensional strategies must be developed to achieve reproductive health and justice (Dixon-Mueller 1993; Germain and Ordway 1989; Hartman 1987; WHO/HRP and IWHC 1991).

Statements and Declarations

One indication of this shift is in international statements, such as the "Statement on Women, Population and Environment: Call for a New Approach" (Committee on Women, Population and the Environment 1993), signed and endorsed by 365 individuals and organizations as of early 1994; the Women's Action Agenda, prepared for UNCED in 1992 (WEDO 1992); and the Women's Declaration on Population Policies (see box on page 31). As of early 1994, the Women's Declaration on Population Policies had been signed by 2,400 individuals and organizations — including grassroots organizations, professional associations, and academic institutions — from over 105 countries and across a range of sectors like health, family planning, environment and development. These statements, along with various regional and national statements generated in 1993 (Carta de Brasília 1993; LACWHN and ISIS 1993), are being used in the press, and to lobby governments as well as international agencies. While these documents differ on whether or not "population" is a significant factor in global survival, they have similar agendas for achieving reproductive health and rights.

While some segments of the movement recognize that women must put forward their agendas in forms that will be persuasive to governments, donors, and international agencies, others are more confrontational (Comilla Declaration 1993). For the most part, such diversity is a source of strength as the various groups and networks work in complementary ways to bring about changes.

Interaction with the Establishment

Similarly, some elements of the women's health movement are prepared to collaborate with and work inside the establishment, maintaining a firm commitment to women's rights and feminist values, while others play an important outside role in monitoring and publicizing the shortcomings of existing policies, programs, and technologies.

Interaction with the establishment has taken the form of "dialogues" between feminist advocates and health and population professionals in, for example, Brazil and Nigeria, as well as at the international level since 1986 (IWHC and the Population Council 1986). Dialogues such as that co-convened by the World Health Organization's (WHO's) Special Programme of Research, Development and Research Training in Human Reproduction and the International Women's Health Coalition in 1991, have identified common ground among participants on some aspects of contraceptive development and introduction, on the role of health infrastructure, and on the participation of women's representatives in all stages of the research process. On other issues, such as definitions and measurement of contraceptive safety, participants agreed that continuing dialogue is needed (WHO/HRP and IWHC 1991).[14]

Dialogues have had direct effects on some agencies. For example, the Human Reproduction Programme at WHO has appointed special staff to help integrate women's perspectives throughout its programs, added women's representatives to several of the steering committees that guide its research, and allocated modest program funds for continuing dialogue about reproductive technologies at the regional level. As a result of this process, and with continuing input from women's health advocates, an international symposium of public-sector agencies and feminists produced the Declaration of the International Symposium, "Contraceptive Research and Development for the Year 2000 and Beyond" (see box on page 231). This declaration recognizes most of women's main concerns about the research, development, and introduction of fertility regulation methods. WHO officially submitted the declaration to the second preparatory committee for the ICPD.

Controversy exists within the movement about the value and risks of these exchanges (Keysers 1993). Some activists are concerned that the result will be small changes at the margin, but no real transformation of policy. Others believe dialogue makes population policies, which they oppose, more acceptable. Many have a deep fear that feminists will be co-opted. Nonetheless, on balance, there is increasing recognition within the movement that dialogue with the establishment

is a critical strategy for change, even though not all women's health advocates may wish to participate.

Another difficult issue is the relationship between feminists working inside the establishment and women working within the movement. Feminists who have chosen to work within institutions in order to change them often face criticism by their colleagues outside. But as Helzner and Shepard (1990: 158–159) point out, "feminist insiders and outsiders need each other...the two paths are complementary, and probably both are indispensable." They suggest that outsiders can generate political pressure for radical change that helps insiders gain acceptance for more moderate actions within their institutions. At the same time, the work of feminists in service provision, research, and advocacy provides examples for the work of insiders.

Lobbying UN Conferences

Drawing on its diversity and strengths, the women's health movement is playing a significant role in reshaping the discourse on population policies at UN meetings by lobbying government delegations and producing its own position papers. At UNCED, for example, feminists effectively lobbied the government conference to maintain appropriate references to population policies, reproductive health and rights, and women's rights in Agenda 21. In the absence of a commitment by the majority of governments to deal with population policies in detail, they countered heavy opposition from fundamentalists and also challenged population control advocates. Feminists lobbied strongly on issues such as global demilitarization, and redistribution of wealth and resources, using the Women's Action Agenda 21 (Kyte 1994; WEDO 1992).

At the second preparatory committee meeting for ICPD, the Women's Caucus was widely agreed to have had a significant influence. It persuaded government delegations to address explicitly reproductive health and rights, access to safe abortion, sexuality and gender equity, and broader socioeconomic development. Four country delegations (those of Canada, Norway, Sweden, and the United Kingdom) indicated in plenary speeches that the Women's Declaration on Population Policies, mentioned earlier, should be considered in the ICPD deliberations, and other governments, including that of the United States, acknowledged the Women's Declaration in working sessions.

Women are continuing to mobilize around the world to ensure that their priorities are reflected in the agreements to be signed by governments at the ICPD, the Social Development Summit, and the UN Women's Conference. But strategies are needed to ensure that this recognition becomes more than just lip service. In the face of shrinking resources and growing needs worldwide, major changes in ideas and attitudes will be needed to ensure that high-quality sexual and reproductive health services for women are available and accessible, particularly in countries with few resources.

Challenges for the Future

The women's health movement faces challenges from two opposing forces, both of which use women's concerns and language to advance their purposes. On the one hand, population control advocates, who have been joined in the last few years by segments of the environmental movement, argue for focusing limited population resources on direct, traditional family planning activities, and argue against extending contraceptive choices, improving the quality of care, and providing broad sexual and reproductive health services, such as safe abortion and STD prevention and treatment (see Aitken and Reichenbach; Germain, Nowrojee, and Pyne; and Zeitlin, Govindaraj, and Chen, in this volume). On the other hand, conservative forces would cut off access to fertility regulation altogether.

Although feminist language has been appropriated by population agencies, the underlying concepts have not yet been widely put into practice (Hartman 1993; WGNRR 1993 a and b). In contrast, conservative movements have used the legitimate concerns of women's health advocates about contraceptive safety to bolster their own arguments against both abortion services and contraception. Correa (1993) makes the point that some feminists seem less aware or wary of the latter kind of co-optation than of the former, but both require careful attention. Both population control advocates and fundamentalists have attempted to trivialize the women's health movement with the sweeping assertions that all women's health advocates are "against family planning" (Mathews 1992), or that the feminist agenda for reproductive rights is culturally imperialistic. We have sought to demonstrate that neither accusation is accurate.

In this context of pressure from both sides, at both national and international levels, women in the movement are seeking solidarity that respects diversity in a common struggle to achieve reproductive health and justice. Building an effective political front to influence the ICPD, as well as national and international policies and programs, will also require increasing numbers of feminists to work inside the establishment, and to make both short-term and long-lasting strategic alliances with other agents such as progressive development organizations, primary health care professionals, human rights groups, and, from time to time, population and family planning organizations open to new ideas. Assessing the relationships between women, development, and environmental NGOs, Sen (in this volume) concludes that there is enough common ground to build such alliances. Some women's groups, while generally wary of such efforts, recognize the key importance of this type of collaboration to affect the ICPD (see, for example, Gabriela 1993).

Women's organizations still run on small budgets with part-time and volunteer staff. Donors need to increase substantially the funds available for women's organizations. This will enable them to strengthen their capacity to do research and advocacy; obtain and assess technical information; document and publicize their experiences systematically; monitor and evaluate their programs; build national, regional, and international networks; initiate alliances with other agents; develop their own agendas; and collaborate with population agencies as equals.

In January 1994, 215 women from 83 countries met in Rio de Janeiro to discuss reproductive health and justice in preparation for the ICPD in Cairo in September 1994. Together they negotiated a statement which highlights women's concerns and their demands for development and for reproductive health and rights (CEPIA and IWHC, 1994). This statement, together with the Women's Declaration on Population Policies, and the Declaration of the International Symposium "Contraceptive Research and Development for the Year 2000 and Beyond" (Mexico City, March 1993; see box on page 231), among other documents, provide clear guidance for policy makers and governments. They also provide the basis for much wider public and political support for reproductive health and rights than has previously been the case.

Notes

1 The women's health movement deals with many other important dimensions of women's health, including malnutrition, occupational health, violence against women, mental health, and aging. For the purpose of this volume, we have singled out the movement's work on population policy, family planning programs, and sexual and reproductive health.

2 For additional information on the women's movement in the United States, see Ryan 1992. On women's movements in the South, see Jacquette 1989; Jayawardena 1986; Mohanty, Russo, and Torres 1991. On women's movements in both North and South, see Rowbotham 1992.

3 The Network is based at Isis International, a NGO created in 1974 as an information and communication channel for women. Isis is part of a global network of about 50,000 contacts in 150 countries.

4 In Indonesia and Bangladesh, only two or three activist groups concerned with women's health exist. Malaysia has fewer than ten activist women's organizations, none of which focuses on women's health, population, or reproductive rights (Abdullah 1993).

5 At least two reasons for slow evolution can be postulated: until recently, few Sub-Saharan countries have encouraged organized political movements after independence, and the overall economic situation poses more urgent priorities and more constraints than in other regions.

Poor infrastructure, communication difficulties, and lack of funds make networking more difficult than in other regions.

6 Reproductive rights, according to WGNRR, include full information about sexuality; reproduction; and the benefits and risks of drugs, devices, medical treatments, and interventions. They also include good-quality comprehensive reproductive health services that meet women's needs; safe, effective contraception and sterilization; safe, legal abortion; safe pregnancy and childbirth; prevention of and safe, effective treatment for the causes of infertility; and freedom from "population policies and social codes that pressure some women to have children and others not to" (WGNRR 1992a).

7 The Boston Women's Health Book Collective was among the first to address women's need for technical information on health and contraception in nontechnical language. It continues to play an important role in disseminating such information to individuals and groups worldwide. Originally a discussion and action group, the Collective published *Our Bodies, Our Selves* in 1973. The book is now in its fifth revision and has been translated and adapted into at least nine languages. It has served as an inspiration and an organizing tool in countries as diverse as Egypt, Indonesia, South Africa, and the Philippines, where women's groups are developing their own publications suited to the local context.

8 The study of sexuality is an extremely rich and growing area, on which there have been a large number of debates within the women's movements. Some establishment organizations have also started to consider how to address sexuality in some of their programs (See Germain, Nowrojee and Pyne in this volume).

9 Perhaps the most articulate group espousing this viewpoint is the Feminist International Network of Resistance to Reproductive and Genetic Engineering (FINRRAGE), whose central office is in Germany.

10 Declaration of People's Perspectives on Population Symposium, 12-15 December, 1993. Comilla, Bangladesh.

11 These "alternative" approaches to health care are women-centered and nonhierarchical. Women are provided with full information and a wide range of services beyond maternal and child health and contraception, including safe abortion, counseling, support in cases of rape or domestic violence, and other gynecological care. Londoño (1991) calls this the "humanistic approach," as compared to the "patriarchal" model (see Toro 1989). Other groups, such as the National Black Women's Health Project in the United States, emphasize "wellness," rather than disease, and the importance of taking responsibility for one's own health.

12 Examples of broader approaches include the Dispensaire des Femmes in Geneva, started in 1978, which inspired and trained many others, such as the Sexuality and

Health Feminist Collective in São Paulo, Brazil. The Collective provides gynecologic and psychological services, including information on the full range of reproductive health issues; trains health care professionals; conducts workshops for women on topics such as AIDS, menopause, and sexuality; and produces training materials. The Bangladesh Women's Health Coalition is a different example of a women-centered service (see box on page 246). The *Qualité* series, published by the Population Council, is an important reference on innovative approaches to women-centered services.

13 The annual global campaigns are coordinated by WGNRR and the Latin American and Caribbean Women's Health Network (WGNRR 1990). Since 1987, the focus of May 28 has been maternal morbidity and mortality (health services and quality of care, 1990 and 1991; adolescent pregnancy, 1992; abortion, 1993).

14 Several other "dialogues" have occurred at the international or regional level, including between WGNRR and WHO on Safe Motherhood, the PanAmerican Health Organization and LACWHN on HIV/AIDS; and a WHO–International Planned Parenthood Federation–United Nations Fund for Population Activities conference on abortion, which gathered feminists, service providers, researchers, and policy makers from Eastern and Western Europe and North America (Newman 1993). Another form of interaction recently started is exchanges or internships between feminist and establishment organizations.

References

Abdullah, R. 1993. Changing population policies and women's lives in Malaysia in population and family planning policies: Women-centered perspectives. *Reproductive Health Matters* 5(1):67–77.

Araujo, M. J. (Founding member of the Feminist Collective for Sexuality and Health). 1993. Personal communication.

Asian and Pacific Women's Resource Collection Network. 1990. *Asian and Pacific women's resource and action series: Health*. Kuala Lumpur: Asian and Pacific Development Centre.

Barroso. 1993. Meeting women's unmet needs: The alliance between feminists and researchers. Remarks at the International Symposium on Contraceptive Research and Development for the Year 2000 and Beyond, March 8–10, in Mexico City.

Bruce, J. 1989. Fundamental elements of the quality of care: A simple framework. Working Paper No. 1. New York: Population Council.

Carta de Brasília. 1993. Conclusions of the National Meeting on Women and Population: Our Rights for Cairo 1994, held on September 28, in Brasília, Brazil.

Cambria, C. (Director of Flora Tristan). 1993. Personal communication.

CEPIA and International Women's Health Coalition (IWHC). 1994 (forthcoming). *Report on reproductive health and justice: International Women's Health Conference for Cairo '94*. Rio de Janeiro.

Chaterjee, M. 1993. Reorienting policy. In *Population Planning: A Symposium on Population, Women, and Development*. October.

Claro, A. 1993. Grupos de mujeres organizadas y activistas feministas y su influencia en la salud reproductiva y la regulación de la fecundidad. Paper presented at the Fourth Latin American Conference on Population: Demographic Transition in Latin America and the Caribbean, March 23–26, in Mexico City.

Colombia Ministry of Health. 1992. *Salud para las mujeres, mujeres para la salud*. Santafé de Bogotá.

Committee on Women, Population and the Environment. 1993. *Women, population and the environment: Call for a new approach*. Newton Centre, Mass.

Correa, S. 1993. DAWN research effort: 1992/94 population and reproductive rights component. Preliminary ideas prepared for DAWN. Unpublished.

Costa, A. M. 1992. *O PAISM: Uma política de assistência integral à saúde da mulher a ser resgatada*. São Paulo, Brazil. Commissão de Cidadania e Reprodução, December 1992.

Declaration of People's Perspectives on "Population." 1993. Symposium organized by UBINIG and Resistance Network (Bangladesh), Research Foundation for Science and Ecology (India), Third World Network (Malaysia), and People's Health Network (India), December 12–15, in Comilla, Bangladesh.

Dixon-Mueller, R. 1993. *Population policy and women's rights: Transforming reproductive choice*. Westport, Conn.: Praeger.

Dixon-Mueller, R., and J. Wasserheit. 1991. *The culture of silence: Reproductive tract infections among women in the third world*. New York: International Women's Health Coalition.

Dixon-Mueller, R., and A. Germain. 1993. Population policy and women's political action in three developing countries. In R. Dixon-Mueller (ed.), *Population policy and women's rights: Transforming reproductive choice*. Westport, Conn.: Praeger.

Fabros, M. (Member of WomanHealth). 1994. Personal communication.

Gabriela (A national coalition of women's organizations). 1993. Resolution on Women's Voices '94. Manila, Philippines.

Germain, A., and J. Ordway. 1989. *Population control and women's health: Balancing the scales.* New York: International Women's Health Coalition.

Germain, A., et al. (eds.). 1992. *Reproductive tract infections: Global impact and priorities for women's reproductive health.* New York: Plenum Press.

Hartman, B. 1987. *Reproductive rights and wrongs: The global politics of population control and contraceptive choice.* New York: Harper & Row.

———. 1993. Old maps and new terrain: The politics of women, population and the environment in the 1990s. Paper presented at the Fifth International Interdisciplinary Congress on Women, February 23, in San José, Costa Rica.

Hélie-Lucas, M. (Coordinator, Women Living Under Muslim Laws). 1994. Personal communication.

Helzner, J., and B. Shepard. 1990. The feminist agenda in population private voluntary organizations. In K. Staudt (ed.), *Women, international development and politics: The bureaucratic mire.* Philadelphia: Temple University Press.

International Women's Health Coalition (IWHC). 1991. Reproductive tract infections in women in the Third World: national and international policy implications. Report of a meeting at the Bellagio Study and Conference Center, April 29–May 3, in Lake Como, Italy.

International Women's Health Coalition (IWHC), and the Population Council. 1986. The contraceptive development process and quality of care in reproductive health services. Rapporteurs' Report of a Meeting Sponsored by the IWHC and the Population Council, October 8–9, in New York.

Isis International. 1992. *Asia-Pacific women and health programs 1992 survey.* Manila, Philippines.

Jaquette, J. S. 1989. *The women's movement in Latin America: Feminism and the transition to democracy.* Boulder, Colo.: Westview Press.

Jayawardena K. 1986. *Feminism and nationalism in the third world.* London: Zed Books.

Keysers, L. 1993. Women and population questions: From Rio to Cairo and beyond. Reflections of a reproductive rights activist. *VENA Journal* 5(2).

Kisekka, M. 1989. Reproductive health research and advocacy: Challenges to women's associations in Nigeria. Paper presented to the Women's Health Research Network in Nigeria panel at the Society of Gynecology and Obstetrics of Nigeria Conference, September 5–8, in Calabar, Nigeria.

Kyte, R. (Consultant, International Environment and Development Policy). 1994. Personal communication.

Latin American and Caribbean Women's Health Network (LACWHN), and Isis International. 1993. *Women and Population Policies.* Proceedings of the meeting on Women and Population Policies in Latin America and the Caribbean, July 5–9, in Oaxtepec, Mexico.

Londoño, M. L. 1991. A humanistic approach to health services for women. *Women's Health Journal* 3(91):4–11.

Matamala, M. 1993. El foro abierto de derechos reproductivos. Paper presented at the meeting on Women and Population Policies in Latin America and the Caribbean, July 5–9, in Oaxtepec, Mexico.

Mathews, J. 1992. Politically correct environmentalists. *Washington Post*, May 12.

Mohanty, C. T., A. Russo, and L. Torres. 1991. *Third World women and the politics of feminism.* Bloomington: Indiana University Press.

Newman, K. (ed.). 1993. *Progress postponed: Abortion in Europe in the 1990s.* London: International Planned Parenthood Federation/Europe Region.

Oakley, A., and J. Mitchell. 1976. *The rights and wrongs of women.* New York: Penguin.

Pitanguy, J. 1994 (forthcoming). Feminist politics and reproductive rights: The case of Brazil. In G. Sen and R. Snow (eds.), *Power and decision: The social control of reproduction.* Cambridge: Department of Population and International Health, Harvard University.

Population Council. 1993. *Day of dialogue on population and feminist perspectives, London, 20 November 1992: Aide-memoire.* New York.

Posada, C. (Executive Director, CERFAMI, Center for Comprehensive Resources for the Family). 1993. Personal communication.

Rede Nacional Feminista de Saúde e Direitos Reprodutivos. 1992. *Nossa fala, nosso espaço hoje PAISM* (Newsletter of the Brazilian National Network of Reproductive Health and Rights), Ano 1, No. 0. Recife, PE, Brazil.

Rowbotham, S. 1992. *Women in movement: Feminism and social action.* London and New York: Routledge.

Ryan, B. 1992. *Feminism and the women's movement: Dynamics of change in social movement, ideology and activism.* London and New York: Routledge.

Sen, G., and C. Grown. 1987. *Development, crises, and alternative visions: Third World women's perspectives.* New York: Monthly Review Press.

Shah, P. 1993. Female Foeticide. *Seminar: The Monthly Symposium* 410 (October):42-44. New Delhi.

Toro, O. L. 1989. Commentary on women-centered reproductive health services. *International Journal of Gynecology and Obstetrics*, suppl. 3:119–123.

Women's Caucus. 1993. Suggested revisions to the proposed conceptual framework. Document produced by the Women's Caucus at the Second Preparatory Committee for ICPD, May 10–21, in New York.

Women's Environment & Development Organization (WEDO). 1992. *Official report of the World Women's Congress for a Healthy Planet*. New York.

Women's Global Network for Reproductive Rights (WGNRR). 1990. *Maternal mortality and morbidity: A call to women for action*, Special issue, May 28. Amsterdam.

———. 1992a. Annual report. Amsterdam.

———. 1993a. *WGNRR Newsletter* 42 (January–March).

———. 1993b. Report of the International Conference, "Reinforcing Reproductive Rights," held in Madras, India, May 5–8, 1993. *WGNRR Newsletter* 43 (April–June). Amsterdam.

Women's Health Project. 1992. *Women's health project newsletter*. Johannesburg: Centre for Health Policy, University of Witts, South Africa.

World Health Organization/Special Programme of Research, Development and Research Training in Human Reproduction (WHO/HRP) and International Women's Health Coalition (IWHC), 1991. Creating common ground: women's perspectives on the selection and introduction of fertility regulation technologies. Report of a meeting between women's health advocates and scientists. February 20–22, Geneva: World Health Organization.

5

Development, Population, and the Environment: A Search for Balance[1]

Gita Sen

Public perceptions, especially among people in Northern countries, of the environmental impact of rapid population growth may have come full circle. Several well-known books (Ehrlich and Ehrlich 1991; Hardin 1993; Kennedy 1993) powerfully express concerns about the implications of rapid population growth for human and planetary health and survival. Their prognoses echo, undoubtedly in new forms, the neo-Malthusian fears that were prominent in mobilizing public support for population programs four decades ago. But, in contrast to the situation in the 1950s and 1960s, other, countervailing and also powerful voices have arisen in the intervening years. Women's health activists have increasingly joined the population debate.

In this chapter, I seek to analyze the origins and distinctions among these voices, focusing in particular on the women's health and environmental movements. In so doing, I argue that the debates on development, population, and the environment should acknowledge the lessons learned from the actual implementation and practices of policies in all three fields. The policies would thereby be better informed, and would take far greater account of humane values than did their counterparts 30 years ago.

Differences in perceptions regarding the linkages between population and environment became particularly prominent during preparations for the United Nations Conference on Environment and Development, known as the Earth Summit, or Rio '92. Disagreement between Southern and Northern countries on the relevance and extent of attention to be accorded to population received considerable publicity. At the nongovernmental level too, the issue of population became a subject of considerable debate among environmentalists (especially those from the North), feminists, and the population community.

My proposition is that although the positions taken in the policy debate have been exaggerated at times, some of the differences have deep roots. They arise from conceptual and paradigmatic differences, rather than from disagreements regarding the validity of particular scientific propositions. These differences shape the protagonists' perceptions of problems, the analytic methods used, and the weights assigned to different linkages and relationships. In particular, varying views regarding development strategies, the linkages between poverty and population growth, and the role of gender relations color the positions taken in the debate.

In this chapter, I attempt to examine the different perspectives on these issues held by mainstream, Northern environmental scientists and activists on the one hand, and women's health researchers and feminist activists from both North and South on the other. The purposes are twofold: to identify the positions taken by these two broad groups within the larger discourses on population and development; and to propose a possible basis for mutual understanding and establishment of common ground.[2]

At first glance, the achievement of common ground may seem impossible because the differences appear to be fundamental. Many environmentalists believe that population growth is a major cause of environmental degradation (for example, see Consortium for Action to Protect the Earth 1992), while many feminists argue that population growth by itself is simply not a significant contributor to global environmental problems (see, for example, Committee on Women, Population and the Environment 1992). An underlying premise of this chapter is that despite apparent divergences of views, environmentalists and women's health advocates have much in common. They share similar critiques of the patterns of economic growth; both believe that currently dominant patterns of economic growth are unsustainable, whether from an ecological standpoint or from a standpoint of human survival and social justice. In addition, important sections of both groups derive their knowledge from grassroots and community activism, share opposition to dominant interests, and rely on methods of popular participation in development action.

Building on the commonalities between environmentalism and the women's health movement will not be easy, but it is possible. It will require clarity of understanding regarding major shifts and controversies in both development and population thinking, as well as the history of the population movement. It will also require the development of a concrete set of commonly shared prescriptions regarding how both women's health and population interests and Northern environ-

mental concerns can be mutually advanced. A recognition of the evolution of controversies in the population field and *how these have been influenced by shifts in development thinking* provides a needed corrective to the belief that population is a simple problem of numbers susceptible to an easy technological fix.

Evolution of the Development Debate

Over the five decades since the end of World War II, public debate about socioeconomic development has undergone many twists and turns. During the 1950s and 1960s, optimism about the possibilities for accelerating the pace of economic growth in the newly decolonized states of Asia, Africa, and Latin America was high. This, combined with sobering assessments of the vicious circles of poverty and backwardness, gave considerable legitimacy to state-led planning for economic growth. The principal task was to raise the stock of physical capital by accelerating investment and mobilizing resources through the use of "surplus" labor domestically, as well as inflows of foreign capital (in different forms) to complement aggregate domestic savings. These early *supply-side* arguments envisioned a leading role for the state and were buttressed by strategies for import substitution and protection of domestic markets.

While there was an emerging counter argument in favor of free trade and private investment during this phase, there was no real challenge to the primacy of the state's role in mobilizing and allocating economic resources.[3] This belief also animated the development assistance provided by most donor agencies.[4]

By the end of the 1960s this approach began to be critiqued as "trickle-down," which not only was ineffective in raising living standards, but had set in motion processes leading to the expropriation of resources by the powerful across and within nations. Criticism of the international economic order by the "dependency" school complemented the rapidly emerging policy arguments in favor of directly targeting poverty alleviation and basic needs provision.

By the mid-1970s, attention shifted from economic growth per se to the entitlements and needs of the poor.[5] Poverty reduction or social equity did not appear to follow automatically from high economic growth, as evidenced by the case of Brazil, which grew very rapidly but inequitably after the mid-1960s. On the other hand, social development, and especially the fulfillment of basic needs such as health, education, housing, sanitation, and a secure livelihood, did not appear to have high rates of economic growth as a prerequisite. The experience of both socialist countries, such as China, and nonsocialist ones, like Sri Lanka and Costa Rica, were presented as cases where basic needs had been improved in the absence of high economic growth. The growing importance of basic needs in the programmatic directions being shaped at the World Bank and the ILO lent strength to the argument that social development ought to be tackled *directly*, and not as an uncertain side effect of economic growth.

In the global political economy, the boom in primary product prices and the spectacular success of the Organization of Petroleum Exporting Countries (OPEC) in capturing a greater share of the rents from oil production created optimism among Third World countries about the possibility of creating a New International Economic Order. The 1970s witnessed considerable experimentation with alternative development paths and models in Third World countries. The experience of Third World socialist states, such as Cuba, China, and Vietnam, in tackling problems of basic needs with equity exerted an influence on countries such as Jamaica, Nicaragua, and Mozambique. These experiments responded to the growth of social movements — comprising different combinations of industrial workers, peasants, students, the "middle classes," and others — which had been fueled by the inequitable patterns of growth in the 1960s. These movements demanded economic change and political participation. An important part of their challenge was the criticism by nongovernmental development practitioners and others of bureaucratic methods of planning and implementation that ignored or excluded the views and needs of people and thereby alienated them.

The 1970s also saw the emergence of an international women's movement. While drawing upon other social movements, it defined its own agendas, in which gender equity was seen as an engine for driving new approaches to development overall (see Sen and Grown 1987). Women's health groups were a vital part of this movement. Their popular base derived from activist work dealing with the health problems of poor women in urban and rural communities.[6] In the process, many of them came to two important conclusions: that women's health can successfully be addressed only within the context of community health generally, taking into consideration such basic needs such as education, sanitation, clean water and nutrition, and secure livelihoods; and that the bureaucratic approach to family planning not only was ineffective in providing services, but often created reproductive health problems for women, violated their basic dignity as human beings, and diverted resources from other primary and preventive health. Strong calls for rethinking population policies and revamping family planning programs began to crystallize (Hartman 1987).

The 1970s was thus a period of considerable ferment and change, with the emergence of new ideas, new actors, and new policy approaches. By contrast, the 1980s witnessed significant reversals in both development thinking and policy. External factors, together with the rigidity of bureaucratic centralism, undermined the capacity and legitimacy of Third World socialist experiments. The slow growth of the world economy and of world trade, combined with the debt crisis, brought social austerity and the economic freedom of market forces to the foreground. Programs of structural adjustment were implemented in country after country, usually accompanied by popular protest, as the cost of living soared and living standards dropped. As in the 1960s, supply-side arguments focused on laying a basis for economic growth became predominant. There were, however, key differences between the growth arguments of the two periods. By the 1980s, the state was no longer viewed as the primary engine of growth; its functions were to be minimized. Growth itself was to be based not on domestic market creation, but on linking up with the global economy on the latter's terms—namely, through competitive exports based on cheap labor, which was seen as the Third World's most available "resource" (see World Bank 1991).

The dominance of such views and the policies based upon them has not gone unchallenged. Among the international development agencies, the views held at the World Bank and the IMF run counter to the positions held at the ILO, UNICEF, and the United Nations Development Programme. The latter group accords greater emphasis to basic needs, to the importance of developing "human resources," and to the problems inherent in promoting structural and institutional changes within inequitable global and national economies.

Internal challenges within countries have also grown, with greater calls for democracy and popular participation. At the same time, social movements within the Third World have linked environmental concerns to the deterioration of the resource base of poor people consequent on inequitable development processes. Many such movements strongly oppose current development patterns (*a fortiori* their structural adjustment variant) as destroying both the environment and the livelihood base of large groups of people.[7] Few, if any, of such groups would agree that population growth is a major reason for local ecological damage. On the basis of grassroots experience, they perceive government policies serving powerful private interests as a major factor. These environmental groups often have strong participation from women who, as those responsible for the household's basic needs, are very aware of both causes and consequences of local environmental degradation (see Agarwal 1991). Along with much of the rest of the Third World women's movements, these organizations criticize current patterns of economic growth and development

policy, and argue for focusing more centrally on the basic needs and rights of the poor.

In Third World contexts of very low per capita incomes, these organizations usually acknowledge the importance of developing the potential for economic growth. They also acknowledge the importance of ecological sustainability. But their understanding is that the dominant crisis for the majority of the world's population is the crisis of survival occasioned by inequitable global and national economic and political structures. They argue, therefore, that strategies to promote either economic growth or ecological sustainability that run counter to the basic needs, livelihoods, or political inclusion of the less powerful are likely to be inequitable and ultimately counterproductive. They believe that development strategies appropriate to the needs of the majority and politically inclusive in their conception *can* be environmentally sustainable.

What lessons can be learned from this description of the evolving development debate? First, development policy is not a simple matter of a supply-side fix, but requires attention to both supply and demand. In particular, policies targeted at improving macroeconomic management or increasing gross national product growth while ignoring or worsening the incomes and livelihoods of the majority are not politically or economically sustainable. Second, supply-side, trickle-down economics (whether at the national or the international level) benefit a few disproportionately while marginalizing many. Third, a direct focus on poverty alleviation and basic needs not only promotes justice and equity, but also lays a firm basis for human resource development, without which no country can hope to progress. Fourth, top-down, bureaucratic development program methods are often ineffective and insensitive, and may even become coercive.

These lessons from development experience need to be borne in mind when we turn to the subject of population. *The population issue is a sub-theme within development and, as such, is continuously framed in the context of one or another approach to development.*

Poverty and Population:
Populationists versus Developmentalists

During the late 1960s and much of the 1970s, the principal debate about population policy centered on the impact of poverty on population growth. Earlier explanations of demographic transitions in different countries stressed the role of per capita income growth in reducing first mortality and then fertility rates. If poverty (in the sense of low per capita incomes) was the main factor in high death rates and birthrates, then the solution was economic growth, aided by strong family planning programs that would make contraceptives and information about them widely available.

On the other side, unchecked growth in population was seen as a drag on economic growth through a variety of mechanisms, such as reduction in domestic savings rates and diversion of funds from productive investment (see, for example, Demeny 1992). This traditional "populationist" view clearly perceived economic growth as both a necessary and a sufficient condition for reduction in population growth, when combined with expanded availability of contraceptive methods through family planning programs. Increases in per capita income would generate the demand for contraception, which would be matched by an increasing supply of family planning services.

By the 1970s, this view came under increasing criticism because of the perceived sluggishness of family planning programs in reducing birthrates. Field evidence of contraceptives' lying unused in rural homes (although family planning officials had expected couples to be willing recipients of birth control technologies) pointed to the urgent need for a fresh look at both policies and programs. Renewed debate on the precise nature of the links between socioeconomic development and population growth culminated in a major challenge to thinking that occurred during the 1974 World Population Conference in Bucharest.

As we have seen, the mid-1970s was a period of considerable rethinking in development policy internationally. The belief in economic growth as a panacea for development problems had been largely discredited. In this climate of ferment and challenge to existing orthodoxies, the aphorism coined at Bucharest that "development is the best contraceptive" became the harbinger of fresh thinking, at least in Southern countries, about the links between population growth and development. Proponents of this view recognized that income increases per se were insufficient. Rather, improvements in general health (children's health in particular) and in education (especially women's education) were viewed as essential to reducing infant and child mortality rates, and thereby laying the basis for reducing the "demand" for children and raising receptiveness to contraceptive technologies. While this "developmentalist" view also recognized the importance of family planning services, it gave higher priority to increasing the *demand* for family planning through improved health and education.

This debate fueled a significant amount of new research on the micro-level foundations of fertility decisions, as well as cross-country analysis of the causes of population change. As a consequence, the 1980s saw the emergence, in some quarters, of a more synthetic view of the links between population and development. Improving people's access to secure incomes, rather than high national economic growth per se, was linked to improvements in health and education, and declines in fertility (see, for example, Krishnan 1992).

The economic realities of the 1980s provided, however, a harsh counterpoint to this emerging synthesis. Many countries in Latin America and Sub-Saharan Africa in particular, and even in Asia (where overall economic growth rates tended to be higher), faced significant declines in real government expenditures on the social sectors (Jolly et al. 1991). The primacy of economic growth as the basis for poverty alleviation and meeting social needs was asserted once again.[8]

International decisionmakers in institutions such as the World Bank appeared to believe in the existence of an implicit trade-off, rather than complementarity, between economic growth and improving social sectors. This belief ignores the dimension of time. Investment in health and education, as in other elements of the social infrastructure, pays off in the medium and longer terms. Likewise, some of the more damaging effects of social sector disinvestment tend to be felt over time. In the longer term, improving health and education, along with meeting other basic needs, raises the quality of a country's labor force, which is critical in determining the economy's growth potential and competitiveness over the long run.

More importantly from the perspective of linkages between population growth and development, real disinvestment in the social sectors, such as occurred during the 1980s and is continuing in a number of countries, might slow down the pace of mortality and fertility declines in the poorest countries. The "developmentalist" thinking that grew after Bucharest and the dominant trends of structural economic reforms appear therefore to be at cross-purposes.[9]

These development debates set the context for the demand side of family planning. They have been matched by equally serious problems on the supply side. On the one hand, population (fertility control) policies and family planning (contraceptive delivery) programs continued apace. On the other hand, concerted attacks on family planning institutions were mounted by religious fundamentalists and right-leaning politicians. Internal political battles over women's reproductive choices and decision-making autonomy in the United States spilled over onto the international arena during the International Population Conference in Mexico City in 1984. The result was relative stagnation in U.S. government funding for family planning assistance (Conly, Speidel, and Camp 1991). Because the U.S. government had been the major source of funds and the main political supporter of international family planning, the U.S. position in Mexico occasioned considerable concern among the population community. Attempts to continue or enhance the rate of increase in U.S. government funds for family planning have become one of the most important items on the agenda of many within the family planning "establishment." Arguments have also been made that such funds should be used only for contraception (rather than reproductive health

more integrally), and that worrying about the *quality* of family planning services is an unaffordable luxury during a time of financial stringency.

This single-minded focus by some institutions on increasing funding for contraceptive services has met with some opposition. As noted earlier, a growing international, grassroots-based women's health movement has, since the 1970s, challenged the quality of traditional family planning programs (see García-Moreno and Claro, in this volume). This challenge has both a theoretical component, rooted in an analysis of gender relations, and an empirical component, based on women's actual experiences with family planning programs.

As a development strategy, the critics see population policies as usually falling within a class of strategies that are top-down in orientation, largely unconcerned with, and often violating, the basic needs or human rights of target populations. Even the developmentalist concern with improving child health and women's education has received little real support from population programs, despite the extensive research and policy debate it has generated (see Germain, Nowrojee, and Pyne in this volume).

The critical perspective argues that ignoring corequisites such as economic and social justice, and women's reproductive health and rights, also makes the overt objective of population policy (namely, a change in birthrates) difficult to achieve. In such conditions, achievement of a fall (or rise) in birthrates is sometimes predicated on highly coercive methods, and is antithetical to women's health and human dignity. Many women's health advocates argue for a different approach to population policy — one that makes women's health and other basic needs central to policy and program focus, and by doing so increases human welfare, transforms oppressive gender relations, and reduces population growth rates (see García-Moreno and Claro, in this volume; Germain and Ordway 1989).

Around the world there is a growing emergence of positive statements about what human rights in the area of reproduction might encompass (Correa and Petchesky in this volume; Petchesky and Weiner 1990). Many of these statements are culturally and contextually specific, but they usually share a critique of existing population programs, and understandings of alternative principles. Many of them give special attention to the perspectives of poor women, although they recognize that the reproductive rights of all women in most societies are less than satisfactory. Their attempt to recast population policies and programs is also an effort to recast development objectives to be more responsive to the needs of the majority.

Enter the Environmentalists

Environmentalist concern with population growth predates the public debate sparked by the Earth Summit. As in the broader field of development and in the parallel field of population policy, opinions vary among environmentalists regarding the links between population and sustainable development. While there are those whose work adopts a global and aggregative perspective, there are others (both researchers and activists) whose approach to sustainable development starts with people and their livelihoods at the ground level. In particular, anthropologists and political economists have worked extensively on the causes and consequences of environmental degradation within specific locales. This has usually been done with systematic regard for the ways in which the interaction of people with their environments is embedded in the (sometimes perverse) logic of economic, political, and cultural systems (see Arizpe, Stone, and Major 1994).

There is, of course, no necessary contradiction between the locale-specific and the global approaches, provided the latter take the results of the former into account while aggregating.[10] Unfortunately the more global approaches have rarely done this when analyzing the interactions between populations and their environments (For exceptions, see Turner et al. 1990). It is useful to remember here that the difference between the two approaches is one not merely of physical scale, but of the extent to which social science analysis is integral to the approach. Part of the problem stems from the fact that behaviorally, much social science is based on individuals or relatively small groups; the analysis does not lend itself easily to large-scale generalization.[11] Another part of the problem arises from the paucity of research at the micro level that links demographic changes to the economic, social, or cultural aspects of ecological changes. Such research would undoubtedly be methodologically complex and difficult; it could take time to generate meaningful or systematic results. In its absence, macro approaches to population-environment linkages have tended to remain innocent of any micro basis.[12]

The paucity of research has not, unfortunately, slowed down popular or even academic writing on the policy implications of presumed population-environment linkages. The interest in global and local carrying capacity vis-à-vis growing human population sizes and densities has spurred a considerable literature, both scientific and popular. Much of the literature, both popular (for example, Blaikie 1985; Little 1992) and activist (for example, Shaw 1989), has ignored important anthropological debates about carrying capacity, as well as assumed away the inconclusiveness of empirical evidence linking environmental change to population growth. It tends to treat population-environment relationships as simple and, indeed, self-evident mathematical ones linking numbers of people to their environments through technology.

However, the argument both of developmentalists in the population field and of women's health and rights advocates has been precisely that population is *not* an issue just of numbers, but of complex social relationships that govern birth, death, and migration. The interactions of people with their environments can be captured only partially by simple mathematical relationships that do not take the distribution of resources, incomes, and consumption into account; such relationships by themselves may therefore be inadequate as predictors of outcomes or as guides to policy.[13]

Furthermore, from a policy point of view, the modeling of population-environment interactions has thus far not given us much better guidance about appropriate population policies or programs. Ignoring the wide disparities in the growth rates of consumption between rich and poor *within* developing countries, and hence their relative environmental impacts, as well as the critiques of women's health advocates outlined in the previous sections, leads to single-minded policy prescriptions directed simply to increasing family planning funding and practice. The leap from overly aggregated population-environmental relations to policy prescriptions favoring increased family planning services becomes then an implicit choice of politics, of a particular approach to population policy, to environmental policy. Because it glosses over fundamental issues of power, gender, and class relations, and of distribution, and because it ignores the historical experience of population programs, it has been viewed by many as a retrograde step in the population-development discourse.

In this context, one might also argue that an urgent need in designing policies for sustainable development is not a single-minded focus on global totals, but a careful, step-by-step improvement in livelihoods and in living conditions in local settings, applying science and technology according to strong ethics and equity guidelines. It is arguable that a central issue for environmental policy, development policy, and population policy in the future will be how to design social and economic systems that will provide for the inevitable doubling of the world's present population at an average income in real terms several times the present one, all on the basis of the present limited supplies of land, water, and air. The failure of much existing environmental science to connect its focus on global warming and loss of habitat to the needs of people for space, land, health, and secure livelihoods has resulted in serious policy omissions and distortions.[14]

Redressing this weakness will also strengthen the links between environmental scientists and grassroots environmental activists, especially in the South, but also among marginalized communities in the North. Many such groups are engaged precisely in active experimentation with methods of sustainable development, often against considerable political odds. But their knowledge of the major role played by inequitable economic and political power in shaping environmental problems on the ground often makes them wary of simplified assumptions regarding the links between population growth and sustainable development.

Shifting environmental policy directions also requires greater recognition that tackling existing relations of gender and power is central to solving the problem of sustainable livelihoods. Peripheral as yet to much of the policy debate on sustainable livelihoods is the acknowledgment that women not only are the long suffering carriers of water and gatherers of fuel, but often hold the key to the preservation and parsimonious use of local resources (see, for example, Dankelman and Davidson 1988; Desai in this volume; Sontheimer 1991). Although feminist environmentalists have been amassing such evidence, it has remained poorly integrated into actual policies that would strengthen rather than hamper women in these roles.

Toward Synergy among Environmentalists and Feminists

Despite the dissonance in the population-environment debate, there is much in common between feminists and environmentalists in their visions of society and in the methods they use. As stated at the outset, both groups (or at least their more progressive wings) have a healthy critical stance toward ecologically profligate and inequitable patterns of economic growth, and have been attempting to change mainstream perceptions in this regard. Both use methods that rely on grassroots mobilization and participation, and are therefore sensitive to the importance of political openness and involvement. As such, both believe in the power of widespread knowledge and in the rights of people to be informed and to participate in decisions affecting their lives and those of nations and the planet. Indeed, there are many feminists within environmental movements (North and South) and environmentalists within feminist movements.

Mutual understanding on the population question can result from a greater recognition that the core problem is development, *within* which population is inextricably meshed. Greater attention to the perspectives of poor women can help ground this recognition in the lives and livelihoods of many within the South.

This means that the population issue must be defined as the right to determine and make reproductive decisions in the context of fulfilling *secure livelihoods, basic needs (including reproductive health), and political participation.* Although the reality in most countries may be far removed from such an ideal, an affirmation of these basic values would provide the needed underpinnings for much-needed changes in policy and action.

Such values carry a number of implications. First, approaches to economic growth and ecological sustainability must be such as to secure livelihoods, basic needs, political participation, and women's reproductive rights, not to work against them. Thus, environmental policies and programs must support and sustain livelihoods and basic needs, not counterpose "nature" against the survival needs of the most vulnerable people in the present. *Where trade-offs among these goals exist or are inevitable, the costs and burdens should not have to be borne by the poorest and most vulnerable. All people must have a voice in negotiating resolutions through open and genuinely participatory political processes.* Strategies that enhance livelihoods and fulfill needs can also lay the basis for mortality and fertility reduction.

Second, population and family planning programs should be framed in the context of health and livelihood agendas, give serious consideration to women's health advocates, and be supportive of women's reproductive health and rights. This has to be more than lip service; it requires reorienting international assistance and national policy, reshaping programs, and rethinking research questions and methodologies. Using the language of

welfare, gender equity, or health while continuing family planning as usual will not meet the need.

Third, reproductive health strategies will succeed in improving women's health and enabling them to make socially viable fertility decisions if they are set in the context of a supportive health and development agenda overall. Where general health and social development are poorly funded or given low priority, as has happened in the development agendas of many major development agencies and countries during the last decade, reproductive rights and health are unlikely to get the funding or attention they need. Reproductive health programs will be more efficacious when general health and development are served. A poor woman agricultural wage laborer, ill nourished and anemic, will respond better to reproductive health care if her nutritional status and overall health improve at the same time.

Fourth, in framing its own strategies, the mainstream Northern environmental movement needs to focus more on gender relations and women's needs, as well as on the issues raised by minority groups. These issues (such as those raised by native peoples and African-Americans in the United States) tend to link environmental issues with livelihoods and basic needs concerns in much the same way as do the people's organizations in the South (Miller 1993). Greater sensitivity to the one, therefore, might bring greater awareness of the other.

Wide discussion and acknowledgment of these principles could help to bridge some of the current gaps between feminists and environmentalists, and make it possible to build coalitions that can move both agendas forward.

Notes

1 A longer and somewhat different version of this essay, entitled "Women, Poverty and Population: Issues for the Concerned Environmentalist," is in L. Arizpe, P. Stone, and D. Major (eds.), 1994, *Population and the Environment: Rethinking the Debate* (Boulder, Colo.: Westview Press, 1994).

2 My own position comes from work on issues of gender and development. The chapter tilts heavily toward the positions taken from within the women's movement. I

do not claim to explicate how the mainstream of the environmental movement (especially in the North) has come to the particular definitions it has of "the population problem."

3 The major development debate of the early and mid-1960s in Asia was around planning methodologies and techniques. In Latin America there was a growing debate between the structuralists, grouped around CEPAL (the UN Economic Commission for Latin America), and the monetarists, headed by the International Monetary Fund (IMF), about the causes and cures of inflation and balance-of-payments problems. While the Latin American debate foreshadowed the neoliberal supply-side arguments propounded by the World Bank in the 1980s, it was not at the time seen as an attack on the state itself.

4 During this period, the only major international agency propounding stricter controls over the state's allocation of economic resources was the IMF; the World Bank did not seriously question the state's role.

5 The International Labour Organization (ILO) in 1972 (in a mission report on Kenya) first defined the concept of basic human needs to include health, education, adequate nutrition, clean water, sanitation, safe housing, and so forth. The concept was adopted by the World Bank and rapidly gained currency in the development thinking of the decade.

6 The social origins of the women's health groups are different, depending on particular country histories and experiences. Many progressive activists came to realize the importance of women's health concerns and of safe reproductive health services only in the process of working with women in base-level popular organizations whose primary concerns were not initially women's health at all. García-Moreno and Claro (this volume) discuss the evolution of the women's health movement.

7 In addition to large movements, such as that against the damming of the Narmada River in India, there are many local settings in which community organizations or nongovernmental organizations are pitted against "development" interests that are often simply private commercial interests. See Rush (1991) for a discussion of such struggles in the context of forests in Asia; and Peluso (1992); Schmink and Wood (1992).

8 For example, see World Bank 1990. Even though that report has been lauded because it seemed to indicate a renewed sensitivity at the World Bank to the problem of poverty after nearly a decade of concentration on structural adjustment, one of its basic messages is that poverty is best addressed by raising economic growth rates, rather than through *direct* antipoverty programs. The latter, the report argues, should be targeted to the destitute.

9 In the World Bank's approach, this contradiction is addressed by focusing on the need to increase the *efficiency* of social sector expenditures through better target-ing and management. Laudable as this may be, it is doubtful whether this has, in practice, countered the effects of reduced per capita real expenditures in countries whose spending on the social sectors was already inadequate.

10 There are more complex issues involved in ensuring compatibility between macro and micro approaches, but I do not deal with them in this discussion. For example, there may be an important time dimension involved; the global population-environment linkages may become valid over much longer (planetary scale) time spans than the local interactions.

11 I would hold this to be true for anthropology, psychology, sociology, political science, and economics, even though each discipline has contended in its own way with the problem of linking macro changes with micro behavior. In economics, for example, the microeconomic foundations of macroeconomic patterns continues to be one of the least resolved theoretical issues ever since the emergence of Keynesian ideas earlier in this century.

12 This is true, for example, for studies such as the well-known National Academy of Sciences (1986) report on population and development linkages.

13 An example is the well-known identity I = PAT, linking environmental impact (I) with population growth (P), growth in affluence or consumption per capita (A), and technological efficiency (T).

14 In this context, one might perhaps laud the refreshing iconoclasm of the World Bank's *World Development Report 1992* in recognizing that the principal environmental problems for most people in developing countries are polluted air and water supplies, and inadequate waste disposal. The World Bank does not, however, present a single or consistent perspective on environmental problems. In particular, there is little acknowledgement of the possible negative environmental consequences of the structural adjustment policies it espouses.

References

Agarwal, B. 1991. Engendering the environment debate: Lessons from the Indian subcontinent. CASID Speaker Series No. 8. Michigan State University.

Arizpe, L., P. Stone, and D. Major (eds.). 1994. *Population and the environment: Rethinking the debate.* Boulder, Colo.: Westview Press.

Blaikie, P. 1985. *The political economy of soil erosion.* London: Longman.

Committee on Women, Population and the Environment. 1992. Women, population and the environment: Call for a new approach. Newton Center, Mass. Unpublished manuscript.

Conly, S., J. Speidel, and S. Camp. 1991. *U.S. population assistance: Issues for the 1990's.* Washington, D.C.: Population Crisis Committee.

Consortium for Action to Protect the Earth. 1992. *Population, environment and development.* Working Paper. Washington, D.C.

Dankelman, I. and J. Davidson. 1988. *Women and environment in the Third World: Alliance for the future.* London: Earthscan.

Demeny, P. 1992. Early postwar perspectives on rapid population growth: Diagnosis and prescription. Paper presented at the Roger Revelle Memorial Symposium, October 20-22, at Harvard University.

Ehrlich, P., and A. Ehrlich. 1991. *Healing the planet: Strategies for resolving the environmental crisis.* Reading, Mass.: Addison-Wesley.

Germain, A., and J. Ordway. 1989. *Population control and women's health: Balancing the scales.* New York: International Women's Health Coalition.

Hardin, G. 1993. *Living within limits: Ecology, economics, and population taboos.* New York: Oxford University Press.

Hartman, B. 1987. *Reproductive rights and wrongs: The global politics of population control and contraceptive choice.* New York: Harper & Row.

Jolly, R., et al. 1991. Rethinking adjustment. *World Development* 19(12):1801-64.

Kennedy, P. 1993. *Preparing for the twenty-first century.* New York: Random House.

Krishnan, T. N. 1992. Population, poverty and employment in India. *Economic and Political Weekly.* 27(46):2479-2498.

Little, P. 1992. *The social causes of land degradation in dry regions.* Binghamton, N.Y.: Institute of Development Anthropology.

Miller, V. (Cofounder of West Harlem Environmental Action, New York) 1993. Personal communication.

National Academy of Sciences. 1986. *Population growth and economic development: Policy questions.* Washington, D.C.: National Academy Press.

Peluso, N. 1992. *Rich forests, poor people: Resource control and resistance in Java.* Berkeley: University of California Press.

Petchesky, R., and J. Weiner. 1990. *Global feminist perspectives on reproductive rights and reproductive health.* Report on the Special Sessions at the Fourth International Interdisciplinary Congress on Women. Hunter College, New York City.

Rush, J. 1991. *The last tree.* New York: Asia Society.

Schmink, M., and C. H. Wood. 1992. *Contested frontiers in Amazonia.* New York: Columbia University Press.

Sen, G., and C. Grown. 1987. *Development, crises, and alternative visions: Third world women's perspectives.* New York: Monthly Review Press.

Shaw, R. P. 1989. Population growth: Is it ruining the environment? *Populi* 16(2):21-29.

Sontheimer, S. (ed.). 1991. *Women and the environment: A reader: Crisis and development in the Third World.* London: Earthscan.

Turner, B. L., and W. C. Clark, R. W. Kates, J. F. Richards, J. T. Mathews, and W. B. Meyer. 1990. *The earth as transformed by human action.* Cambridge: Cambridge University Press.

World Bank. 1990. *World development report 1990.* New York: Oxford University Press.

———. 1991. *World development report 1991.* New York: Oxford University Press.

———. 1992. *World development report 1992.* New York: Oxford University Press.

6

Population, Well-being, and Freedom

Sudhir Anand

Traditional approaches to population policy have viewed the number, or "stock," of people *instrumentally* — as a means of achieving some desirable goal, such as growth in aggregate income per head or environmental conservation. In this chapter, I examine the implications of viewing "population" *intrinsically* — as people — and not as an instrument to serve some impersonal economic objective. As Immanuel Kant (1785) observed two centuries ago, "So act as to treat humanity, whether in thine own person or in that of any other, in every case as an end withal, never as means only." This perspective sees a concern with *people and their lives* as the real end of "population" policies. It involves protecting people's liberty (negative freedom) in their "personal spheres," and promoting their well-being and opportunities for wider choice (positive freedom). It also involves reducing the sharp inequalities that exist among them, especially between women and men. It leads us in the direction of rethinking "population policy," away from traditional demographic objectives and targets, and toward individual well-being and freedom, including the right of reproductive choice.

To explore the relationship of these concepts to population policy, I briefly review the recent economic and philosophic literature on well-being and freedom. The deficiency of traditional income-based assessments of well-being is illustrated through some international comparisons, and the instrumental role of private incomes relative to publicly provided services is discussed. Against this background, I examine one of the most pervasive intergroup differentials to be found in developing countries: gender inequality in well-being and freedom. Next, I investigate the likely demographic consequences of redressing such inequalities. I also look at the claims of liberty and rights of existing people in reproductive decisions in terms of their implications for "population" policy.

Income, Well-being, and Freedom
Income and Well-being

There has been growing recognition of the inadequacy of equating development with the growth of average income in a society. The dissatisfaction has begun to be expressed in works dealing with "basic needs," "social indicators," and "quality of life." These alternative approaches all move away from income per se in assessing the living standard. Yet they settle on distinctly different types of space in which (or variables by which) to measure development. For example, the basic-needs approach is centered on the possession of vitally important commodities, such as food and housing, while social indicators measure a population's access to education, health, safe water, and adequate sanitation.

The concept of capabilities and functionings proposed by Amartya Sen (1985a, 1987) — what people can actually do and be — argues that a basic distinction should be made between the means and the ends of development. This was recognized at least as far back as Aristotle in his *Nicomachean Ethics*, where he clearly distinguished the means from the ends: "The life of money-making is one undertaken under compulsion, and wealth is evidently not the good we are seeking; for it is merely useful and for the sake of something else" (Barnes 1984). Although income, wealth, and commodities have instrumental importance in enhancing well-being, they do not constitute a direct measure of the living standard. Likewise, happiness or utility might provide evidence of achievement, but cannot be equated with well-being. A thoroughly deprived person who sees no way out of her adversity may, as a strategy of living, be reconciled to her condition and take pleasure from small mercies in life. In a direct sense, "well-being" has to do with *being* well, not with having income — to which it is posterior — or with having utility — to which it is, generally, prior. What is valued intrinsically are a person's achievements — her "beings" and "doings" — or her "capabilities" to function (Sen 1987).

The capabilities approach focuses directly on the lives that people lead, on what they succeed in doing and being. Do they live long? Do they escape preventable morbidity? Do they avoid mortality during infancy and childhood? Do they achieve literacy? Are they free from hunger and undernourishment? Do they enjoy personal liberty? Do they participate in the life of the community? Do they possess the social bases for self-respect? These are living standard achievements that have *intrinsic* value; income, by contrast, has only *instrumental* value in terms of what it does, and sometimes does not, allow one to purchase or achieve (for example, a longer life).

The capabilities approach should also be contrasted with the basic-needs and physical-quality-of-life approaches. The former, advocated by the International Labour Office (1976), is centered on commodity possession (minimum requirements of food and the like), rather than on people's achievements. The latter, proposed by

Morris (1979), combines three indicators — infant mortality, life expectancy at age one, and basic literacy — into a composite Physical Quality of Life Index (PQLI).

The concept of human development advocated by the United Nations Development Programme (UNDP) also takes a broader view of living standards than that captured by income alone (UNDP 1990). It focuses attention on the "space" of people's achievements, and proposes a human development index (HDI). The HDI can be seen as an evolution of Morris's PQLI. It relies upon three key indicators for its construction: life expectancy at birth (not age one), adult literacy, and "command over resources needed for a decent living." The last indicator continues to be based on income, even though various adjustments are made to it, such as purchasing-power-corrected real gross domestic product (GDP) per capita, and a logarithmic transform applied to reflect diminishing returns in converting income into a decent living standard. For this reason, it is not directly an indicator of any achievement or functioning, but rather a measure of what can be done with income (Anand 1991).

UNDP (1990) measures progress in each dimension not in terms of the level attained, but in terms of the shortfall from some desired value or target. HDI calibrates each component indicator from 0 to 1 as an index of shortfall from a "desirable" or "adequate" value, reflecting the degree of deprivation. The target values used are Japan's 1987 life expectancy at birth, 78 years; an adult literacy rate of 100 percent; and the average official "poverty line" income in nine industrial countries, adjusted by purchasing power parities, $4,861 (or 3.69 in logarithmic terms). The minimum values of life expectancy in 1987, adult literacy, and the logarithm of real GDP per capita in the sample of countries were 42 years, 12 percent, and 2.34, respectively. A deprivation index between 0 and 1 is then calculated for each component indicator.[1] Finally, a simple unweighted average is taken to obtain an average deprivation index, and this is subtracted from 1 to give the HDI (UNDP 1990).

Well-being and Freedom[2]

Most would agree that freedom of choice is central to leading a good life. But is its importance merely *instrumental*—a means of achieving other ends — or does it have *intrinsic* significance? What are the content and role of freedom, and how can they be assessed? I will briefly address these questions in the context of the capabilities approach to well-being, which is noteworthy for its emphasis on freedoms.

In a famous essay entitled "Two Concepts of Liberty," Isaiah Berlin (1969) makes an important distinction between "negative" and "positive" freedom. The "positive" view, which is closely connected to the capabilities approach, sees freedom in terms of what a person can actually do or be, or as the *opportunities* that are available to her. From the set of possible "functionings" within the person's reach, she typically chooses one (described as a vector or as an *n*-tuple). In appraising the well-being of the person, it is important to pay attention to the capability *set,* and not just to the chosen functioning vector.[3] This allows us to assess the overall, or positive, freedoms that the individual has.

The "negative" view of freedom, on the other hand, focuses exclusively on the absence of interference or restrictions by others, including the state, other institutions, and individuals.[4] A person's freedom to choose one commodity over another, or one activity over another, obviously influences the living standard she can enjoy and the goals of her life she can fulfill. Any interference with her ability to choose valued functionings within her reach can lead directly to a loss of well-being. Negative freedom is, therefore, certainly important as a means to other ends.[5]

But there also exists a powerful defense of the intrinsic value of negative freedom. According to this view, freedom is not just a means of achieving a good life, it is *constitutive* of the good life. Rawls's (1971) case for the "priority of liberty" derives from attaching such intrinsic importance to negative freedom, as does Nozick's (1974) "entitlement theory" of justice, involving the requirement to obey certain "constraints" against interference. Nozick's theory proceeds from the premise that "individuals have rights, and there are things that no person or group may do to them (without violating their rights)." In examining the concept of a person's "agency," Sen (1985b) argues that the status of individual rights can be linked, ultimately, to the importance of freedom, which is a central aspect of being a person.

It is not just the demands of "agency freedom" — the liberty to choose for oneself certain basic features of one's personal existence — that can lead to rights. Some positive freedoms can also yield straightforward notions of rights. Minimal demands of "well-being freedom"—in the form of having the capability to avoid hunger and starvation, for example — can also be seen as rights that command attention (Sen 1985b).

International Comparisons

International comparisons of capabilities must take note of certain basic features of well-being. Because a prerequisite to well-being is "being," the most elementary capability would appear to be that of survival. Hence, the discussion here concentrates on life expectancy and survival,[6] although one other indicator, adult literacy, is also considered.

How well do differences in income, which has only instrumental importance, account for the levels of these indicators across countries? In general, the higher the average income of a country, the more likely it is to have a higher average life expectancy (see Figure 1 on next page) and adult literacy rate, and thus also a higher HDI value. But the fits are far from perfect. In regression analyses, income per capita typically accounts for about 50 percent of the variation in life expectancy and adult literacy (see Anand 1991; Anand and Ravallion 1993; and the references cited there).

Such regressions suggest, of course, that there is a large residual variation that is not explained by income per capita. These regressions have been used to identify "outliers" from the general pattern, especially countries — like China and Sri Lanka — with low gross national product (GNP)

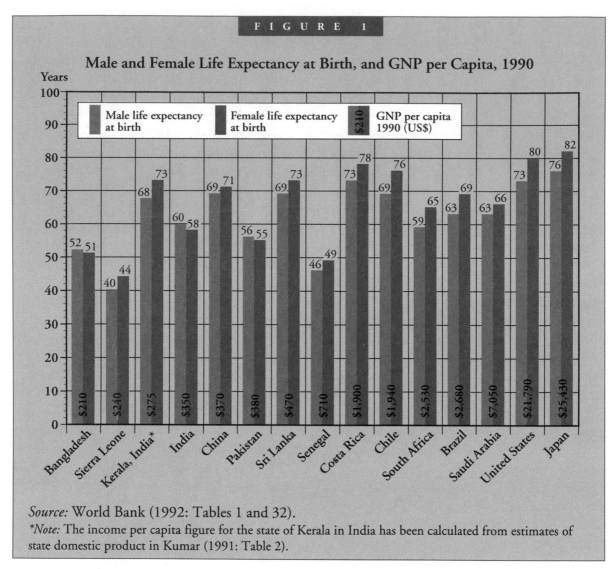

FIGURE 1

Male and Female Life Expectancy at Birth, and GNP per Capita, 1990

Years

| | Male life expectancy at birth | Female life expectancy at birth | $210 | GNP per capita 1990 (US$) |

Bangladesh: 52, 51, $210
Sierra Leone: 40, 44, $240
Kerala, India*: 68, 73, $275
India: 60, 58, $350
China: 69, 71, $370
Pakistan: 56, 55, $380
Sri Lanka: 69, 73, $470
Senegal: 46, 49, $710
Costa Rica: 73, 78, $1,900
Chile: 69, 76, $1,940
South Africa: 59, 65, $2,530
Brazil: 63, 69, $2,680
Saudi Arabia: 63, 66, $7,050
United States: 73, 80, $21,790
Japan: 76, 82, $25,430

Source: World Bank (1992: Tables 1 and 32).

*Note: The income per capita figure for the state of Kerala in India has been calculated from estimates of state domestic product in Kumar (1991: Table 2).

per capita but high levels of life expectancy, literacy, and other living standard achievements. (Countries typically falling *below* such a fitted relationship include Brazil, South Africa, and Saudi Arabia.) Much research has attempted to explain the exceptional performance of China and Sri Lanka relative to their income levels: life expectancies in China and Sri Lanka exceed by 12 and 11 years, respectively, those of typical countries at their per capita GNP levels in the Asia and Pacific region. Similarly, adult literacy rates in China and Sri Lanka are 15 and 27 percentage points higher, respectively, than those predicted for their income levels (Anand 1991).

These achievements owe much to government intervention in the health, education, and social services sectors over a long period of time. In Sri Lanka, for example, intervention in most areas predates independence in 1948; in some areas it even predates the granting of universal adult suffrage in 1931. The first health unit in Sri Lanka was established in 1926 to provide primary health care, including control of infectious diseases. In education, government intervention began even earlier, in 1920.[7]

Identifying such outliers in cross-country regressions with GNP per capita as the independent variable does not, in fact, reveal the role played by income in influencing these achievements, because the countries are isolated by their large residuals at different levels of GNP per capita. However, higher levels of aggregate income can allow both the financing of improved social services (such as public health care, disease prevention, clean drinking water, and basic education) *and*, if the income is well distributed, command over basic goods and services (such as food, sanitation, and housing) — especially by poor people, for whom the instrumental importance of additional private income is likely to be greater than it is for rich people. This suggests that we should control both for the public provisioning of social services and for the incidence of absolute (income) poverty in such cross-country regressions.

Once one controls for public spending on social services and for the incidence of absolute poverty, there is *no* significant partial correlation between life expectancy and average income (Anand and Ravallion 1993); the significantly positive relationship between life expectancy and income vanishes entirely in a regression of life expectancy against poverty incidence, public health spending, and average income. This does not imply that aggregate income levels are unimportant in enhancing life expectancy. Rather, it says that the importance of aggregate income lies in the way that its benefits are distributed among people, and the extent to which it allows the support of public health services.

Although there are a number of caveats to this sort of cross-country analysis, the results do provide provisional support for the view that social expenditures and reduction in income poverty, rather than economic growth per se, are the major forces driving improvements in life expectancy. This suggests that policy intervention can play a role independent of the promotion of aggregate economic growth in developing countries.

Gender Inequalities in Well-being and Freedom

In developing countries, one of the most pervasive intergroup inequalities is that between the genders.[8] Not only does this take the form of unequal access to the labor market, and hence to income-earning opportunities, but once employed, women appear to receive lower wages than men. Bias against girls also exists in access to

food, health care, and education, and may be experienced both inside and outside the household (Chen, Huq, and D'Souza 1981). This unequal treatment is reflected in the differential achievements of women and men in many parts of the world.

Indicators based on income or on the possession and use of commodities are not particularly well suited to examining gender, or other interindividual, inequalities. This is because information on resource use or availability is typically available only at the household level, and cannot be easily used to uncover allocation *within* the household (see, however, Deaton 1987). By contrast, the consequences of female disadvantage and gender bias, both within and outside the household, are reflected in the life expectancy, literacy, and other achievements of the individuals concerned. Data on these achievements are collected not at the household level, through household income and expenditure surveys, but at the individual level, through demographic surveys and population censuses.[9] There is, thus, a strong practical reason — apart from concern for what is intrinsically important — to focus on strictly personal features of well-being to examine gender and other interindividual disparities.

We can illuminate some gender inequalities straightforwardly by considering the differential adult literacy rates of women and men in many developing nations. Looking at female-male differences in literacy, and in educational attainments more generally, is critical not only for the intrinsically important question of gender justice, but also because of the instrumental importance of women's education to the long-term well-being of both women and men (Schultz 1992; Summers 1992; among others).

The female adult literacy rate is less than half the male rate in many poor countries. In Mozambique, Bangladesh, Pakistan, and Senegal, for example, the rate of female literacy in 1990 was about 20 percent, while the male rate was 45–50 percent. In Sierra Leone, the female literacy rate was only 11 percent, whereas the male rate was 31 percent. Notable exceptions to the general pattern observed in developing countries are found in Sri Lanka, China, Jamaica, Costa Rica, and Chile, where the overall literacy rates are higher and the gender disparities somewhat lower. Although the average rates for the last three countries are in excess of 90 percent and essentially the same for women and men, China has an overall rate of 73 percent and a significant disparity between females and males (62 percent and 84 percent, respectively). Sri Lanka has an overall rate of 88 percent, split between a female rate of 84 percent and a male rate of 93 percent (UNDP 1993: Table 5). For most developed countries there are no recent surveys on adult literacy, but according to UNESCO, less than five percent of their populations are illiterate (in World Bank 1992: Table 1).

Next we move on to a consideration of life expectancy differentials between women and men. There is strong evidence that the maximal potential life expectancy for women is greater than for men — given symmetry of treatment in nutrition, health care, and other conditions of living, including the duration and intensity of work (see Waldron 1983 and the references cited there). Indeed, this biological advantage of females is reflected in lower mortality rates at every age, including the fetal stage. Hence, we should expect a higher life expectancy for females than for males.

That is indeed what we observe in the developed nations, where women typically outlive men by five to seven years. It is also the case in most developing countries, even though the overall life expectancy is lower and the gap between the genders smaller. But there are some notable exceptions, especially among South Asian countries. In Bangladesh, India, and Pakistan, female life expectancy is *lower* than male life expectancy by one to two years (see Figure 1). This would appear to be *prima facie* evidence of antifemale bias in these countries.

However, for countries where female life expectancy is higher than male life expectancy, it is more difficult to assess the relative performance of the genders because of the difference in their maximal potential life expectancies. Should one simply take the ratio of female to male life expectancy in each developing country and compare it with the ratio for the developed nations as a group — where the gender bias, if any, in nutrition and health care is likely to be much smaller (despite the existence of gender bias in other areas)? Should one look at the absolute shortfalls in life expectancy from the maximum levels achieved in the advanced nations by females and males, respectively? The complex issues posed in comparing achievement by looking at attainment versus shortfall (either absolute or as a proportion of the respective maximal values) are discussed in Sen (1992) and Anand (1993).

Another approach to assessing relative female disadvantage in survival, even for countries where female life expectancy exceeds male life expectancy, is through the simple ratio of total females to males in the population. In the most advanced nations, the female-to-male ratio is about 105 in percentage terms. In South Asian countries the ratio is below 100: 92 in Pakistan, 93 in India, and 94 in Bangladesh. But in China, where life expectancy for females is higher than for males, the female-to-male ratio is only 94 percent (UNDP 1993: Table 9). This is despite the fact that everywhere, about 5 percent more boys than girls are born. Drèze and Sen (1989) estimate the number of "missing women" in Asia and North Africa by applying the female-to-male ratio of 102.2 percent for Sub-Saharan Africa as a standard, rather than the higher ratio for the developed nations. The purpose of using the Sub-Saharan standard for comparison is essentially to control for the age distribution of the population, given lower female mortality rates in the developed nations; in Sub-Saharan Africa, by contrast, fertility rates are no lower than those in Asia and North Africa, and there is little female disadvantage in terms of relative mortality rates of females and males (as witnessed by higher levels of female life expectancy there). Drèze and Sen come up with startling statistics: 100 million women missing worldwide, including 44 million in China and 37 million in India.[10] They attribute this to the low status of females in these countries, which results in a relative neglect of women, and especially of female children, in the areas of health care and nutrition.

For a different sort of comparison, one can look at the situation within a large country, such as India. The state of Kerala, which has a below-average income per capita among the Indian states, has a much higher average life expectancy at birth than the country as a whole (70 years, as compared with 59 years). The level of female life expectancy in Kerala is 73 years, and that of male life expectancy is 67.5 years (see Figure 1). Moreover, the female-to-male ratio is 104 percent, and adult literacy rates exceed 90 percent. Drèze and Sen (1989) attribute this to a long history of state intervention in education, especially female education, dating back to the early 19th century. There is also a wide network of health services for the population and a tradition of matrilineal inheritance of land and property in a substantial section of the community (the Nairs); further, the women of Kerala participate significantly in paid work.[11] These features have helped to raise the social standing of women, and to curb the antifemale bias that prevails in many other parts of India.

Demographic Consequences of Policies to Promote Well-being and Freedom

What would be the long-term demographic consequences of a population policy based on promoting the well-being and freedom of people living now? One immediate consequence follows from the discussion in the previous section. There, it was suggested that enhancing the well-being of all people requires redressing the pervasive inequalities that exist between women and men. If the elimination of gender bias leads to the addition of 100 million women in the world, that consequence cannot be considered undesirable simply because it increases the world population. The issue of gender justice — protecting women's right to equal treatment as men — would surely appear to take precedence over impersonal aggregate demographic goals.

This view derives in part from a lack of convincing moral justification for particular demographic targets. The literature on "optimum population size," based on ethical formulas such as the maximization of total or average utility (or income), is beset with difficulties.[12] These concern not only the use of very specific, and often quite arbitrary, formulas that have little intrinsic significance and are hard to defend, but also limitations arising from the framework of "consequential welfarism." That framework is based on an engineering approach to reproductive behavior, which fails to pay adequate attention to nonutilitarian notions of individual well-being and freedom (both positive and negative); the claims of liberty and rights in personal lives; and the asymmetry in the status of existing and potential people (Sen 1991). Not surprisingly, the demographic objectives embodied in the concept of "optimum population" provide little help in guiding policy.

How do considerations of liberty, privacy, and autonomy in personal lives affect the assessment of reproductive decisions of individuals? If individual liberties and rights have intrinsic importance — as powerfully argued by Rawls (1971), Nozick (1974), and others — and if the rights of an individual over her "personal domain" are guaranteed, then the bearing of these considerations on the population problem can be profound. An individual's decisions regarding reproductive choice are deeply private, and cannot be easily overridden on grounds of their adverse effects on, say, the utility of others. Any compulsion in this sphere — a violation of her negative freedom — would be held as unacceptable, unless there were very strong reasons to the contrary. Moreover, such reasons would have to be properly established, not assumed, and would have to be evaluatively sustainable.

Two points might be adduced against such an unconditional right. The first suggests that the rights in question include those of people who would or would not come into existence *directly as a result* of these choices. But there is clearly a lack of parity between people already in existence and possible people (who could exist but do not); in other words, it is hard to argue in favor of potential people's rights (namely, to come into existence or not) over the rights of actual people who are here now (Sen 1991).

The second point warns that a large population resulting from unrestricted birthrates may cause adverse effects on the well-being and freedom of others — for example, of present and future generations, through environmental degradation. It is noteworthy that this argument warns against a large population not on grounds that it is intrinsically bad, but because of the "externalities" imposed on others. This extrinsic argument, however, depends on a tenuous distinction between two groups of people: those whose well-being is the object of our concern, and those whose presence is assessed purely in terms of what it does for the first group.

To be sure, even if one weights the interests of future people less than those of present people, there might still be a good case for intervention. Voluntary birth control subsidized by government would be fully justified on the basis of advancing individual well-being and freedom, but it does not follow that compulsory birth control is the way to deal with the problem. There are other instruments and policies, standardly considered in the economics literature, that address the issue of externalities, public goods (bads), market imperfections, and defective price signals. Public policy can adapt the incentive structure in a number of ways to protect the global environment and "resource base" for people yet to be born; various interventions can help reduce the divergence between private and social costs (benefits) (Dasgupta 1993; Sen 1993b). Thus, it does not necessarily follow from the "stewardship" argument that population growth should be restricted through coercive methods.[13] As Sen (1991) puts it:

> There is a real disanalogy here between (1) arguments for compulsory birth control and other authoritarian means of influencing population growth (varying from regulations for "one child family" to involuntary sterilization), and (2) the case for public intervention in promoting health services,

educational opportunities, social security, and other facilities that expand people's capability to lead the kind of life they have reasons to value. Liberty and freedom are threatened by the former programmes in a way they are not by the latter.

Moreover, the evidence that is emerging from study after study in developing countries shows that expanding health services and educational opportunities — for women, especially — leads ultimately to significant reductions in fertility (see, for example, Dasgupta 1993; Schultz 1994; Summers 1992; and the references cited there). Also, the means of family planning and voluntary birth control become more readily available as health facilities are expanded. Fortunately, the infringement of individual liberties and rights is not the only way of arresting the rate of population growth.[14]

Conclusion

In this chapter, I have suggested that traditional approaches to population policy, including theorics of "optimum population size," have viewed people instrumentally to serve some impersonal objective, such as total income or utility per head, or environmental conservation. I have examined the implications of an intrinsic concern for people and their lives, and have argued that income is not the right space for assessing people's well-being. I have reviewed the recent literature on quality of life, and argued that the capabilities approach offers a firmer foundational base for systematic study of well-being and freedom.

These concepts of individual well-being and freedom push us in the direction of rethinking "population policy." The reappraisal calls not only for the protection of liberty (negative freedom) in people's "personal spheres," but for active policies to promote their well-being (positive freedom) and to reduce the sharp inequalities that prevail among them, especially between women and men.

Such a shift in population policy may well turn out to be effective in reducing fertility (for example, through advances in women's education and autonomy); much recent evidence suggests that this would be the case. But even if it is not, and adverse effects on the environment can be demonstrated to ensue, these should be addressed through standard economic policies, such as prices, taxation, and regulation, that alter the incentive structure in desired directions. Restricting reproductive choice through compulsion is, happily, not the only, or necessarily the most effective, way of dealing with environmental externalities. The intrinsic importance of gender justice, and of expanding people's overall freedoms through policies that promote health and education, cannot be seen on a par with the instrumental rationale for coercion, in the alleged interest of the social good, in the deeply private domain of reproductive behavior.

Unlike conventional approaches to population policy, the perspective described in this chapter views people as agents in their own right, with goals, achievements, and freedoms that they have reasons to value. Attaching priority to these claims provides policy makers with a focus different from the earlier concentration on aggregate population numbers. It is essential that population policies and programs respect the legitimate well-being and agency objectives of people.

Notes

1   Thus a country's life expectancy deprivation is given by the formula: (78-life expectancy at birth)/(78-42). Similarly, a country's GDP deprivation is given by the formula: (3.69-logarithm of real GDP per capita)/(3.69-2.34).

2   This discussion draws heavily on Sen (1985a, b; 1987; 1988).

3   Sen (1985b) provides the example of two persons with identical functioning vectors in terms of undernourishment: one starving out of choice, because of his religious beliefs, and the other because she is very poor and lacks the means to command food. Even though both persons' achieved level of well-being (in terms of being undernourished) is the same, there is an important difference in their respective capability sets: the first person *could have* chosen not to starve, while the second person did not have that choice. In a straightforward sense, the first person's well-being freedom, and hence advantage, is greater than the second person's.

4   Thus, if a person is starving because she is poor and lacks the means to command food, her positive freedom from hunger is clearly compromised. But her negative freedom may be perfectly intact, if her failure to acquire sufficient food is not the result of interference or restraints imposed by others.

5   A defense of the instrumental role of negative freedom is provided by Milton Friedman, among others. He refers to the "fecundity of freedom," and argues in its favor precisely because it is so productive. For example, see Friedman and Friedman (1980).

6   Although life expectancy and survival are measures of achievement rather than capability (or positive freedom), they can nevertheless be seen as an important indicator of the *freedom* to live long. People tend to exercise the option to live as long as they can; thus, the metric of life expectancy will be a good indicator of the corresponding capability.

7   For a detailed account of Sri Lanka's achievements, see Anand and Kanbur (1991). The case of China is analyzed in some detail in Drèze and Sen (1989).

8   Of all such inequalities, gender inequalities (along with racial ones, and those associated with physical handicap) are the least justifiable. The reason is that these biological traits cannot be altered, so the inequalities cannot be instrumentally defended in terms of incentives (altering behavior to increase aggregate efficiency).

9   The quality of data obtained from demographic surveys and censuses, which form the basis of estimates of life expectancy, is sometimes not very good. The same is true of national income data for many developing countries.

10 Even using somewhat different bases for the calculation that take into account actual life expectancy and fertility rates in these countries yields an estimate of excess female mortality of 60 million (see Sen 1993a).

11 The same is also true in many countries of Sub-Saharan Africa.

12 For illuminating discussions of the difficulties involved, see Broome (1993), Parfit (1984; 1986), and Sen (1991). Parfit rejects the utilitarian framework on grounds that it leads to a "repugnant conclusion" (see his discussion of "the mere addition paradox").

13 Note that the question of limiting the aggregate world population is an issue quite distinct from how this total population should be distributed between the rich and poor countries of the world.

14 Sen (1993b) illustrates this point forcefully by contrasting the experience of China and the state of Kerala in India. China has followed a coercive "one-child policy" and managed to reduce its crude birthrate to 21 per 1,000. On the other hand, Kerala, by following a voluntary family planning policy accompanied by expansion

of health facilities, female education, and so on (see previous section), has succeeded in cutting down its crude birthrate to 20 per 1,000.

References

Anand, S. 1991. Poverty and human development in Asia and the Pacific. In *Poverty alleviation in Asia and the Pacific*. New York: United Nations Development Programme.

————. 1993. Inequality between and within nations. Cambridge, Mass.: Center for Population and Development Studies, Harvard University.

Anand, S., and S. M. R. Kanbur. 1991. Public policy and basic needs provision: Intervention and achievement in Sri Lanka. In J. P. Drèze and A. K. Sen (eds.), *The political economy of hunger, vol. 3*. Oxford: Clarendon Press.

Anand, S., and M. Ravallion. 1993. Human development in poor countries: On the role of private incomes and public services. *Journal of Economic Perspectives* 7(1):133–150.

Barnes, J. (ed.). 1984. *The complete works of Aristotle*. Revised Oxford Translation, Bollingen Series LXXI.2. Princeton, N.J.: Princeton University Press.

Berlin, I. 1969. *Four essays on liberty*. Oxford: Oxford University Press.

Broome, J. 1993. The welfare economics of population. Discussion Paper No. 93/360, Department of Economics, University of Bristol.

Chen, L., E. Huq, and S. D'Souza. 1981. Sex bias in the family allocation of food and health care in rural Bangladesh. *Population and Development Review* 7(1):55–70.

Dasgupta, P. 1993. The population problem. Cambridge: University of Cambridge.

Deaton, A. S. 1987. The allocation of goods within the household: Adults, children and gender. Living Standards Measurement Study Working Paper No. 39. World Bank.

Drèze, J. P., and A. K. Sen. 1989. *Hunger and public action*. Oxford: Clarendon Press.

Friedman, M., and R. Friedman. 1980. *Free to choose*. London: Secker and Warburg.

International Labour Office. 1976. *Employment, growth and basic needs: A one-world problem*. Geneva.

Kant, I. 1785. *Foundations of the metaphysics of morals*. Trans. L. W. Beck 1959. Indianapolis, Ind.: Bobbs-Merrill Co.

Kumar, A. K. S. 1991. UNDP's human development index: A computation for Indian states. *Economic and Political Weekly*. October 12, Bombay.

Morris, M. D. 1979. *Measuring the condition of the world's poor: The physical quality of life index*. New York: Pergamon.

Nozick, R. 1974. *Anarchy, state and utopia*. Oxford: Basil Blackwell; and New York: Basic Books.

Parfit, D. 1984. *Reasons and persons*. Oxford: Clarendon Press.

————. 1986. Overpopulation and the quality of life. In P. Singer (ed.), *Applied ethics*. Oxford: Oxford University Press.

Rawls, J. 1971. *A theory of justice*. Cambridge, Mass.: Harvard University Press; and Oxford: Clarendon Press.

Schultz, T. P. 1992. The benefits of educating women. In E. King and M. A. Hill (eds.), *Women's education in developing countries*. Baltimore, Md.: Johns Hopkins University Press.

————. 1994. Human capital, family planning and their effects on population growth. Paper presented at the American Economic Association meetings, January 5, in Boston, Mass. Forthcoming in *American Economic Review* (Papers and Proceedings), May 1994.

Sen, A. K. 1985a. *Commodities and capabilities*. Amsterdam: North-Holland.

————. 1985b. Well-being, agency and freedom: The Dewey Lectures 1984. *Journal of Philosophy* 82(4):169–221.

————. 1987. *The standard of living*. The Tanner Lectures. Cambridge: Cambridge University Press.

————. 1988. Freedom of choice: concept and content. *European Economic Review* 32:269–294.

————. 1991. Welfare economics and population ethics. Paper presented at the Nobel Jubilee Symposium on Population, Development and Welfare, December 5–7, in Lund, Sweden.

————. 1992. *Inequality reexamined*. Oxford: Clarendon Press; and Cambridge, Mass.: Harvard University Press.

————. 1993a. The economics of life and death. *Scientific American* 268(5):40–47.

————. 1993b. Population and reasoned agency: Food, fertility and economic development. Paper presented at the Royal Swedish Academy of Sciences and the Beijer Institute, November 11, in Stockholm.

Summers, L. H. 1992. Investing in *all* the people. Policy Research Working Paper WPS 905. World Bank.

United Nations Development Programme (UNDP). 1990. *Human development report 1990.* New York: Oxford University Press.

————. 1993. *Human development report 1993.* New York: Oxford University Press.

Waldron, I. 1983. The role of genetic and biological factors in sex differences in mortality. In A. D. Lopez and L. T. Ruzicka (eds.), *Sex differences in mortality.* Canberra: Department of Demography, Australian National University.

World Bank. 1992. *World development report 1992: Development and the environment.* New York: Oxford University Press.

SECTION TWO

Human Rights
and Reproductive Rights

7

Honoring Human Rights in Population Policies: From Declaration to Action

Reed Boland, Sudhakar Rao, and George Zeidenstein

International documents, treaties, and declarations from three interrelated fields — population, women's rights, and human rights — address both directly and tangentially the treatment of human and reproductive rights in population policies. Although these documents arc rhetorically strong on human rights, our assessment is that fundamental ambiguities and conflicts have been glossed over in favor of political consensus. Human rights have gained increasing prominence in debates over population policies and programs, and most documents dealing with population policy contain provisions on human rights or reproductive rights. Nonetheless, discussion of human rights in population documents is often inadequate. Furthermore, while signatories acknowledge human rights, they ultimately downplay them in actual policies.

This ambivalence has developed in part because of the narrow concept of population policies held by many donors, as well as some governments that have adopted strong fertility control policies. It may also emanate from the historical nature of the human rights debate, which has emphasized civil and political rights and minimized social, economic, and cultural rights, including women's rights. The undervaluing of these "second-generation" rights has affected debates about the balance between individual choice and the collective needs of society. Ambiguity has made it difficult to stop violations of human rights during the implementation of population policies.

In this chapter, we review the relevant aspects of major international documents on human rights, population, and women's rights. We then propose an alternative approach to population policies which places human rights at the center and emphasizes full sexual and reproductive rights for women, their empowerment, and their exercise of social and economic rights. Such an approach, we argue, could transform the essence of population policies, shifting the primary focus toward improving directly the social welfare and quality of people's lives. In our view, this is also the most effective way to lower population growth rates.

Basic Human Rights Documents

Concerns for individual human welfare in the international arena emerged 200 years ago as countries debated the abolition of slavery and the treatment of prisoners of war. Concepts of human rights and equality originated during the period of the French and American revolutions. These concerns grew significantly in the years following the First World War and influenced the formation of the League of Nations. The United Nations Charter, adopted in 1945, encoded international human rights in international law, and was followed by the Universal Declaration on Human Rights in 1948. These two documents provide the modern foundation for establishing the relationship between individuals and the nation-state.

The United Nations Charter (1945)

The charter was the first international treaty to enunciate the principle of equality in specific terms. It reaffirmed "fundamental human rights,…. the dignity and worth of the human person,…. equal rights of men and women" as aims of the UN. It listed, among the purposes and principles of the international body, the promotion and encouragement of respect by member countries for "human rights and fundamental freedom for all without distinction as to race, sex, language or religion."

The Universal Declaration of Human Rights (1948)

The principle of equality and nondiscrimination was formalized as the central theme of the declaration. Article 1 states that "all human beings are born free and equal in dignity and rights." The declaration spells out specifically the fundamental human rights that member states of the UN have pledged to protect and promote, including several that have a close bearing on population issues: life, liberty, and security of person; equality before law; freedom from arbitrary interference with privacy, family, and home; social security and the realization of economic, social, and cultural rights indispensable for dignity and the free development of personality; and work, rest, leisure, and education, including the prior right of parents to choose the kind of education to be given to their children. Article 16 states that "men and women of full age, without any limitation due to race, nationality or religion, have the right to marry and to found a family," and that "marriage shall be entered into only with the free and full consent of the intending spouses." Article 25 speaks of every person's right "to a standard of living adequate for the health and well being of himself and of his family" and states that "motherhood and childhood are entitled to special care and assistance. All children, whether born in or out of wedlock, shall enjoy the same social protection." The declaration designates the family as the "natural and fundamental group unit of society" entitled to protection by society and the state.

The Political and Economic Covenants (1966)

In 1966, the UN General Assembly adopted and opened for signature two instruments designed to implement the human rights provisions of the charter and the declaration — the International Covenant on Civil and Political Rights (the Political Covenant), and the International Covenant on Economic, Social and Cultural Rights (the Economic Covenant). Together with the declaration, the covenants constitute the International Bill of Rights. Even though differing in emphasis, both covenants stress their mutuality and the importance of civil, political, economic, social, and cultural rights (United Nations 1966). Although the original intention of the drafters was to have a single covenant, two covenants emerged because some argued that it would be impossible to develop a single system of implementation for both sets of rights. Protection of political and civil rights requires only that governments refrain from proscribed action, but realization of economic, social, and cultural rights depends on affirmative action and resource commitments by governments (Scott 1993). The distinction has continued to cause heated debate (Scott 1993; Trubek 1984). Nonetheless, both groups of rights were reaffirmed at the Human Rights Conference in Vienna in 1993.

A fundamental tension between the UN Charter and the human rights documents is the simultaneous assertion of unconditional national sovereignty and of universal individual human rights. The UN itself is based upon the sovereignty of nation-states; yet human rights is an individual entitlement that does not recognize national boundaries. These two apparently conflicting principles have surfaced in debates over Northern countries, promotion of population control in Southern countries, and over coercive reproductive policies within sovereign member states of the UN.

Another ambiguity in these international documents concerns women's rights. As Correa and Petchesky in this volume show, women's rights have generally been neglected because these rights have been treated as social or second-generation rights. Furthermore, the declaration and the covenants have been faulted for lack of gender sensitivity, unqualified endorsement of "the family" as the most important social group, and failure to articulate reproductive rights (Holmes 1983). Because of such shortcomings, the equality prescribed in international instruments has limited significance for women in the real world. For example, discriminatory practices that hold women in a subservient position and lead to their exclusion from public life have generally not been seen as violations of the human rights and fundamental freedoms of women. The principal international organs established for the promotion and protection of human rights have dealt with violations of women's rights, if at all, in a marginal way (Correa and Petchesky in this volume; Reanda 1981). Customary law, traditional institutions and cultural practices, and the biases they lead to, have generally remained outside the purview of these organs, and discriminatory practices arising from the biological and reproductive differences between men and women remain unaddressed (Law and Rackner 1987). Furthermore, reluctance to "violate the privacy of the family" has perverse consequences when forcible confinement, domestic violence, child abuse, and torture take place within it. Since patriarchy and other traditional hierarchies result in the domination of the family by men, it is women's and children's rights that are violated within the privacy of the household, despite the special consideration accorded to motherhood and childhood in the international instruments.

Silence about reproductive freedom and rights in the basic human rights instruments must be understood in this context. As the women's movement has long argued, economic and political rights, important as they are, have little meaning for women without the freedom to control their reproductive capacity. By omitting this basic right, the International Bill of Rights has overlooked one of the most fundamental freedoms for women. Nonetheless, the first time reproductive freedom or choice was mentioned by the international community was at a human rights meeting. In 1968, 20 years after the adoption of the declaration, the International Conference on Human Rights, held at Teheran, passed resolution 18, which stated: "Parents have a basic human right to determine freely and responsibly the number and spacing of their children and a right to adequate education and information in this respect" (United Nations 1968).[1]

Human Rights in International Population Policy Documents

The two major population documents are the World Population Plan of Action (WPPA), adopted at the 1974 World Population Conference, held in Bucharest, and the Recommendations for the Further Implementation of the Plan of Action, adopted at the 1984 International Conference on Population, held in Mexico City. These documents embody the consensus of most governments on a framework for population policies and the means to be used to attain population goals. The WPPA reflects a significant political compromise. Whereas the original draft prepared by the organizers was unidimensional, devoted solely to the need to limit fertility, the WPPA is a much more comprehensive statement, explicitly addressing development, population, status of women, and human rights. A similar view was expressed by John D. Rockefeller 3rd in his speech at the conference (see Box 1 on next page). In its analysis of population programs, the WPPA asserts four times that such programs must be "consistent" with, or must not violate, international standards of human rights embodied in the charter and the declaration. The 1984 recommendations incorporate similar statements. Both documents also make specific reference to reproductive rights. Drawing on language originally formulated at the 1968 Teheran conference, they provide, several times apiece, in these or similar words, that "all couples and individuals have the basic right to decide freely and responsibly the number and spacing of their children and to have the information, education, and means to do so."

At first glance, both documents appear to require that population policies be carried out with full respect for human rights, and to establish women's unrestricted right to control their own fertility. The 1984 recommendations even declare that this control "forms an important basis for the enjoyment of other rights." Scrutiny of these statements, however, reveals a number of problems. The first is language, which is ambiguous. One example is the repeated linkage of "individuals and couples." Although this language is preferable to that of the Teheran conference's final document, which referred only to the right of "parents" to determine the spacing and number of children, it still avoids an unencumbered focus on individual reproductive rights. Implicitly, it suggests that when couples, particularly married couples, are involved in reproductive decisions, partners should make the decisions jointly, not individually. In practical terms the documents do not guarantee women, the persons who bear most of the reproductive burden, the right to decide by themselves. At best, they oblige women to consult with their husbands or other partners; at worst, given gender inequalities, they leave women susceptible to being strongly swayed, even forced, to do what their husbands or partners tell them.

B O X   1

Excerpts from John D. Rockefeller 3rd's Address at the World Population Conference, 1974

Mr. Rockefeller was an early and very influential leader in the development of the population field. In 1974, reflecting on his involvement of 20 years, he sensed that the field had moved in directions that jeopardized its central concern with human well-being. Indeed, his speech at Bucharest posed a major challenge to the field to return to this central concern.

"The basis of my interest from the first has been the individual, not his or her relationship to some demographic tabulation, important as this is. To me, interest in population means interest in the problems, well-being and future of people. There are four elements of reappraisal which I believe are essential to the attainment of effective results.

"The first is the relationship between population policy and economic and social development....

"The second...is the need to revise our concept of economic growth.... Whether in the industrialized nations or the developing nations, growth should be pursued not for its own sake, but to meet basic human needs for jobs, food, shelter, health, education.

"The third key element of reappraisal is active recognition of the growing interdependence of all peoples and nations. In an interdependent world, the internal task of the developed nations is clear — to stabilize their own populations and moderate their levels of consumption in a sensible and orderly way.

"The final element...is the role of women in society.... new and urgent attention to the role of women must be a vital characteristic of any modern development program.... In my opinion, if we are to make genuine progress in economic and social development, if we are to make progress in achieving population goals, women increasingly must have greater freedom of choice in determining their roles in society."

Source: Rockefeller 1974.

Equally confusing is the repeated use of the phrase *freely and responsibly* in describing reproductive rights. One is left to wonder just what *responsibly* means, in particular when yoked with the word *freely*. One answer to this question is provided by the 1984 recommendations, which contain the following explication:

> Any recognition of rights also implies responsibilities; in this case it implies that couples and individuals should exercise this right, taking into consideration their own situation, as well as the implications of their decisions for the balanced development of their children and of the community and the society in which they live.

This complements language in the WPPA stating that, in exercising reproductive rights, individuals and couples "should take into account the needs of their living and future children and their responsibilities towards the community." In other words, the right to decide on the number of children is a limited right, balanced by significant responsibilities to others.

Although it is difficult to disagree in principle with the sentiments behind the theory of responsibility described here, such a theory raises a second troubling question: Who is to decide whether persons are acting responsibly? A partial answer is found in additional language — that used to describe the term human rights. First, this language is overwhelmingly general, with vague references to unspecified standards and treaties. Second, it is often qualified: both documents state that while population policies should be consistent with human rights, they should also be consistent with "national goals and values" and recognize the "national sovereignty" of each nation to establish its own population policy. The WPPA is most insistent on this point. It provides that the right of each nation to formulate population policy "is to be exercised in accordance with national objectives and needs and without external interference." This language, in effect, undermines the concept of universal reproductive freedom expressed in the documents by making in-dividual human rights subordinate to national objectives and values, and thereby insulating national policy from outside scrutiny.

Despite their references to human rights, the two documents are not in any sense human rights documents. Rather, they responded to international perceptions that developing countries face overpopulation and, to a lesser extent, social and economic underdevelopment (Finkle and Crane 1975, 1985). Although both documents purport to take a neutral stance with respect to overpopulation, most of their specific recommendations are directed toward lowering rates of population growth, not toward ensuring that individuals are free to determine their fertility.

Equal status for women is accorded high priority in the WPPA language, but "status" is not defined and does not necessarily include rights (see also Correa and Petchesky; and Mahmud and Johnston, in this volume). "Equal status of men and women in the family and in society improves the overall quality of life. This principle should be fully realized in family planning where each spouse should consider the welfare of the other members of the family... Improvement of the status of women in the family and the society can contribute, where desired, to smaller family size, and the opportunity for women to plan births also improves their individual status..." As in the declaration, the family is recognized as the basic unit of society, requiring protection by appropriate legislation and policy. However, implicitly recognizing that the family may not be a loving and caring entity, the WPPA suggests that "family ties be strengthened by giving recognition to the importance of love and mutual respect within the family unit."

The 1984 conference noted that in developing countries, on average, over half of the women who wanted no more children and were exposed to the risk of pregnancy did not have access to family planning. The ability of women to control their fertility is essential for the exercise of other rights, the participants agreed. They urged governments to adopt measures to enable women to take greater responsibility for their reproductive lives. The preeminence of the family as the main institution through which social, political, economic, and cultural change affects fertility was reiterated, and the rights of adolescents and their unique needs came in for special mention.

The formulators of human rights and population documents have overwhelmingly been men, who have often underrecognized women's concerns. For example, until very recently, international human rights organizations focused almost exclusively on the investigation and reporting of violations of the civil and political rights of men, involving such issues as torture, unjust imprisonment, and political persecution, rather than on the equally serious abuses that are perpetrated against women in less-public settings (Bunch 1990; Cook 1993; Martin 1993). Moreover, human rights as a whole have in some sense been a casualty of international power struggles between competing national blocks. For years they were merely another arena of battle for Leninist and capitalist states, which expended enormous energy debating, first, whether the concept of individual human rights was only an invention of capitalism and, then, whether the only true rights were social and economic ones (Murphy 1981; Robertson and Merrills 1989). Similarly, at the international population conferences, human rights issues were secondary to questions of whether control of population growth should be emphasized at all (1974), as developed countries wished, or whether socioeconomic development was more significant, as most socialist and developing countries argued; and whether population control should be emphasized (1984), as many developing countries had become convinced in the interim, or whether free markets and prohibitions on abortion should be stressed, as the United States argued (Finkle and Crane 1975, 1985).

Basic Women's Rights Documents
The Women's Convention (1981)

It was only in 1981, with the UN General Assembly's adoption of the Convention on the Elimination of All Forms of Discrimination Against Women (Women's Convention or CEDAW), that the first international treaty designed specifically to address the concerns and rights of women was codified. Even though the movement for international human rights had articulated the importance of equality between men and women from its inception, in practice women's rights had received little attention. CEDAW is the first legally binding international treaty in which states assume the duty to eliminate all forms of discrimination against women, but only those states that ratify are bound by the treaty.[2]

CEDAW provisions are specific and direct. Discrimination against women is defined in article 1 as "any distinction, exclusion or restriction made on the basis of sex which has the effect or purpose of impairing or nullifying the recognition, enjoyment or exercise by women, irrespective of their marital status, on a basis of equality of men and women, of human rights and fundamental freedoms in the political, economic, social, cultural, civil or any other field." Article 2 calls on governments to "embody the principle of the equality of men and women in their national constitutions or other appropriate legislation." Article 3 requires that states parties take, in all fields, "all appropriate measures, including legislation, to ensure the full development and advancement of women."

The right of reproductive choice figures prominently in the Women's Convention. Article 16 requires that "States Parties shall take all appropriate measures to eliminate discrimination against women in all matters relating to marriage and family relations." The article goes on to list several aspects of marriage and family relations wherein the basis of equality should operate and, in the context of reproductive choice, makes a subtle but significant departure from the Teheran and Bucharest formulations by stating that men and women should have the "same rights to decide."

Article 17 requires all ratifying countries to submit periodic reports, through the secretary-general of the UN to "a Committee on the Elimination of Discrimination against Women," on "legislative, judicial, administrative or other measures which they have adopted to give effect to the provisions of the present Convention and on the progress made in this respect."

As an international instrument prescribing normative standards, the Women's Convention has far-reaching implications. It covers a vast range of issues relevant to women and deals with hitherto uncovered areas, such as inequalities within the family and in marriage, and cultural, religious, and social practices that have a bearing on gender discrimination. Take, for instance, the right to equal access to family planning services and, to information and counseling in this respect (articles 12 and 14). Some countries allow husbands, but not wives, to obtain contraceptives without the spouse's authorization. Some make access to voluntary sterilization conditional on the number of cesarean sections that a woman has undergone, or her age and the number of children that she has. Both are practices that discriminate on the basis of sex and violate the principle of equal rights, in this case the equal right to family planning services. Other examples of discrimination are laws prescribing a lower minimum age at marriage for women than for men; ostracizing pregnant unmarried girls, but not their partners; and refusing adolescents access to family planning services.

CEDAW recognizes, similarly, that the prominence given to the family as the basic unit of the society can work against women's equality. In many societies, women are stereotyped into childbearing and service roles, and the value of their work is neither recognized nor given due respect. Equal status within marriage and family life and elimination of stereotyped roles for men and women are therefore among CEDAWS's stated goals (Cook and Haws 1986) but there are gaping holes in implementation.

Documents from International Conferences on Women (1975, 1980, and 1985)

In 1972, the UN General Assembly adopted a resolution proclaiming 1975 the International Women's Year (IWY), "to be devoted to intensified action with a view to: promoting equality

between men and women, to ensuring the full integration of women in the total development effort, and increasing the contribution of women to the strengthening of world peace" (United Nations 1976). In 1975, the General Assembly proclaimed 1976–1985 the United Nations Decade for Women: Equality, Development and Peace.

The IWY, the Decade for Women, and the three conferences held during the decade were all inspired by the desire to "end discrimination against women and to ensure their equal participation in society" (United Nations 1985). A world conference was convened in Mexico City in 1975 to commemorate IWY. "For the first time in Mexico City the eyes of the world focused on that half of its population who carried out two-thirds of the world's work, received one-tenth of the world's income, and owned less than one-hundredth of its property" (Galey 1986). The conference adopted without a vote the World Plan of Action, a set of guidelines for governmental and private groups to promote equality, development, and peace. It also adopted the Declaration of Mexico on the Equality of Women and Their Contribution to Development and Peace, 1975. The conference looked at a broad spectrum of issues concerning women and development, and the status of women. The family, population, maternal and child health, and family planning were among the issues specifically considered. Reproductive choice was looked at in a perspective markedly different from those of Teheran and Bucharest, a perspective that reflected the thinking of the women's movement on the subject and linked it to the notion of bodily integrity and control (Freedman and Isaacs 1993). Thus, articles 11 and 12 of the Mexico declaration state, respectively, that "the human body, whether that of woman or man, is inviolable and respect for it is a fundamental element of human dignity and freedom," and that "every couple and every individual has the right to decide freely and responsibly whether or not to have children" (United Nations 1976).

The conference on Human Rights, held in Vienna in June 1993, expressed deep concern about the "various forms of discrimination and violence, to which women continue to be exposed all over the world" and dealt extensively with the "equal status and human rights of women" in its concluding declaration. This declaration represents a major advance for the human rights field.

Human Rights and Population Policy and Programs to Date

The weakness of human rights language in the WPPA and the 1984 recommendations has had several results. One is that many subsequent population policy documents have contained little on human rights other than the reiteration of this language or broad statements about ensuring equality for women. A second is the emergence (without express debate on the subject) of a view of human rights and population in which individual rights are required to be subordinated to perceptions (usually elite) of the generalized social and economic welfare rights of the society. This view focuses on economic development of the nation-state and argues it can be enhanced by influencing the behavior of individuals so as to change the rate of population growth. Individual injustices that may be caused by limiting reproductive freedom, or by the use of incentives and coercion, are seen as less important than the future collective injustice and denial of economic and social rights that would result if stern population measures were not adopted.

This view has manifested itself in many forms. It has been the implicit position not only of promoters of traditional population policies, but also, paradoxically, of those who have supported an increase in the rate of population growth (Berelson and Lieberson 1979; Lee 1990; World Bank 1984). Both have looked primarily toward long-term economic goals to be achieved, rather than the moral legitimacy of means used to achieve them (Bok in this volume). Some have explicitly equated compulsory contraceptive use with other forms of government coercion; at the extreme, compulsory education has been cited (Lee 1990; UNESCO 1977).

Various nations have used this view to justify both pronatalist and antinatalist population policies. For example, in a detailed human rights document, the government of China condones coercive means such as group pressure, incentives, and heavy propaganda (China 1991). It stresses efforts to raise living standards, enhance the quality of life, and safeguard the well-being of future generations, asking the question: Is it better to have fewer children who grow up healthy and live a decent life, or unlimited fertility, producing many people who are short of food and clothing and who die young? Similarly, the government of Romania for years used the need for more people to achieve socioeconomic development as justification for its policy of prohibiting most abortions and contraceptives (Boland 1990).

The burgeoning environment and population movement has argued that overpopulation poses one of the greatest environmental threats, undermining health, threatening life systems, and making increased economic and social welfare impossible for the future (Brown et al. 1984; Ehrlich and Ehrlich 1990; Shelton 1991–1992). The logical conclusion is that in order to sustain the environment and protect future generations, limiting population growth may be more important than the protection of individual rights. Supporters of this view often rely on the argument that human rights are relative (Callahan 1981; China 1991). According to this argument, the entire concept of human rights is a Western invention deriving from Enlightenment ideals that are unsuitable or alien to other parts of the world. As a result, the concept has focused excessively on individual rights and autonomy, rather than on society and family. It has also mistakenly stressed individual happiness, self-fulfillment, and growth, rather than collective responsibility, cooperation, consensus, interdependence, restraint, and communal welfare. For those espousing this argument, human rights must be looked at in the context of social, religious, and cultural customs and beliefs prevailing in a community, not from the perspective of individual well-being. Their conclusion is that different societies have different values and ways of safeguarding those values; practices that seem to constitute human rights violations in one part of the world may, in their view, be acceptable elsewhere (Brennan 1988–1989; Cobbah 1987; Donnelly 1989; Renteln 1985).

On the surface, this view of human rights and population has considerable appeal. When examined closely, however, it has serious flaws. First, the idea that individuals in the present generation will not, left to their own free desires, make sound decisions, and therefore should be persuaded or forced to sacrifice for the good of future generations, rests on several faulty assumptions (see Anand in this volume). One is that the only way to lower population growth is through authoritarian enforcement of harsh measures. Another is that imposition of harsh measures will lead to slower population growth and improved socio-economic development. Given that so little is known about the impact of present behavior on the future, neither notion justifies serious interference with human rights respecting reproductive choice. Indeed, it is truly a cynical proposition to subordinate the value of existing people to that of people who have not been born, and may never be born, and to make the former suffer in very real ways when there is no assurance that their suffering will produce real future benefit. The environmental version of this argument is especially weak, for what is really being argued is that the present generation in developing, rather than developed, countries should be the ones to sacrifice — a doubtful proposition when, thus far, consumption in developed countries is far more responsible for environmental problems than is the growth of population in developing countries.

Similarly, the argument that human rights are relative and largely dependent on local culture and tradition is flawed. Such an argument wrongly assumes that societies are static, internally homogeneous entities where all citizens lead contented lives governed by the same communal ideals. This assumption is hardly consistent with the reality of societies anywhere, particularly in recent years, with the dramatic increase in urbanization and "modernization." Further, this argument denies the basic premise that, whether called human rights or not, there exist ethical norms in all societies that embody universal concepts of human dignity and tolerance — especially when it comes to matters of bodily integrity (see Correa and Petchesky in this volume).

The most forceful argument, however, against the view that the generalized social and economic welfare of society is more important than individual rights is the devastating effect this view has had on the lives of individuals, particularly women. At the same time that some countries have proclaimed their adherence to human rights, they have carried out repressive population policies — policies that have not conformed to even minimal human rights standards. One notorious example is Romania. Even as it was hosting the 1974 population conference, Romania was implementing a draconian campaign to raise the rate of population growth, purportedly to ensure socio-economic development. The campaign included the prohibition of abortion and contraception. It even forced gynecologic examinations of women in the workplace and monitoring of pregnant women until delivery to ensure that they would not attempt abortions. The result of these measures was the second-highest infant mortality rate in Europe; a maternal mortality rate eight times the next highest in Europe; 500 deaths a year associated with illegal abortions; and by 1989, some 20,000 women hospitalized for complications of unsafe, mostly illegal abortions. Moreover, tens of thousands of children, who were unwanted or whose parents could not afford to care for them, were placed in state orphanages and lived in almost unimaginable conditions of loveless squalor (Boland 1990; David 1992).

Similar flagrant human rights abuses have occurred and continue to occur in countries that, in contrast to Romania, have pursued aggressive antinatalist policies. In the 1970s, the government of India established mass sterilization camps;

subjected individuals to fines, imprisonment, and withdrawal of government benefits for failure to meet demographic objectives; and made the salaries of public servants contingent on their recruiting a certain number of sterilization acceptors (Banerji 1980; Chadney 1987; Gwatkin 1979; Ledbetter 1984). At the height of India's sterilization program the state of Maharashtra enacted compulsory sterilization legislation (Maharashtra 1976), and in a six-month period millions of people were sterilized in the country as a whole, many rounded up by police against their will. Although some of the most flagrant violations of human rights have been corrected, many abuses remain, among them widespread harassment and the application of psychological pressure (Larsen 1987; Singh 1990). Sterilization camps still exist where health conditions are substandard; financial incentives are offered to both sterilization recruiters and the persons, mostly women, who agree to be sterilized; and villages have sterilization quotas to be filled (Guha 1990; Kabra and Narayanan 1990; Singh 1990). In addition, because vasectomies were emphasized during the period of greatest coercion, vasectomy rates have since plummeted, with the result that most sterilizations are now performed on women, even though female sterilizations involve more risk and expense than do vasectomies (Basu 1985).

In China, despite official denials, coercion plays an even larger part in the population program (Aird 1990; Banister 1987; Saith 1984; White 1990; Wong 1984). (See Box 2.) Much of this coercion is psychological, with implicit or explicit threats of physical force. Typically, party members, local officials, coworkers, and neighbors bring intense pressure to bear on individuals to enforce the one-child policy, which, although relaxed in the mid-1980s for rural families and minorities, is still in effect in urban areas and in fact has been strengthened (Kristof 1993a; Schmetzer 1993). Such pressure ensures that women use contraceptives, primarily the outmoded steel ring IUD, which they are forbidden to remove; are sterilized; or, if they are pregnant and already have one child, undergo an abortion.

BOX 2

Population Policies in China

Central Policy

"In no case is coercion allowed as a means of implementing family planning policy" (Family Planning Minister Peng Peiyun April 1990, cited in Tyson 1990).

"It is a firm policy of the Chinese government to prohibit coercive action in implementing family planning" (Family Planning Minister Peng Peiyun December 1992, cited in China 1992).

Provincial Policies

"Couples who have serious hereditary diseases including psychosis, mental deficiency, and malformation must not be allowed to bear children. Those who are already pregnant must terminate the pregnancy" (Sichuan Family Planning Regulations, article 14, 1987, cited in Sichuan 1987).

"Fertile couples must use reliable birth control according to the provisions. In case of pregnancies in default of the plan, measures must be taken to terminate them." (Zhejiang Family Planning Ordinance, article 20, 1989, cited in Zhejiang 1990).

"All fertile couples who are conformable to the criteria of child-bearing must adopt birth control measures without exception. Birth control should be practiced by contraception as a principle. Conceptions against family planning caused by the failure of contraceptive measures must be ended" (Jilin Family Planning Regulations, article 18, 1988, cited in Jilin 1991).

In addition, the government withholds various privileges, including medical, educational, and housing benefits, or imposes fines to force compliance with state policy. In a number of cases, forced abortions and sterilizations have occurred; indeed, a number of local laws call for such measures when individuals have failed to adhere to family planning guidelines (Henan 1990; Sichuan 1987; Zhejiang 1990). Local laws also call for the forced sterilization of the mentally retarded (Henan 1990; Kristof 1989). One by-product of the one-child policy is an increase in cases of female infanticide and the abortion of female fetuses. When couples are limited to having one child, many would prefer to have a son (Kristof 1993b; Schmetzer 1993; Wasserstrom 1984). By 1992, the sex ratio of newborn children was 118.5 boys for every 100 girls, leading to estimates that some 1.7 million girls are missing each year (Kristof 1993b).

Technology designed to increase contraceptive options, when used improperly, can also be abused. Oral contraceptives, IUDs, and injectable or implantable contraceptives all have potential adverse side effects; education, counseling, screening, good technical care, and follow-up care must be provided if these methods are to be safely prescribed and used. Unfortunately, in many parts of the developing world, good-quality care is often not available. The experience of Indonesia with Norplant® offers an instructive example. A report issued by the National Family Planning Coordinating Board in 1993 indicated that: only one-half of the doctors and midwives, and few field-workers, involved with Norplant® had received training in its use; the level of knowledge regarding Norplant® among most providers and fieldworkers was low; most acceptors were unaware of possible side effects and many were unaware that Norplant® could be removed before five years; prior to receiving Norplant®, only one-half of acceptors had their medical history taken, and some had no physical examination; adequate information about Norplant® was not available to patients; recommended aseptic conditions were not consistently maintained, with reuse of disposable syringes and use of unsterilized instruments a particular problem; some providers encouraged women to continue using Norplant® despite complaints or fears; not all doctors and midwives considered screening and counseling as mandatory procedures; those who wanted Norplant®

removed before five years had to pay for removal; and a small number of acceptors had their requests for removal refused (Indonesia 1993).

In addition, Norplant® has been administered in part by means of "safaris" — operations in which family planning personnel, accompanied by soldiers, enter a village, gather the populace together, and expound upon the advantages of family planning, often with an implied threat that the village will be punished if family planning methods are not adopted. These safaris have historically played an important part in Indonesia's family planning program, typically resulting in village women's mass acceptance of contraception — often of the one method being promoted at that particular moment by the government (Caplan 1991; Makabenta 1992; Todd 1991; Tweedie 1985). The government has moved to correct many of the deficiencies in its Norplant® program, but we must ask why the program was not properly planned at the start. The characteristics of the contraceptive were well known, and the service recommendations of its developers were unambiguous.

When women are treated as objects of demographic policies, whose fertility is to be manipulated, their rights will be compromised. Indeed, failure to observe human rights, and in particular reproductive rights, has been an important factor in the nonuse of contraceptives and in political resistance to population programs (Banerji 1980; Bose 1989; Wong 1984). Denial of individual choice and refusal to listen to the views of users, combined with the provision of substandard services, have resulted in the alienation of the very populations that governments wish to convince of the need to practice birth control. Once alienated, people are skeptical of further family planning efforts, no matter how humane, and some have actively opposed them.

Proposal for a New Population Policy

In our view, human rights, particularly women's reproductive rights, must be moved from the periphery to the center of concern. Moreover, the language used to describe human rights must be altered to remove ambiguities and generalities that have allowed abuses. A policy incorporating these changes would, above all, explicitly grant full reproductive rights to women —that is, it would acknowledge that each woman has a right to liberty and security of person, including an absolute right to bodily integrity and to decide herself on matters of sexuality and childbearing with no interference from her partner, family, health care professionals, religious groups, the state, or any other actor. *Coercion* would be expressly defined to include forced abortion, sterilization, or contraceptive use; the denial of safe abortion; and more subtle activities, such as the imposition of psychological pressure and incentives that compromise voluntary choice. When, for example, a woman who is desperately poor is offered a significant amount of money or social benefits, or is denied them on the basis of dictated reproductive choices, she who is most in need of help is harmed instead.

To achieve these reproductive rights, the policy would guarantee access to a wide range of family planning choices, including barrier methods, such as diaphragms, condoms, and spermicides; IUDs; hormonal methods, such as the birth control pill; traditional methods; and sterilization. It would also guarantee access to safe and affordable abortion, so that women would not be forced to make the choice between bearing unwanted children and undergoing an illegal and unsafe procedure. Finally, it would ensure the availability of sex education, preventive treatment for subfertility, and treatment for sexually transmitted diseases and reproductive tract infections.

The policy would mandate that family planning programs work from the ground up, focusing primarily on the users. Programs would solicit the opinions of users and respond to their expressed needs and preferences, respecting local cultural and community concerns in the way services are offered. They would ensure that persons receiving services are provided complete care, including family planning education and information, nondirective counseling, continued supervision, and adequate follow-up. In cases where complications occur, they would provide necessary treatment. In particular, they would require that women who wish to be sterilized or agree to participate in the testing of new contraceptive technologies give their informed consent only after being made aware of all possible alternatives and possible harmful effects. Quality of care, rather than demographic targets and numbers of acceptors, would be the central concern.

In addition to reproductive rights, the policy would guarantee broad equal rights for women with respect to other spheres of life, such as education, training, employment, family relations, property rights, political life, land tenure, and inheritance. It would also ensure that women are free from harassment, abuse, genital mutilation, and gender-based violence. Moreover, the policy would emphasize social and economic rights that, although included in major human rights instruments, have often been ignored in deference to civil and political rights. Among these are rights to adequate primary health care, housing, social security, education, and nutrition.

This approach to population policy could have a number of important benefits. First, it would both improve the general welfare of the population and aid in lowering the rate of population growth without the violation of human rights inherent in narrow efforts at fertility control. It would also promote more democratic societies and encourage individual initiative so as to permit individuals, in particular, women to view the fulfillment of their own rights as contributing to the general welfare. Moreover, there is evidence that emphasis on such factors as the status of women and improved education and health are the most important factors in reducing fertility, not the single-minded provision of family planning services (Isaacs 1981; Jain 1985; Jain and Nag 1986).

Implementation

The difficulties in implementing such a new policy would be formidable. The policy would face stiff opposition from the entrenched interests of international donors and governments, such as

China's, that are wedded to the idea of fertility control enforced from above; from international economic institutions that have recently required "structural adjustments;" and from governments uninterested in social investments. Similarly, it could expect strong resistance from powerful nongovernmental groups, such as religious fundamentalists of all persuasions, social conservatives, those espousing patriarchal notions of women and the family, and those holding economic power.

Nonetheless, some strategies might be helpful. One is greater use of the existing international treaties on human rights to advocate a new conception of population policy centered on reproductive and women's rights. Rather than relying on the weak human rights provisions of the 1974 and 1984 population documents, which are not legally binding on governments, supporters of this new conception could draw on relevant provisions of human rights treaties that are legally binding, as reviewed earlier. These treaties could be used as a tool for argument and persuasion in discussions with donor governments and nongovernmental agencies on the content of proposed family planning programs; with national governments on the programs being carried out in their countries or on actual or proposed national legislation; with international agencies on the specifics of population policies and guidelines; and with the media. The treaties could also be used as a means of mobilizing grassroots advocacy by giving such action a clear point of focus and standards that have internationally recognized legitimacy.

Theoretically, treaties also provide the base for legal action, but such action is difficult at the international level because of the lack of adequate enforcement mechanisms and resources. All three treaties provide for monitoring bodies to which countries are required to make reports, and which have the power to make recommendations on how the treaties should be applied and respected. These monitoring bodies should be furnished by nongovernmental organizations with accurate information on human rights abuses, and per-

suaded to make critical statements when they question countries on the reports. They should also be encouraged to make strong statements as to the applicability of the treaties to issues of population and reproductive health. In addition, individual cases of human rights violations may be brought by citizens of any country before the Human Rights Committee, the monitoring body established by countries that are parties to the Covenant on Political and Civil Rights, as well as several regional human rights bodies, such as the European Commission and Court of Human Rights and the Inter-American Commission of Human Rights. More practical, probably, would be efforts at the national level. Here the strategy would be to make countries that have ratified treaties and incorporated treaty guarantees into their domestic laws legally accountable for their actions. Local laws and customs that violate these treaty provisions should be challenged through the court and administrative systems (Cook 1993).

Mechanisms for enforcement of existing treaties should be enhanced. For example, the international monitoring committee established under the Women's Convention has limited powers; it is authorized only to receive the individual countries' mandatory periodic reports on compliance and to issue general recommendations on how to interpret various provisions of the convention. The UN General Assembly should give the committee additional authority and resources to investigate individual complaints and to censure countries that fail to respect their obligations, including that to submit reports (Galey 1984; Meron 1986). The United Nations High Commissioner for Human Rights, mandated by the 1993 Vienna conference, should help widen awareness of human rights violations and monitor enforcement of human rights treaties. In addition, countries that have not ratified the Women's Convention should be persuaded to do so, and countries that have introduced reservations should be persuaded to withdraw them. The nongovernmental sector, too, can make an enormous difference in establishing more effective accountability under the existing treaties. Existing human rights groups need to broaden their horizons (Martin 1993), and those in population and related fields must add human rights to their agendas.

International law, however, provides little more than moral support for concrete action in the effort to achieve widespread change at the local level. In some sense, treaties are only what people are willing to make of them. Thus, the most effective strategy will probably remain the mobilization of forces that can bring pressure to bear on the various actors, both national and international, to modify their behavior. In many countries, such mobilization has started at the local level by women's health activists and other groups within the feminist community, who are the natural constituencies for a human rights–centered population policy (see García-Moreno and Claro in this volume). These groups are reaching out to enlist the aid of health professionals, including family planning program administrators and sympathetic government officials; they are listening to the users of family planning services to ascertain their needs, desires, and problems, so as to empower them to help themselves. At the same time, these groups are establishing links, formal and informal, with other organizations involved in related struggles, including progressive development groups; sympathetic governments, such as those in Scandinavia; and nongovernmental organizations that are in a position to influence donor agencies, the UN, and governments.

A major part of these efforts should be the use of information networks and the media. One important strategy is to broaden the dissemination of information on human rights abuses and on the shortcomings of current population policies. Facts about harmful practices and stories of individual suffering should be supplied to those who, persuaded by alarmist views of the dangers of overpopulation, overlook injustices committed in the name of population control. The arena of public argument should not be ceded to those who see limitation of reproduction *by any means* as the only solution to the problems of countries with high population growth rates.

An excellent example of how to utilize some of these methods on an international level is provided by the work of women's groups at the 1993 Vienna conference. Planning by these groups began several years before the conference, with the creation by the Global Campaign for Women's Human Rights of an alliance of close to 1,000 nongovernmental organizations from around the world. With support from the campaign, local nongovernmental organizations in 123 countries circulated petitions demanding that the conference act to end violence against women. They also held local and regional hearings to document human rights abuses committed against women, forwarded evidence of abuses to the UN Human Rights Commission, and lobbied their governments to support measures to end abuses. At the conference, the campaign was the most articulate and effective lobbying group. As a climax to its efforts, the campaign presented hundreds of thousands of the petitions to the conference and held a tribunal, at which women from around the world testified about the violence committed against them (Moseley 1993; Reifenberg 1993a,b; Riding 1993). Despite major disagreements at the conference over other issues, the campaign got much of what it wanted; the final document of the conference contains a forceful statement that "the human rights of women and of the girl-child are an inalienable, integral and indivisible part of universal rights."

In preparation for the 1994 International Conference on Population and Development, women, and sympathetic men, are mobilizing at national and international levels in similar ways. The Women's Declaration on Population Policies (see Germain, Nowrojee, and Pyne in this volume; see box on page 31) prepared by more than 100 women's groups, is a potentially powerful tool, similar to the petition on violence against women. The women's caucus at the Second Preparatory Committee for the conference had a significant impact on deliberations and on the annotated outline for the new WPPA (see Correa and Petchesky; and García-Moreno and Claro, in this volume).

Even if these efforts succeed, however, hard work will remain. Time and again, countries have undertaken obligations at international conferences, only to ignore them later. Pressure will have to be maintained on donors and international agencies that devise and provide the means to implement many population policies, as well as on governments that impose the policies. They must be reminded continually that human rights are at the heart of population policy, and that the international community will not tolerate policies that violate these rights.

Notes

1 The Teheran conference took place just as rapid population growth was becoming recognized as an international problem of serious dimensions, particularly by the developed countries. In the light of demographic projections, population literature of the time predicted fearful global food shortages and environmental degradation caused by uncontrolled fertility in poor countries. The conference participants noted that the "rapid rate of population growth in some areas of the world hampers the struggle against hunger and poverty...thereby impairing the full realization of human rights" (Freedman and Isaacs 1993).

2 By 1993, 122 countries had ratified the convention, but as of 1990, these ratifications included 113 reservations that seriously undermine the core objective (Cook 1993).

References

Aird, J. S. 1990. *Slaughter of the innocents*. Washington, D.C.: AEI Press.

Banerji, D. 1980. Political economy of population control in India. In L. Bonderstam and S. Bergstrom (eds.), *Poverty and population control*. New York: Academic Press.

Banister, J. 1987. *China's changing population*. Stanford, Calif.: Stanford University Press.

Basu, A. M. 1985. Family planning and the emergency: An unanticipated consequence. *Economic and Political Weekly* 20:422–425.

Berelson, B., and J. Lieberson. 1979. Government efforts to influence fertility: The ethical issues. *Population and Development Review* 5:609.

Boland, R. 1990. Recent developments in abortion law in industrialized countries. *Law, Medicine & Health Care* 18:404–418.

Bose, A. 1989. India's quest for population stabilization: Progress, pitfalls and policy options. *Demography India* 18(1–2):261–273.

Brennan, K. 1988–1989. The influence of cultural relativism on international human rights law: Female circumcision as a case study. *Law and Inequality* 7:367–398.

Brown, L. R., et al. 1984. *State of the world 1984: A World-Watch Institute report on progress toward a sustainable society*. New York: W. W. Norton and Co.

Bunch, C. 1990. Women's rights as human rights: Toward a revision of human rights. *Human Rights Quarterly* 12:486–498.

Callahan, D. 1981. Population policy, universal rights and national sovereignty. In D. Callahan and P. G. Clark (eds.), *Ethical issues of population aid: Culture, economics and international assistance*. New York: Irvington Publishers.

Caplan, A. 1991. The Norplant® safaris: Birth-control implant leads to population control by governments. *Seattle Times*, July 7.

Chadney, J. G. 1987. Family planning: India's Achilles Heel? *Journal of Asian and African Studies* 22:218–231.

China. 1991. *White paper on human rights in China*. Xinhua General Overseas News Service, November 2.

———. 1992. *China's family planning relies on education and services*. Xinhua General Overseas News Service, December 23.

Cobbah, J. A. M. 1987. African values and the human rights debate: An African perspective. *Human Rights Quarterly* 9:309–331.

Cook, R. J. 1993. International human rights and women's reproductive health. *Studies in Family Planning* 24:73–86.

Cook, R. J., and J. M. Haws. 1986. The United Nations convention on the rights of women: Opportunities for family planning providers. *International Family Planning Perspectives* 12:49–53.

David, H. P. 1992. Abortion in Europe, 1920–91: A public health perspective. *Studies in Family Planning* 23:1–22.

Donnelly, J. 1989. *Universal human rights in theory and practice*. Ithaca, N.Y.: Cornell University Press.

Ehrlich, P. R., and A. H. Ehrlich. 1990. *The population explosion*. New York: Simon & Schuster.

Finkle, J. L., and B. B. Crane. 1975. The politics of Bucharest: Population, development, and the new international economic order. *Population and Development Review* 1:87–114.

———. 1985. Ideology and politics at Mexico City: The United States at the 1984 International Conference on Population. *Population and Development Review* 11:1–27.

Freedman, L. P., and S. L. Isaacs. 1993. Human rights and reproductive choice. *Studies in Family Planning* 24:18–30.

Galey, M. E. 1984. International enforcement of women's rights. *Human Rights Quarterly* 6:463–490.

———. 1986. The Nairobi conference: The powerless majority. *PS* 19:255–265.

Guha, A. 1990. Population programs: The national scene. In B. Sengupta, A. Guha, and P. P. Talwar (eds.), *Corporate sector and family welfare problems in India.* Delhi: Council of Indian Employers.

Gwatkin, D. R. 1979. Political will and family planning: The implications of India's emergency experience. *Population and Development Review* 5:29–59.

Henan. 1990. Henan provincial rules and regulations on family planning. *Foreign Broadcast Information Service* FBIS-CHI-90-106, June 1.

Holmes, H. 1983. A feminist analysis of the Universal Declaration of Human Rights. In C. C. Gould (ed.), *Beyond domination: New perspectives on women and philosophy.* Totowa, N.J.: Rowman & Allanheld.

Indonesia: National Family Planning Coordinating Board. 1993. *1992 Indonesia Norplant® use dynamics study: Final report.* Jakarta.

Isaacs, S. L. 1981. *Population law and policy: Source materials and issues.* New York: Human Sciences Press.

Jain, A. K. 1985. The impact of development and population policies on fertility in India. *Studies in Family Planning* 16:181-198.

Jain, A. K., and M. Nag. 1986. Importance of female primary education for fertility reduction in India. *Economic and Political Weekly* 21:1602-1608.

Jilin. 1991. Family Planning Regulations of Jilin. In Y. Hayase and S. Kawamata (eds.), *Population policy and vital statistics in China.* Tokyo: Institute of Developing Economies.

Kabra, S. S., and R. Narayanan. 1990. Sterilization camps in India. *Lancet* 335:224–225.

Kristof, N. D. 1989. Chinese region uses new law to sterilize mentally retarded. *New York Times*, November 21.

———. 1993a. China's crackdown on births: A stunning, and harsh, success. *New York Times*, April 25.

———. 1993b. Peasants in China discover a new way to weed out girls. *The New York Times*, July 21.

Larsen, T. 1987. Of policies and actions. *People* 14(1):22–23.

Law, S. A., and L. F. Rackner. 1987. Gender equality and the Mexico City policy. *New York University Journal of International Law and Politics* 20:193-228.

Ledbetter, R. 1984. Thirty years of family planning in India. *Asian Survey* 24:736–768.

Lee, L. T. 1990. Law, human rights, and population policy. In G. Roberts (ed.), *Population policy: Contemporary issues.* New York: Praeger.

Maharashtra Family (Restriction on Size) Act. 1976. In United Nations, *Annual Review of Population Law.* New York.

Makabenta, L. 1992. Indonesia: Population success story has its shady side. *Inter Press Service*, November 2.

Martin, I. 1993. *The new world order: Opportunity or threat for human rights.* Cambridge, Mass.: Harvard Human Rights Program.

Meron, T. 1986. *Human rights law-making in the United Nations.* Oxford: Clarendon Press.

Moseley, R. 1993. Vision of liberation: Women gain as UN forum attends to their issues. *Chicago Tribune*, June 27.

Murphy, C. F. 1981. Objections to Western conceptions of human rights. *Hofstra Law Review* 9:433–447.

Reanda, L. 1981. Human rights and women's rights: The united approach. *Human Rights Quarterly* 3:11-31.

Reifenberg, A. 1993a. Women appear primed for success at human rights meeting. *Dallas Morning News*, June 14.

———. 1993b. World rights conference urged to end violence against women. *The Dallas Morning News*, June 18.

Renteln, A. D. 1985. The unanswered challenge of relativism and the consequences for human rights. *Human Rights Quarterly* 7:515–540.

Riding, A. 1993. Women seize focus at rights forum. *New York Times*, June 16.

Robertson, A. H., and J. G. Merrills. 1989. *Human rights in the world.* Manchester: Manchester University Press.

Rockefeller, J. D. 1974. *Population growth: The role of the developed world.* Geneva: International Union for Scientific Study of Population.

Saith, A. 1984. China's new population policies. In K. Griffin (ed.), *Institutional reform and economic development in the Chinese countryside.* London: Macmillan.

Schmetzer, U. 1993. In controlling China's population, girls "disappear." *Chicago Tribune*, April 27.

Scott, D. 1993. *Human Rights.* Philadelphia, Pa.: Open University Press.

Shelton, D. 1991–1992. Human rights, environmental rights, and the right to environment. *Stanford Journal of International Law* 28:103–138.

Sichuan. 1987. Family planning regulations. *Joint Publications Research Service* JPRS-CHI-87-044, September 8.

Singh, H. 1990. India's high fertility despite family planning: An appraisal. In G. Roberts (ed.), *Population policy: Contemporary issues*. New York: Praeger.

Todd, D. 1991. Expert sounds alarm on Indonesian birth-control program. *Gazette* (Montreal), November 26.

Trubek, D.M.. 1984. Economic, social and cultural rights in the Third World: Human rights law and human needs programs. In T. Meron (ed.), *Human Rights in International Law*. Oxford: Clarendon Press.

Tweedie, J. 1985. *Women: A world report*. New York: Oxford University Press.

Tyson, A. S. 1990. Chinese charge zealous officials with abuses in enforcing birth plan. *The Christian Science Monitor*, October 31.

United Nations. 1966. *The international covenant on economic, social and cultural rights*. New York.

————. 1968. *Final act of the international conference on human rights*. New York.

————. 1974. *Report of the United Nations world population conference*. New York.

————. 1976. *Report of the world conference of the international women's year*. New York.

————. 1985. *Report of the world conference to review and appraise the achievements of the United Nations decade for women: Equality, development, and peace*. New York.

————. 1993. *Adoption of the final documents and report of the conference*. New York.

United Nations Educational, Scientific, and Cultural Organization (UNESCO). 1977. *Human rights aspects of population programs with special reference to human rights law*. Paris.

Wasserstrom, J. 1984. Resistance to the one-child family. *Modern China* 10:345–374.

White, T. 1990. Post-revolutionary mobilization in China: The one-child policy reconsidered. *World Politics* 43:53–76.

Wong, S. 1984. Consequences of China's new population policy. *China Quarterly* 98:220–240.

World Bank. 1984. *World development report 1984*. Washington, D.C.

Zhejiang. 1990. 1989 Family planning ordinance. *Verfassung und Recht in Üabersee* 23:112–126.

8

Reproductive and Sexual Rights: A Feminist Perspective

Sônia Correa and Rosalind Petchesky

In current debates about the impact of population policies on women, the concept of reproductive and sexual rights is both stronger and more contested than ever before. Those who take issue with this concept include religious fundamentalists, as well as opponents of human rights in general, who associate human rights with individualist traditions deriving from Western capitalism. Some feminists, too, are skeptical about the readiness with which advocates of fertility reduction programs, whose primary concern is neither women's health nor their empowerment, have adopted the language of reproductive rights to serve their own agendas.

As a Southern and a Northern feminist who have written about and organized for women's reproductive health for many years, we are conscious of the tensions and multiple perspectives surrounding this conceptual territory. Our purpose in this chapter is not to impose a concept, but to explore a different way of thinking about it in order to advance the debate. We define the terrain of reproductive and sexual rights in terms of power and resources: power to make informed decisions about one's own fertility, childbearing, child rearing, gynecologic health, and sexual activity; and resources to carry out such decisions safely and effectively. This terrain necessarily involves some core notion of "bodily integrity,"

or "control over one's body." However, it also involves one's relationships to one's children, sexual partners, family members, community, caregivers, and society at large; in other words, the body exists in a socially mediated universe.

Following a review of the epistemological and historical underpinnings of this concept, we address several fundamental problems that critics have raised about rights discourse: its indeterminate language, its individualist bias, its presumption of universality, and its dichotomization of "public" and "private" spheres. We argue that rather than abandoning rights discourse, we should reconstruct it so that it both specifies gender, class, cultural, and other differences and recognizes social needs. Our principal point is that sexual and reproductive (or any other) rights, understood as private "liberties" or "choices," are meaningless, especially for the poorest and most disenfranchised, without *enabling conditions* through which they can be realized. These conditions constitute *social rights* and involve social welfare, personal security, and political freedom. Their provision is essential to the democratic transformation of societies to abolish gender, class, racial, and ethnic injustice.

We then analyze the ethical bases of reproductive and sexual rights, and propose four component principles: bodily integrity, personhood, equality, and respect for diversity. In examining each of these principles, we emphasize the broader social implications that ethicists, legal scholars, and demographers often ignore. All four principles, as we interpret them, both derive from and further society's interest in empowered and politically responsible citizens, including all women. By thus linking reproductive and sexual rights to development, we challenge legalistic notions of civil and political rights that still dominate the human rights field.

Throughout this discussion, we raise a number of policy-related issues. When are reproductive and sexual decisions freely made and when coerced? What is the relationship between women's reproductive and sexual rights and responsibilities and men's, and should women's social and biological positioning in reproduction give us a privileged voice in the construction of rights? Is there a "right to procreate" or a "socially responsible" way to make procreative decisions? What conditions predicate "socially responsible" decisionmaking? What are the obligations of state governments and international organizations to provide the necessary conditions for "free and responsible choices"?

We are suggesting not that reproductive and sexual rights are absolute or that women have the right to reproduce under any circumstances, but that policies to enforce those rights must address existing social conditions and begin to change them. We conclude by proposing a feminist social rights approach to population and development policies.

Epistemological and Historical Premises

Contrary to many social critics, we are not convinced that reproductive and sexual rights (or human rights) are simply a "Western" concept. As Kamla Bhasin and Nighat Khan (1986) have argued with regard to feminism in South Asia, "an idea cannot be confined within national or geographic boundaries." Postcolonial writers and Southern governments have readily adopted, and adapted, the theories of Marx, Malthus, or Milton Friedman to suit their own purposes. Democracy

movements in postcolonial societies easily invoke rights when it comes to voting, or forming political parties or trade unions. Why should concepts like "reproductive rights," "bodily integrity," and women's right to sexual self-determination be any less adaptable?

Second, we assume that ethical norms and language itself are always subject to historical variation and political contestation. Feminist engagement in the debate over the meanings of rights, including reproductive and sexual rights, is a necessary part of our efforts to transform women's situation as citizens, nationally and internationally. Changing the rhetoric of legal instruments or official policies can be one strategic step toward transforming the conditions of people's lives.

The term "reproductive rights" is of recent — and probably North American[1] — origin, but its roots in ideas of bodily integrity and sexual self-determination have a much older and culturally broader genealogy. The idea that women in particular must be able "to decide whether, when, and how to have children" originated in the feminist birth control movements that developed at least as early as the 1830s among the Owenite socialists in England and spread to many parts of the world over the course of a century (Chesler 1992; Gordon 1976; Huston 1992; Jayawardena 1993; Ramusack 1989; Weeks 1981). Leaders of these movements in Western countries, like Margaret Sanger in North America and Stella Browne in England, linked "the problem of birth control" not only with women's struggle for social and political emancipation, but also with their need to "own and control" their bodies and to obtain sexual knowledge and satisfaction (Sanger 1920). Their counterparts among women's rights advocates in 19th-century Europe and America and among the early birth control pioneers in 20th-century Asia, North Africa, and Latin America were more reticent about women's sexuality, emphasizing instead a negative right: that of women (married or single) to refuse unwanted sex or childbearing.

Underlying both the defensive and the affirmative versions of these early feminist prototypes of reproductive rights language were the same basic principles of *equality, personhood,* and *bodily integrity.* They held a common premise: in order for women to achieve equal status with men in society, they must be respected as full moral agents with projects and ends of their own; hence they alone must determine the uses — sexual, reproductive, or other — to which their bodies (and minds) are put.[2]

In the late 1970s and early 1980s, women's health movements emerged throughout Asia, Latin America, Europe and North America (DAWN 1993; García-Moreno and Claro in this volume). These movements aimed at achieving the ability of women, *both* as individuals *and* in their collective organizational forms and community identities, to determine their own reproductive and sexual lives in conditions of optimum health and economic and social well-being. They did not imagine women as atoms completely separate from larger social contexts; rather, they consciously linked the principle of "women's right to decide" about fertility and childbearing to "the social, economic and political conditions that make such decisions possible" (Women's Global Network for Reproductive Rights 1991).

Increasingly, as women of color in Northern societies and women from Southern countries have taken leadership in developing the meanings of sexual and reproductive rights for women, these meanings have expanded. They have come to encompass both a broader range of issues than fertility regulation (including, for example, maternal and infant mortality, infertility, unwanted sterilization, malnutrition of girls and women, female genital mutilation, sexual violence, and sexually transmitted diseases); and a better understanding of the structural conditions that constrain reproductive and sexual decisions (such as reductions in social sector expenditures resulting from structural adjustment programs; lack of transportation, water, sanitation, and child care; illiteracy; and poverty). In other words, the concept of sexual and reproductive *rights* is being enlarged to address the *social needs* that erode reproductive and sexual choice for the majority of the world's

women, who are poor (Desai in this volume; Petchesky and Weiner 1990).

In the past decade, the integral tie between reproductive rights and women's sexual self-determination, including the right to sexual pleasure, has gained recognition not only in the North, but in Latin America, Africa and Asia.[3] As the Women's Resource and Research Center (WRRC) in the Philippines states in its Institutional Framework and Strategies on Reproductive Rights (Fabros 1991), "self-determination and pleasure in sexuality is one of the primary meanings of the idea of 'control over one's body' and a principal reason for access to safe abortion and birth control." Anchoring the possibility of women's *individual* right to health, well-being, and "self-determined sexual lives" to the *social* changes necessary to eliminate poverty and empower women, this framework dissolves the boundary between sexuality, human rights, and development. It thus opens a wider lens not only on reproductive and sexual rights, but on rights in general.

Rights Discourse: Rethinking Rights as Individual and Social

The discourse of (human) rights has come under heavy assault in recent years, from, among others, feminist, Marxist, and postmodernist sources (Olsen 1984; Tushnet 1984; Unger 1983). Critics point out, first, that the value and meaning of rights are always contingent upon the political and social context; even the most traditional, authoritarian, patriarchal regimes will have some notion of correlative rights and duties that may be turned to the advantage of the state or corporate powers and made to perpetuate the burdens of citizens or the powerless. Second, rights language is indeterminate; if women demand their sexual and reproductive rights, male partners can demand theirs, fetuses (or fetal advocates) can demand theirs, clinicians and pharmaceutical companies theirs, and so forth. Finally there is the problem of abstract individualism and universality typically ascribed to rights language. In the classical liberal model of supposedly equal individuals choosing and bargaining to get satisfaction of their rights, differences of economic condition, race, gender, or other social circumstance that structure real people's lack of choice are rendered invisible (Rosenfeld 1992).

While these criticisms are theoretically compelling, they offer no alternative discourse for social movements to make collective political claims. Whatever its theoretical weaknesses, the polemical power of rights language as an expression of aspirations for justice across widely different cultures and political-economic conditions cannot easily be dismissed (Heller 1992). In practice, then, the language of rights remains indispensable but needs radical redefinition.

Feminist theorists and activists have figured prominently in efforts to shed the abstract universality, formalism, individualism and antagonism encumbering rights language (Bunch 1990; Crenshaw 1991; Friedman 1992; Nedelsky 1989; Petchesky 1994; Schneider 1991; Williams 1991). Allying themselves with worldwide struggles for democratization among indigenous peoples, ethnic minorities, sexual minorities, immigrant groups, and oppressed majorities — all of whom invoke the language of "human rights" — they seek to recast rights discourse in a more inclusive "referential universe" (Williams 1991). The purpose is to transform the classical liberal rights model in order: (1) to emphasize the *social*, not just individual, nature of rights, thus shifting the major burden of correlative duties from individuals to public agencies; (2) to acknowledge the *communal* (relational) *contexts* in which individuals act to exercise or pursue their rights; (3) to foreground the *substantive* basis of rights in human needs and a redistribution of resources; and (4) to recognize the bearers of rights in their self-defined, multiple identities, including their gender, class, sexual orientation, race, and ethnicity.

Classical liberal rights discourse has traditionally assumed a sharp division between "public" and "private" spheres and a tendency of individuals to act only with reference to narrow self-interests rather than any concept of public good. According to this dualistic vision of society, rights exist in a "private" domain where "individuals" ought to be pretty much left alone by the state to maximize their self-interests according to market demands. Feminist political theorists have amply criticized this presumed public-private division, pointing out that both domains in most societies tend to be dominated by men and that male dominance in one sphere reinforces it in the other (Eisenstein 1983; Elshtain 1981; Kelly 1984; Okin 1979). Thus the construction of a legal and normative boundary between "public" and "private" insulates the daily, routine practices of gender subordination — in the home, the workplace, the streets, and religious institutions. It masks the ways in which women's labor and services as caretakers and reproducers provide the material and emotional basis for "publics" to survive:

> For many girls and women, the most severe violations of their human rights are rooted deeply within the family system, bolstered by community norms of male privilege and frequently justified by religious doctrines or appeals to custom or tradition. These hidden injuries of gender are rarely addressed in public policies and international assemblies because they threaten collective beliefs in the "sanctity, harmony, and stability" of the family unit. (Dixon-Mueller 1993)

Feminist writings and actions in defense of women's human rights build on these critiques to challenge the customary reluctance of states and international agencies to intervene in traditionally defined "family matters." Through vigorous international campaigns leading up to and beyond the United Nations Human Rights Conference in Vienna in 1993, they have called for national and international sanctions against gender-based violations of human rights, and they have shown how such violations occur most frequently in the supposedly private realms of family, reproduction, and sexuality (for example, through endemic violence against women). Inaction by public authorities in response to such violations — whether at the hand of state officials, nongovernmental organizations (NGOs), or spouses — constitutes, they argue, a form of acquiescence (Bunch 1990; Cook 1993b; Copelon 1994; Freedman and Isaacs 1993; Heise 1992).

By prying open the "citadel of privacy," feminist legal and political theory offers a wedge with which to challenge the claims of "tradition" and "local culture" used to defeat domestic application of international human rights norms (see Boland, Rao and Zeidenstein, in this volume). Feminist deconstructions of the public-private division also point to a model of reproductive and sexual behavior that is socially contextualized, contrasting sharply with the assumption of the classical liberal model and of many family planners and demographers (echoing Malthus) that women's reproductive decisions reflect only narrow self-interest. Supported by sociological and anthropological data, they show, on the contrary, that such decisions are usually made under enormous pressures from family, community, and society to comply with prevailing gender and reproductive norms, as well as internalized commitments to act responsibly toward others.

A social model of human behavior does not assume that individuals make decisions in a vacuum or that "choices" are equally "free" for everyone. Group identities that are complex and "intersectional" (across gender, class, ethnicity, religion, age, nationality) pull women's decisions in multiple directions. Moreover, because of existing social inequalities, the resources and range of options women have at their disposal differ greatly, affecting their ability to exercise their rights (Crenshaw 1991; Eisenstein 1994; Williams 1991).

How does this interactive, socially embedded model of personal decisionmaking apply to the realm of sexual and reproductive rights? Qualitative data across a variety of cultural and historical settings suggest that the extent to which reproductive and sexual decisions are "freely" made eludes easy classification; but "free" or "voluntary," whatever its meaning, is not the same as isolated or individualistic. In each concrete case

we must weigh the multiple social, economic, and cultural factors that come to bear on a woman's decision and constitute its local meaning. Women's decisions about whether or not to bring a pregnancy to term are most frequently made in consultation with, under the constraint of, and sometimes in resistance against networks of significant others — mothers, mothers-in-law, sisters, other kin, neighbors; sometimes husbands or male partners, sometimes not (Adams and Castle in this volume; Ezeh 1993; Gilligan 1982; Jeffery, Jeffery, and Lyon 1989; Khattab 1992; Petchesky 1990). While some communities or female kin networks may function as sites of support for women's reproductive freedom — for example, facilitating clandestine abortion or contraception, or refusal of unwanted sex — others may present direct barriers or antagonisms. Jealous or violent husbands or vigilant in-laws may prevent women from visiting clinics, using condoms, getting abortions, or attending workshops on women's health, thus not only constricting their "choices" but increasing their risks of unwanted pregnancy, maternal mortality, sexually transmitted diseases (STDs), and AIDS (Heise 1992; Protacio 1990; Ramasubban 1990). Indeed, right-wing religious movements to restore "family values" and "community traditions" may harbor some men's distrust of the communities women make and their aim to refortify the conjugal dyad, where women are isolated from natal and friendship bonds.

Here we confront the nagging problem, always a dilemma for feminist advocates, of how to critique the kinds and range of choices available to women without denigrating the decisions women do make for themselves, even under severe social and economic constraints.[4] The debate concerning sterilization prevalence rates in Brazil provides a striking illustration. In a context of rapid fertility decline, female sterilization has become a "preferred" method in Brazil, used by 44 percent of current contraceptors. In some regions, the sterilization rate reaches more than 64 percent, as in the case of the Northeast, and the average age of sterilization has rapidly declined since the early

1980s (15 percent of sterilized women in the Northeast are under 25 years of age). A complex mix of factors explains this trend: concerns about the side effects or effectiveness of reversible contraception, failure of the public health system to provide adequate information about and access to other methods, severe economic conditions, women's employment patterns, and cultural and religious norms making sterilization less "sinful" than abortion (Correa 1993; Lopez 1993; Petchesky 1979).

In their analysis of the sterilization trends, Brazilian feminists are caught between the urgent need to denounce the inequities in sterilization rates — particularly among black women — and the evidence of research findings that many women have consciously chosen and paid for the procedure and are satisfied with their decision. On the one hand, this is a clear example of the "constrained choices" that result from circumstances of gender, poverty, and racism; the very notion that women in such conditions are exercising their "reproductive rights" strains the meaning of the term (Lopez 1993). On the other hand, the call for criminal sanctions against sterilization by some groups in Brazil seems a denial of women's moral agency in their search for reproductive self-determination.

We need to develop analytical frameworks that respect the integrity of women's reproductive and sexual decisions, however constrained, while also condemning social, economic, and cultural conditions that may force women to "choose" one course over another. Such conditions prevail in a range of situations, curtailing reproductive choices and creating dilemmas for women's health activists. Women desperate for employment may knowingly expose themselves to reproductively hazardous chemicals or other toxins in the workplace. Women hedged in by economic dependence and the cultural preference for sons may "choose" abortion as a means of sex selection. Where female genital mutilation is a traditional practice, women must "choose" for their young daughters between severe health risk and sexual loss on the one hand, and unmarriageable pariah status on the other.

For reproductive decisions to be in any real sense "free," rather than compelled by circumstance or desperation, requires the presence of certain *enabling conditions*. These conditions constitute the foundation of reproductive and sexual rights and are what feminists mean when they speak of women's "empowerment." They include material and infrastructural factors, such as reliable transportation, child care, financial subsidies, or income supports, as well as comprehensive health services that are accessible, humane, and well staffed. The absence of adequate transportation alone can be a significant contributor to higher maternal mortality and failure to use contraceptives (see Asian and Pacific Women's Resource Collection Network 1990; and McCarthy and Maine 1992). They also include cultural and political factors, such as access to education, earnings, self-esteem, and the channels of decisionmaking. Where women have no education, training, or status outside that which comes from bearing sons, childbearing may remain their best option (Morsy 1994; Pearce 1994; Ravindran 1993).

Such enabling conditions, or social rights, are integral to reproductive and sexual rights and directly entail the responsibility of states and mediating institutions (for example, population and development agencies) for their implementation. Rights involve not only *personal liberties* (domains where governments should leave people alone), but also *social entitlements* (domains where affirmative public action is required to ensure that rights are attainable by everyone). They thus necessarily imply public responsibilities and a renewed emphasis on the linkages between personal well-being and social good, including the good of public support for gender equality in all domains of life.

This is not meant to suggest a mystical "harmony of interests" between individual women and public authorities, nor to deny that conflicts between "private" and "public" interests will continue to exist. In societies governed by competitive market values, for example, middle-class couples and entrepreneurs may raise serious ethical questions by exploiting reproductive technologies to produce the "right sex" or the "perfect child." Meanwhile, under repressive or dictatorial regimes, the reproductive desires of individuals may be sacrificed altogether to an ethics of public expediency: witness the harsh antinatalist campaign in China. These realities prompt us to rethink the relationship between the state and civil society, and to map out an ethical framework for reproductive and sexual rights in the space where the social and the individual intersect.

The Ethical Content of Reproductive and Sexual Rights

We propose that the grounds of reproductive and sexual rights for women consist of four ethical principles: *bodily integrity, personhood, equality,* and *diversity.* Each of these principles can be violated through acts of invasion or abuse — by government officials, clinicians and other providers, male partners, family members, and so on — or through acts of omission, neglect, or discrimination by public (national or international) authorities. Each also raises dilemmas and contradictions that can be resolved only under radically different social arrangements from those now prevailing in most of the world.

Bodily Integrity

Perhaps more than the other three principles, the principle of bodily integrity, or the right to security in and control over one's body, lies at the core of reproductive and sexual freedom. As suggested in our introduction, this principle is embedded in the historical development of ideas of the self and citizenship in Western political culture. Yet it also transcends any one culture or region, insofar as some version of it informs all opposition to slavery and other involuntary servitude, torture, rape, and every form of illegitimate assault and violence. As the Declaration of the International Women's Year Conference in Mexico City put it in 1975, "the human body, whether that of women or men, is inviolable and respect for it is a fundamental element of human dignity and freedom" (quoted in Freedman and Isaacs 1993).

To affirm the right of women to "control over" or "ownership of" their bodies does not mean that women's bodies are mere things, separate from themselves or isolated from social networks and communities. Rather, it connotes the body as an integral part of one's self, whose health and wellness (including sexual pleasure) are a necessary basis for active participation in social life. Bodily integrity, then, is not just an individual but a social right, since without it women cannot function as responsible community members (Freedman and Isaacs 1993; Petchesky 1990, 1994). Yet in its specific applications, the bodily integrity principle reminds us that while reproductive and sexual rights are necessarily social, they are also irreducibly *personal.* While they can never be realized without attention to economic development, political empowerment, and cultural diversity, ultimately their site is individual women's bodies (DAWN 1993; Petchesky 1990).

Bodily integrity includes both "a woman's right *not to be alienated from her sexual and reproductive capacity* (e.g., through coerced sex or marriage,...[genital mutilation], denial of access to birth control, sterilization without informed consent, prohibitions on homosexuality) and...her right to the *integrity of her physical person* (e.g., freedom from sexual violence, from false imprisonment in the home, from unsafe contraceptive methods, from unwanted pregnancies or coerced childbearing, from unwanted medical interventions)" (Dixon-Mueller 1993). Such negative abuses occur at multiple levels or sites, including not only relations with sexual partners and kin, clinicians and other providers, but also state or military campaigns (for example, coercive fertility reduction programs or the rape of women as a tool of "ethnic cleansing").

But bodily integrity also implies *affirmative* rights to enjoy the full potential of one's body — for health, procreation, and sexuality. Each of these raises a host of complex questions we can only touch upon here. In regard to health, the very term "integrity" connotes *wholeness* — treating the body and its present needs as a unity, not as piecemeal mechanical functions or fragments.

Dr. Rani Bang in India found that in one district in Maharashtra State, 92 percent of the women who used local family planning clinics suffered from untreated gynecologic infections or diseases (Bang 1989, cited in Bruce 1990). How can this happen if clinicians are treating women's bodies and reproductive health as a whole? Similarly, family planning programs that emphasize so-called medically efficacious methods of contraception at the cost or even to the exclusion of barrier methods fail to offer women protection against STD and Human Immunodeficiency Virus (HIV) infection, thus exposing them to morbidity, infertility, or death.

The question of whether there is a "fundamental right to procreate" based in one's biological reproductive capacity is clearly more complicated than whether one has a right, as a matter of bodily integrity, to prevent or terminate a pregnancy. Yet we can recognize that childbearing has consequences for others besides an individual woman, man, or lineage without subscribing to the claim that women have a duty to society (or the planet!) to abstain from reproducing. Such a duty could begin to exist only when all women are provided sufficient resources for their well-being, viable work alternatives, and a cultural climate of affirmation outside of childbearing so that they no longer depend on children for survival and dignity (Berer 1990; Freedman and Isaacs 1993). And even then, antinatalist policies that depend on coercion or discriminate against or target particular groups would be unacceptable.

Our hesitancy about a "right to procreate" is not based on any simple correlation between population growth, environmental degradation, and women's fertility, persuasively refuted elsewhere in this volume. Rather, it comes from apprehensions about how patriarchal kinship systems throughout history have used such claims to confine and subordinate women, who alone have bodies that can be impregnated. Procreative rights are, however, an important part of reproductive and sexual rights. They include the right to participate in the basic human practice of raising and nurturing children; the right to bring wanted

pregnancies to term in conditions of safety, decency, and good health, and to raise one's children in such conditions; and the right of gay and lesbian families to bear, foster, or adopt children in the same dignity as other families. They also include a transformation in the prevailing gender division of labor so that men are assigned as much responsibility for children's care as women.

Finally, what shall we say of the body's capacity for sexual pleasure and the right to express it in diverse and nonstigmatized ways? If the bodily integrity principle implies such a right, as we believe, its expression surely becomes more complicated and fraught with dangers for women and men in the context of rising prevalence of HIV and STD infection (Berer 1993a; DAWN 1993). In addition to these immediate dangers — compounded by the now well-documented fact that many STDs increase women's susceptibility to HIV — there is the "vicious cycle" in which "women suffering the consequences of sexually transmitted disease find themselves in a social circumstance that further increases their risk of exposure to sexually transmitted infections and their complications" (Elias 1991). This cycle currently affects Sub-Saharan African women most drastically, but is rapidly becoming a worldwide phenomenon. It includes women's lack of sexual self-determination; the high risk they incur of infertility and ectopic pregnancy from STD infection; their dependence on men and in-laws for survival; the threat of ostracism or rejection by the family or male partner following infection or infertility; then the threat of unemployment, impoverishment, and prostitution, followed by still greater exposure to STD and HIV infection (Elias 1991; Wasserheit 1993).

The global crisis of HIV and AIDS complicates but does not diminish the right of all people to responsible sexual pleasure in a supportive social and cultural environment. For women and men of diverse sexual orientations to be able to express their sexuality without fear or risk of exclusion, illness, or death requires sex education and male and female resocialization on a hitherto unprecedented scale. This is why bodily integrity has a necessary social rights dimension that, now more than ever, is a matter of life and death.

Personhood

Listening to women is the key to honoring their moral and legal personhood — that is, their right to self-determination. This means treating them as principal actors and decision makers in matters of reproduction and sexuality — as subjects, not merely objects, and as ends, not only means, of population and family planning policies. As should be clear from our earlier discussion emphasizing a relational-interactive model of women's reproductive decisions, our concept of decisionmaking autonomy implies respect for how women make decisions, the values they bring to bear, and the networks of others they choose to consult; it does not imply a notion of solitude or isolation in "individual choices." Nor does it preclude full counseling about risks and options regarding contraception, prenatal care, childbearing, STDs and HIV, and other aspects of gynecologic health.

At the clinical level, for providers to respect women's personhood requires that they trust and take seriously women's desires and experiences, for example, concerning contraceptive side effects. When clinicians trivialize women's complaints about such symptoms as headaches, weight gain, or menstrual irregularity, they violate this principle. Qualitative studies of clinical practices regarding the use of Norplant® in the Dominican Republic, Egypt, Indonesia, and Thailand found that women's concerns about irregular bleeding were often dismissed, and their requests for removal of the implant not honored (Zimmerman et al. 1990).

Respect for personhood also requires that clients be offered a complete range of safe options, fully explained, without major discrepancies in cost or government subsidization. When some contraceptive methods are *de facto* singled out for promotion (for instance, long-acting implants or sterilization), or clinical practices manifest strong pronatalist or antinatalist biases (as in programs governed by demographic targets), or safe legal

abortion is denied, respect for women's personhood is systematically abused. "Quality of care" guidelines, which originated in women's health activism and were codified by Judith Bruce, reflect not only good medical practice but an ethic of respect for personhood (Bruce 1990; DAWN 1993; Jain, Bruce and Mensch 1992; Mintzes 1992).

At the level of national and international policies and programs, treating women as persons in sexual and reproductive decisionmaking means assuring that women's organizations are represented and heard in the processes where population and health policies are made and that effective mechanisms of public accountability, in which women participate, are established to guard against abuses. It also means abandoning demographic targets in the service of economic growth, cost containment, or ethnic or nationalist rivalries and replacing them with reproductive health and women's empowerment goals (see Jain and Bruce in this volume). Demographic targeting policies that encourage the use of material incentives or disincentives often work to manipulate or coerce women, particularly those who are poor, into accepting fertility control methods they might otherwise reject, thus violating their decisionmaking autonomy.

The question of "incentives" is clearly a complicated one, since in some circumstances they may expand women's options and freedom (Dixon-Mueller 1993). Feminists and human rights activists have justly criticized programs that promote particular fertility control methods or antinatalist campaigns through monetary inducements or clothing to "acceptors," fines or denials of child care or health benefits to "offenders," or quotas reinforced with "bonuses" for village officials or clinic personnel (Freedman and Isaacs 1993, Ravindran 1993). What would be our reaction, however, to a system of women-managed comprehensive care clinics that provided child care or free transportation to facilitate clinic visits? A distinct difference exists between these two cases, since the former deploys the targeting and promotional strategies that undermine women's personhood, whereas the latter incorporates the kinds of enabling conditions we earlier found necessary for equalizing women's ability to exercise their reproductive rights. To distinguish *supportive* or *empowering* conditions from *coercive* incentives or disincentives, we need to assure that they respect all four ethical principles of reproductive rights (bodily integrity, personhood, equality, and diversity). When poor or incarcerated women are expected to purchase other rights "for the price of their womb" (for example, a job for sterilization or release from prison for Norplant®), "incentives" become corrupted into bribes (Williams 1991). Women's social location determines whether they are able to make sexual and reproductive decisions with dignity.

Equality

The principle of equality applies to sexual and reproductive rights in two main areas: relations between men and women (gender divisions), and relations among women (conditions such as class, age, nationality, or ethnicity that divide women as a group). With respect to the former, the impetus behind the idea of reproductive rights as it emerged historically was to remedy the social bias against women inherent in their lack of control over their fertility and their assignment to primarily reproductive roles in the gender division of labor. "Reproductive rights" (or "birth control") was one strategy within a much larger agenda for making women's position in society equal to men's. At the same time, this notion contains the seeds of a contradiction, since women alone are the ones who get pregnant, and in that sense, their situation — and degree of risk — can never be reducible to men's.

This tension, which feminists have conceptualized in the debate over equality versus "difference," becomes problematic in the gender-neutral language of most United Nations documents pertaining to reproductive rights and health. For example, article 16(e) of the Convention on the Elimination of All Forms of Discrimination against Women (CEDAW) gives men and women "*the same rights* to decide freely and responsibly on

the number and spacing of their children and to have access to the information, education and means to enable them to exercise these rights [emphasis added]." Might this article be used to mandate husbands' consent to abortion or contraception? Why should men and women have "the same" rights with regard to reproduction when, as not only child-bearers but those who in most societies have responsibility for children's care, women have so much greater stake in the matter — when, indeed, growing numbers of women raise children without benefit of male partners? (The language of "couples" in family planning literature raises the same kinds of questions.)

If we take the issue of contraception as an illustration, the principle of equality would seem to require that, where contraceptive methods carry risks or provide benefits, those risks and benefits must be distributed on a fair basis between women and men, as well as among women. This would suggest a population policy that puts greater emphasis on encouraging male responsibility for fertility control and scientific research into effective "male" contraceptives. In fact, many women express a sense of unfairness that they are expected to bear nearly all the medical risks and social responsibility for avoiding unwanted pregnancies (Pies n.d.). But such a policy might also conflict with the basic right of women to control their own fertility and the need many women feel to preserve that control, sometimes in conditions of secrecy and without "equal sharing" of risks.

On the surface, this dilemma seems to be a contradiction within feminist goals, between the opposing principles of equality and personhood. The feminist agenda that privileges women's control in reproductive rights would seem to reinforce a gender division of labor that confines women to the domain of reproduction. Yet exploring the problem more deeply reveals that women's distrust of men's taking responsibility for fertility control and reluctance to relinquish methods women control are rooted in other kinds of gendered power imbalances that work against a "gender equality" approach to reproductive health policies. These include social systems that provide no educational or economic incentives toward men's involvement in child care and cultural norms that stigmatize women's sexuality outside the bounds of heterosexual monogamy. Thus, while a reproductive health policy that encourages the development and use of "male methods" of contraception may increase the total range of "choices," in the long run it will not help to realize women's social rights nor gender equality until these larger issues are also addressed.

Applying the equality principle in the implementation of sexual and reproductive rights also requires attention to potential inequalities *among* women. This means, at the least, that risks and benefits must be distributed on a fair basis and that providers and policy makers must respect women's decision-making authority without regard to differences of class, race, ethnic origin, age, marital status, sexual orientation, nationality, or region (North-South). Returning to our example of contraception, there is certainly ample evidence that access to safe methods of fertility control can play a major role in improving women's health, but some contraceptive methods can have negative consequences for some women's health (National Research Council 1989). Issues of equal treatment may arise when certain methods — particularly those that carry medical risks or whose long-term effects are not well known — are tested, targeted, or promoted primarily among poor women in Southern or Northern countries. Indeed, when clinical trials are conducted among poor urban women, who tend to move frequently or lack transportation, the necessary conditions for adequate medical follow-up may not exist, and thus the trials themselves may be in violation of the equality principle. Meanwhile, issues of discrimination arise when safe, beneficial methods such as condoms or diaphragms, low-dose hormonal pills, or hygienic abortion facilities are available only to women with the financial resources to pay for them.

For governments and international organizations to promote sexual and reproductive rights in ways that respect equality among women requires addressing at least the most blatant differences in power and resources that divide women within countries and internationally. In the case of safe, effective methods of contraception, laws that guarantee the "freedom" of all women to use whatever methods they "choose" are gratuitous without geographic access, high-quality services and supplies, and financing for all women who need them. We are saying that the economic and political changes necessary to create such conditions are a matter not just of development, but of (social) *rights;* indeed, they are a good example of why development *is* a human right and why women's reproductive rights are inseparable from this equation (Sen 1992).

Diversity

While the equality principle requires the mitigation of inequities among women in their access to services or their treatment by health providers and policy makers, the diversity principle requires respect for differences among women — in values, culture, religion, sexual orientation, family or medical condition, and so on. The universalizing language of international human rights instruments, reflecting a Western liberal tradition, needs to be reshaped to encompass such differences (see Freedman and Isaacs 1993; Cook 1993 a, b). While defending the universal applicability of sexual and reproductive rights, we must also acknowledge that such rights often have different meanings, or different points of priority, in different social and cultural contexts.

Differences in cultural or religious values, for example, affect attitudes toward children and childbearing, influencing how diverse groups of women think about their entitlements in reproduction. In her study of market women in Ile-Ife, Nigeria, anthropologist Tola Olu Pearce (1994) found that the high value placed on women's fertility and the subordination of individual desires to group welfare in Yoruba tradition made the notion of a woman's individual right to choose alien. Yet Yoruba women in Ile-Ife have also used methods of fertility control to space their children and "avoid embarrassment" for untold generations and no doubt consider it part of their collective "right" as women to do so. A similar communal ethic governing women's reproductive decisions emerges in a study of Latina single mothers in East Harlem (New York City), who consider their "reproductive rights" to include the right to receive public assistance in order to stay home and care for their children (Benmayor, Torruellas, and Juarbe 1992).

Local religious and cultural values may also shape women's attitudes toward medical technologies or their effects, such as irregular menstrual bleeding. Clinic personnel involved in disseminating Norplant® have not always understood the meanings menstrual blood may have in local cultures and the extent to which frequent bleeding — a common side effect of Norplant® — may result in the exclusion of women from sex, rituals, or community life (Zimmerman et al. 1990). Imposing standards of what is "normal" or "routine" bleeding (for example, to justify refusal to remove the implant upon request) could constitute a violation of the diversity principle, as well as the bodily integrity and personhood principles.[5]

It is important to distinguish between the feminist principle of respect for difference and the tendency of male-dominated governments and fundamentalist religious groups of all kinds to use "diversity" and "autonomy of local cultures" as reasons to deny the universal validity of women's human rights.[6] In all the cases cited above, women's assertion of their particular needs and values, rather than denying the universal application of rights, clarifies what those rights mean in specific settings. Women's multiple identities — whether as members of cultural, ethnic, and kinship groups, or as people with particular religious and sexual orientations, and so forth — challenge human rights discourse to develop a language and methodology that are pluralistic yet faithful to the core principles of equality, personhood, and bodily integrity. This means that the diversity principle is never absolute, but always conditioned upon a conception of human rights that promotes women's development and respects their self-determination. Traditional patriarchal practices

that subordinate women — however local or time-worn, or enacted by women themselves (for example, genital mutilation) — can never supersede the social responsibility of governments and intergovernmental organizations to enforce women's equality, personhood, and bodily integrity, through means that respect the needs and desires of the women most directly involved.

Bringing a Feminist Social Rights Approach to Population and Development Policies

The above analysis has attempted to show that the individual (liberty) and the social (justice) dimensions of rights can never be separated, as long as resources and power remain unequally distributed in most societies. Thus the affirmative obligations of states and international organizations become paramount, since the ability of individuals to exercise reproductive and sexual rights depends on a range of conditions not yet available to many people and impossible to access without public support. In this respect, the language of "entitlement" seems to us overly narrow, insofar as it implies claims made by individuals on the state without expressing the idea of a mutual *public* interest in developing empowered, educated, and politically responsible citizens, including all women. Likewise, the language of "choosing freely and responsibly" still contained in most international instruments that address family planning and reproductive rights is at best ambiguous and at worst evasive (see Boland, Rao, and Zeidenstein in this volume). What does it mean to choose "responsibly"? Who, in fact, is responsible, and what are the necessary conditions — social, economic, cultural — for individuals to act in socially responsible ways? The correlative duties associated with sexual and reproductive rights belong not only to the bearers of those rights, but to the governmental and intergovernmental agencies charged with their enforcement.

Health policies and programs that treat reproduction and women holistically, across the life cycle and through means appropriate to women's social situations, require comprehensive services with well-trained staff and adequate facilities for all women. If women are to be empowered to speak out in clinical settings and to make claims about their sexual and reproductive health needs — particularly where the quality of care is inadequate — they must have "a culture of health awareness," which may in turn rest on their having opportunities for economic independence and political self-determination (Basu 1990). Ultimately such ends are a question not so much of economic transformations as of political priorities and values. As the participants in the Expert Group Meeting on Population and Women, held in Botswana in 1992, stated: "Equality for women depends not on the level of development or the economic resources available but on the political will of Governments and on the cultural setting in which women have to live" (1992).

The necessary conclusion is that governments and population agencies professing to uphold women's reproductive and sexual rights must do a lot more than avoid abuses. They must do more even than enforce "quality of care" guidelines, which reach only to conditions in the clinic and not to local communities and the larger society. Beyond this, they must seek a reordering of international economic policies (including so-called structural adjustment programs), national budgetary priorities, and national health and population policies to deemphasize debt servicing and militarism in favor of social welfare and primary health care. And they must adopt affirmative programs that promote "a culture of health aware-ness" and empowerment among women and an attitude of respect, nonviolence, and responsibility toward women and children among men.

Documents developed in preparation for the 1994 International Conference on Population and Development (ICPD), in Cairo, have begun to reflect the vision of reproductive and sexual rights as social rights that we have presented here. This is true not only of documents produced by women's NGOs, but also of official conference preparatory meetings and summaries, where for the first time in international population discourse, issues of gender equality and women's empowerment overshadow demographic targets

and economic growth and are recognized as part of "sustainable development." In both the topical outline adopted for the new World Population Plan of Action and the Second Preparatory Committee chairman's summary, issues of gender equality, women's rights, and reproductive rights cut across all sections, rather than being limited to the customary one or two token references. In sharp contrast to the previous World Population Plan of Action, the Preparatory Committee chairman's summary emphasizes the importance, in relation to family planning and reproductive health, of sexuality, sexual health, and STD and HIV/AIDS prevention. Unlike most UN documents, moreover, it includes "sexual orientation" in listing conditions that "many delegations" recognized should not be discriminated against in women's "access to information, education and services to exercise their reproductive and sexual rights."

We need to see this marked shift from the emphases of the plans of action adopted in 1974 and 1984 as a direct consequence of the strength and global impact of the women's health and rights movements during the last decade (see García-Moreno and Claro in this volume). Years of organizing and advocacy by women's health groups throughout the world have clearly had an important effect *at the level of official rhetoric* on intergovernmental forums concerned with "population" issues. To what extent are we likely to see governments, UN agencies, and international population organizations move from awareness to action to translate this rhetoric into concrete policies and programs that truly benefit women?

Many women's health groups, in both the South and the North, are concerned that feminist-sounding rhetoric is being used by international population agencies to legitimate and gloss over what remain instrumentalist and narrowly quantitative ends. Perceiving the history of population control policies and programs as all too frequently oblivious to women's needs and the ethical principles outlined above, they fear the language of reproductive rights and health may simply be co-opted by the Cairo process to support business as usual.

Our position is slightly more optimistic but nonetheless cautious. Feminists are putting pressure on population and family planning agencies to acknowledge women's self-defined needs and our conceptions of reproductive and sexual rights. This should move us closer to social and policy changes that empower women, but whether it does will depend on even more concerted action by women's NGOs, including alliances with many other groups concerned with health, development, and human rights. One such action should be to insist on full participation by women's rights and health groups in all relevant decision-making bodies and accountability mechanisms. In the long run, however, it is not enough that we call population agencies to account. To bridge the gap between rhetoric about reproductive and sexual rights and the harsh realities most women face demands a much larger vision. We must integrate, but not subordinate, those rights with health and development agendas that will radically transform the distribution of resources, power, and wellness within and among all the countries of the world (DAWN 1993; Sen 1992). These are the enabling conditions to transform rights into lived capacities. For women, Cairo is just a stop along the way.

Notes

1 The term seems to have originated with the founding of the Reproductive Rights National Network (R2N2) in the United States in 1979. R2N2 activists brought it to the European-based International Campaign for Abortion Rights in the early 1980s; at the International Women and Health Meeting in Amsterdam in 1984, the Campaign officially changed its name to the Women's Global Network for Reproductive Rights (Berer 1993b). Thereafter, the concept rapidly spread throughout women's movements in the South (for example, in 1985, under the influence of feminist members who had attended the Amsterdam meeting, the Brazilian Health Ministry established the Commission on the Rights of Human Reproduction). See also García-Moreno and Claro in this volume.

2 In fact, the principle of "ownership of one's body and person" has much deeper roots in the history of radical libertarian and democratic thought in Western Europe. Historian Natalie Zemon Davis traced this idea to 16th-

century Geneva, when a young Lyonnaise girl, brought before the Protestant elders for sleeping with her fiancé before marriage, invoked what may have been a popular slogan: "*Paris est au roi, et mon corps est à moi.*" (Paris is the king's, and my body is mine). The radical Levellers in 17th-century England developed the notion of a "property in one's person," which they used to defend their members against arbitrary arrest and imprisonment (Petchesky 1994). But the principle is not only of European derivation. Gandhi's concept of *Brahmacharya*, or "control over the body," was rooted in Hindu ascetic traditions and the Vedas' admonition to preserve the body's vital fluids. Like that of 19th-century feminists and the Catholic church, Gandhi's concept was theoretically gender-neutral, requiring both men and women to engage in sexual restraint except for purposes of procreation (Fischer 1962; O'Flaherty 1980). Islamic law goes further toward a sexually affirmative concept of self-ownership. Quranic provisions not only entitle women to sexual satisfaction in marriage, as well as condoning abortion and contraception; they also allow that, upon divorce — which wives as well as husbands may initiate — a woman regains her body. (Ahmed 1992; Musallam 1983; Ruthven 1984)

3 In Latin America, a new resolution of the Colombian Ministry of Public Health "orders all health institutions to ensure women the right to decide on all issues that affect their health, their life, and their sexuality, and guarantees rights 'to information and orientation to allow the exercise of free, gratifying, responsible sexuality which cannot be tied to maternity'" (quoted in Cook 1993a). In North Africa, Dr. Hind Khattab's field research among rural Egyptian women has revealed strong sentiments of their sexual entitlement to pleasure and gratification from husbands (Khattab 1993).

4 Feminist theory and practice have witnessed a long history of division over this question. Whether with regard to protective labor legislation, prostitution, pornography, or providing contraceptive implants to teenagers or poor women, conflicts between "liberals" (advocates of "freedom to choose") and "radicals" (advocates of social protection or legal prohibition) have been bitter and protracted.

5 Not only clinicians but feminist activists may be guilty of imposing their own values and failing to respect diversity. Feminist groups that condemn all reproductive technologies (for example, technologies that artificially assist fertility) as instruments of medical control over women and against "nature" ignore the ways that such technologies may expand the rights of particular women (for example, lesbians seeking pregnancy through artificial insemination or in vitro fertilization).

6 It seems crucial to us to recognize that religious fundamentalist movements are on the upswing in all the world's regions and major religions — Catholicism, Protestantism, Judaism, and Hinduism as well as Islam. Despite vast

cultural and theological differences, these fundamentalisms share a view of women as reproductive vessels that is antipathetic to any notion of women's reproductive rights. In an otherwise excellent discussion of the clash between religious and customary law and human rights, Lynn Freedman and Stephen Isaacs (1993) place undue emphasis on Muslim countries and Islamic law.

References

Ahmed, L. 1992. *Women and gender in Islam*. New Haven: Yale University Press.

Asian and Pacific Women's Resource Collection Network. 1990. *Asia and Pacific women's resource and action series: Health*. Kuala Lumpur: Asia and Pacific Development Centre.

Bang, R. 1989. High prevalence of gynecological diseases in rural Indian women. *Lancet* 337:85–88.

Basu, A. M. 1990. Cultural influences on health care use: Two regional groups in India. *Studies in Family Planning* 21:275–286.

Benmayor, R., R. M. Torruellas, and A. L. Juarbe. 1992. *Responses to poverty among Puerto Rican women: Identity, community, and cultural citizenship*. New York: Centro de Estudios Puertorriqueños, Hunter College.

Berer, M. 1990. What would a feminist population policy be like? *Women's Health Journal* 18:4–7.

———. 1993a. Population and family planning policies: Women-centered perspectives. *Reproductive Health Matters* 1:4–12.

———. 1993b. Personal communication.

Bhasin, K., and N. Khan. 1986. *Some questions on feminism for women in South Asia*. New Delhi: Kali.

Bruce, J. 1990. Fundamental elements of the quality of care: A simple framework. *Studies in Family Planning* 21:61–91.

Bunch, C. 1990. Women's rights as human rights: Toward a re-vision of human rights. *Human Rights Quarterly* 12:486–498.

Chesler, E. 1992. *Woman of valor: Margaret Sanger and the birth control movement in America*. New York: Simon & Schuster.

Cook, R. J. 1993a. International human rights and women's reproductive health. *Studies in Family Planning* 24:73–86.

———. 1993b. Women's international human rights law: The way forward. *Human Rights Quarterly* 15:230–261.

Copelon, R. 1994. Intimate terror: Understanding domestic violence as torture. In R. J. Cook (ed.), *International women's human rights*. Philadelphia: University of Pennsylvania.

Correa, S. 1993. Sterilization in Brazil: Reviewing the analysis. Unpublished.

Crenshaw, K. 1991. Demarginalizing the intersection of race and sex: A black feminist critique of anti-discrimination doctrine, feminist theory, and anti-racist politics. In K. T. Bartlett and R. Kennedy (eds.), *Feminist Legal Theory*. Boulder, Colo.: Westview Press.

Development Alternatives with Women for a New Era (DAWN). 1993. Population and reproductive rights component: Platform document/preliminary ideas. Unpublished.

Dixon-Mueller, R. 1993. *Population policy and women's rights: Transforming reproductive choice*. Westport, Conn.: Praeger.

Eisenstein, Z. 1983. *The radical future of liberal feminism*. Boston: Northeastern University.

———. 1994. *The color of gender*. Berkeley: University of California.

Elias, C. 1991. *Sexually transmitted diseases and the reproductive health of women in developing countries*. New York: Population Council.

Elshtain, J. B. 1981. *Public man, private woman*. Princeton, N.J.: Princeton University.

Expert Group Meeting on Population and Women. 1992 (October). *Substantive preparations for the conference — recommendations*. New York: United Nations Economic and Social Council.

Ezeh, A. C. 1993. The influence of spouses over each other's contraceptive attitudes in Ghana. *Studies in Family Planning* 24:163–174.

Fabros, M. L. 1991. The WRRC's institutional framework and strategies on reproductive rights. *Flights* 4. Official publication of the Women's Resource & Research Center, Quezon City, Philippines.

Fischer, L. 1962. *The essential Gandhi*. New York: Vintage.

Freedman, L. P., and S. L. Isaacs. 1993. Human rights and reproductive choice. *Studies in Family Planning* 24:18–30.

Friedman, M. 1992. Feminism and modern friendship: Dislocating the community. In S. Avineri and A. de-Shalit (eds.), *Communitarianism and individualism*. New York: Oxford University Press.

Gilligan, C. 1982. *In a different voice: Psychological theory and women's development*. Cambridge, Mass.: Harvard University Press.

Gordon, L. 1976. *Woman's body, woman's right: A social history of birth control in America*. New York: Penguin.

Heise, L. 1992. Violence against women: The missing agenda. In M. A. Koblinsky, J. Timyan, and J. Gay (eds.), *Women's health: A global perspective*. Boulder, Colo.: Westview Press.

Heller, A. 1992. Rights, modernity, democracy. In D. Cornell, M. Rosenfeld, and D. G. Carlson (eds.), *Deconstruction and the possibility of justice*. New York: Routledge.

Huston, P. 1992. *Motherhood by choice: Pioneers in women's health & family planning*. New York: Feminist Press.

Jayawardena, K. 1993. *With a different voice: White women and colonialism in South Asia*. London: Zed.

Jain, A., J. Bruce, and B. Mensch. 1992. Setting standards of quality in family planning programs. *Studies in Family Planning* 23:392–395.

Jeffery, P., R. Jeffery, and A. Lyon. 1989. *Labour pains and labour power: Women and childbearing in India*. London: Zed.

Kelly, J. 1984. *Women, history, and theory*. Chicago: University of Chicago Press.

Khattab, H. 1992. *The silent endurance: Social conditions of women's reproductive health in rural Egypt*. Amman: UNICEF; and Cairo: Population Council.

———. 1993. Personal communication.

Lopez, I. 1993. *Constrained choices: An ethnography of sterilization and Puerto Rican women in New York City*. Unpublished manuscipt.

McCarthy, J., and D. Maine. 1992. A framework for analyzing the determinants of maternal mortality. *Studies in Family Planning* 23:23–33.

Mintzes, B., ed. 1992. *A question of control: Women's perspectives on the development and use of contraceptives*. Amsterdam: WEMOS, Women & Pharmaceuticals Project.

Morsy, S. 1994. Maternal mortality in Egypt: Selective health strategy and the medicalization of population control. In F. D. Ginsburg and R. Rapp (eds.), *Conceiving the new world order: The global stratification of reproduction*. Berkeley: University of California.

Musallam, B. F. 1983. *Sex and society in Islam: Birth control before the nineteenth century*. Cambridge: Cambridge University Press.

National Research Council. 1989. *Contraception and reproduction: Health consequences for women and children in the developing world*. Washington, D.C.: National Academy Press.

Nedelsky, J. 1989. Reconceiving autonomy. *Yale Journal of Law and Feminism* 1:7–36.

O'Flaherty, W. D. 1980. *Women, androgynes, and other mythical beasts*. Chicago: University of Chicago.

Okin, S. M. 1979. *Women in Western political thought*. Princeton, N.J.: Princeton University.

Olsen, F. 1984. Statutory rape: A feminist critique of rights analysis. *Texas Law Review* 63:387–432.

Pearce, T. O. 1994. Women's reproductive practices and biomedicine: Cultural conflicts and transformations. In F. D. Ginsburg and R. Rapp (eds.), *Conceiving the new world order: The global stratification of reproduction*. Berkeley: University of California.

Petchesky, R. P. 1979. Reproductive choice in the contemporary United States: A social analysis of female sterilization. In K. Michaelson (ed.), *And the poor get children*. New York: Monthly Review.

———. 1990. *Abortion and woman's choice: The state, sexuality and reproductive freedom*. Revised ed. Boston: Northeastern University.

———. 1994. The body as property: A feminist revision. In F. D. Ginsburg and R. Rapp (eds.), *Conceiving the new world order: The global stratification of reproduction*. Berkeley: University of California.

Petchesky, R. P., and J. Weiner. 1990. *Global feminist perspectives on reproductive rights and reproductive health*. New York: Reproductive Rights Education Project, Hunter College.

Pies, C. n.d. *Creating ethical reproductive health care policy*. San Francisco: Education Programs Associates, Inc.

Protacio, N. 1990. From womb to tomb: The Filipino women's struggle for good health and justice. Paper presented at the Fourth International Interdisciplinary Congress on Women, June 12, at Hunter College, New York.

Ramasubban, R. 1990. Sexual behaviour and conditions of health care: Potential risks for HIV transmission in India. Paper prepared for the International Union for the Scientific Study of Population Seminar on Anthropological Studies Relevant to the Sexual Transmission of HIV, in Sonderborg, Denmark.

Ramusack, B. N. 1989. Embattled advocates: The debate over birth control in India, 1920-40. *Journal of Women's History* 1:34–64.

Ravindran, T. K. S. 1993. Women and the politics of population and development in India. *Reproductive Health Matters* 1:26–38.

Rosenfeld, M. 1992. Deconstruction and legal interpretation: Conflict, indeterminacy and the temptations of the new legal formalism. In D. Cornell, M. Rosenfeld, and D. G. Carlson (eds.), *Deconstruction and the possibility of justice*. New York: Routledge.

Ruthven, M. 1984. *Islam in the world*. New York: Oxford University Press.

Sanger, M. 1920. *Woman and the new race.* New York: Truth.

Schneider, E. M. 1991. The dialectic of rights and politics: Perspectives from the women's movement. In K. T. Bartlett and R. Kennedy (eds.), *Feminist legal theory.* Boulder, Colo.: Westview Press.

Sen, G. 1992. *Women, poverty and population: Issues for the concerned environmentalist.* Cambridge, Mass.: Center for Population and Development Studies, Harvard University.

Tushnet, M. 1984. An essay on rights. *Texas Law Review* 62:1363–1403.

Unger, R. 1983. The critical legal studies movement. *Harvard Law Review* 96(3):561–675.

Wasserheit, J. 1993. The costs of reproductive tract infections in women. In M. Berer and S. Ray (eds.), *Women and HIV/AIDS: An international resource book.* London: Pandora.

Weeks, J. 1981. *Sex, politics and society: The regulation of sexuality since 1800.* New York: Longman.

Williams, P. J. 1991. *The alchemy of race and rights.* Cambridge, Mass.: Harvard University.

Women's Global Network for Reproductive Rights. 1991. *Statement of Purpose.* General leaflet.

Zimmerman, M., et al. 1990. Assessing the acceptability of Norplant® implants in four countries: Findings from focus group research. *Studies in Family Planning* 21:92–103.

SECTION THREE

Gender and Empowerment

9

The Meaning of
Women's Empowerment:
New Concepts from Action[1]

Srilatha Batliwala

Since the mid-1980s, the term *empowerment* has become popular in the field of development, especially in reference to women. In grassroots programs and policy debates alike, *empowerment* has virtually replaced terms such as *welfare, upliftment, community participation,* and *poverty alleviation* to describe the goal of development and intervention. In spite of the prevalence of the term, however, many people are confused as to what the empowerment of women implies in social, economic, and political terms. How empowerment strategies differ from or relate to such earlier strategies as integrated rural development, women's development, community participation, conscientization, and awareness building is even less clear.

Nonetheless, many large-scale programs are being launched with the explicit objective of "empowering" the poor and "empowering" women. Empowerment is held to be a panacea for social ills: high population growth rates, environmental degradation, and the low status of women, among others.[2]

The attention given here to women's empowerment is based on the premise that it is an enabling condition for reproductive rights (Correa

and Petchesky, this volume). This chapter attempts an operational definition of women's empowerment, and delineates the components and stages of empowerment strategies, on the basis of insights gained through a study of grassroots programs in South Asia. Undoubtedly, the nature and priorities of the women's empowerment process in South Asian countries are shaped by the historical, political, social, and economic conditions specific to that region. Still, there are sufficient commonalities with other regions — such as an extended period of colonial rule; highly stratified, male-dominated social structures; widespread poverty and vulnerable economies; and fairly rigid gender- and class-based divisions of labor — to render the definition and analytic framework for empowerment presented in this essay more widely relevant.

The Concept of Empowerment

The concept of women's empowerment appears to be the outcome of several important critiques and debates generated by the women's movement throughout the world, and particularly by Third World feminists. Its source can be traced to the interaction between feminism and the concept of "popular education" developed in Latin America in the 1970s (Walters 1991). The latter had its roots in Freire's theory of "conscientization," which totally ignored gender, but was also influenced by Gramscian thought, which stressed the need for participatory mechanisms in institutions and society in order to create a more equitable and nonexploitative system (Forgacs 1988; Freire 1973).

Gender subordination and the social construction of gender were a priori in feminist analysis and popular education. Feminist popular educators therefore evolved their own distinct approach, pushing beyond merely building awareness and toward organizing the poor to struggle actively for change. They defined their goals in the following terms:

…To unambiguously take the standpoint of women; [and]…demonstrate to women and men how gender is constructed socially,…and…can be changed…[to show] through the lived experience of the participants, how women and men are gendered through class, race, religion, culture, etc.;…to investigate collectively… how class, [caste], race and gender intersect…in order to deepen collective understanding about these relationships…

…To build collective and alternative visions for gender relations…and…deepen collective analysis of the context and the position of women…locally, nationally, regionally and globally,…To develop analytical tools…to evaluate the effects of certain development strategies for the promotion of women's strategic interests… [and develop strategies] to bring about change in their personal and organizational lives…

…To help women develop the skills to assert themselves…and to challenge oppressive behavior…to build a network of women and men nationally, [and internationally]…[and] to help build demo-

cratic community and worker organizations and a strong civil society which can pressurize for change (Walters 1991).

Meanwhile, in the 1980s feminist critiques emerged of those development strategies and grassroots interventions that had failed to make significant progress toward improving the status of women. They attributed the failure mainly to the use of welfare, poverty alleviation, and managerial approaches, for example, that did not address the underlying structural factors that perpetuate the oppression and exploitation of poor women (Moser 1989). These approaches had made no distinction between the "condition" and the "position" of women (Young 1988). Young defined *condition* as the material state in which poor women live — low wages, poor nutrition, and lack of access to health care, education, and training. *Position* is the social and economic status of women as compared with that of men. Young argues that focusing on improving the daily conditions of women's existence curtailed women's awareness of, and readiness to act against, the less visible but powerful underlying structures of subordination and inequality.

Molyneux (1985) made a similar distinction between women's "practical" and "strategic" interests. While women's practical needs — food, health, water, fuel, child care, education, improved technology, and so forth — must be met, they cannot be an end in themselves. Organizing and mobilizing women to fulfill their long-term strategic interests is essential. This requires

…analysis of women's subordination and…the formulation of an alternative, more satisfactory set of arrangements to those which exist…such as the abolition of the sexual division of labor, the alleviation of the burden of domestic labor and child care, the removal of institutionalized forms of discrimination, the establishment of political equality, freedom of choice over childbearing and…measures against male violence and control over women (Molyneux 1985).

It is from these roots that the notion of empowerment grew, and it came to be most clearly articulated in 1985 by DAWN[3] as the "empowerment approach" (Sen and Grown 1985). Empowerment, in this view, required transformation of structures of subordination through radical changes in law, property rights, and other institutions that reinforce and perpetuate male domination.

By the beginning of the 1990s, women's empowerment had come to replace most earlier terms in development jargon. Unfortunately, as it has become a buzzword, the sharpness of the perspective that gave rise to it has been diluted. Consequently, its implications for macro- and micro-level strategies need clarification. The key question is: How do different approaches to women's "condition," or practical needs, affect the possibility or nature of changes in women's "position," or strategic interests?

This question is most pertinent to the whole issue of women's reproductive rights. Many of the existing approaches to contraception and women's reproductive health, for example, focus entirely on improved technologies and delivery systems for birth control, safe delivery, prenatal and postnatal care, and termination of fertility. But none of these addresses the more fundamental questions of discrimination against girls and women in access to food and health care; male dominance in sexual relations; women's lack of control over their sexuality; the gender division of labor that renders women little more than beasts of burden in many cultures; or the denial by many societies of women's right to determine the number of children they want. These issues are all linked to women's "position," and are not necessarily affected by reduced birthrates or improvements in women's physical health. This is one of the dichotomies that an empowerment process must seek to address.

What is Empowerment?

The most conspicuous feature of the term *empowerment* is that it contains the word *power*, which, to sidestep philosophical debate, may be broadly defined as control over material assets, intellectual resources, and ideology. The material assets over which control can be exercised may be physical, human, or financial, such as land, water, forests, people's bodies and labor, money, and access to money. Intellectual resources include knowledge, information, and ideas. Control over ideology signifies the ability to generate, propagate, sustain, and institutionalize specific sets of beliefs, values, attitudes, and behavior — virtually determining how people perceive and function within given socioeconomic and political environments.[4]

Power thus accrues to those who control or are able to influence the distribution of material resources, knowledge, and the ideology that governs social relations in both public and private life. The extent of power held by particular individuals or groups corresponds to the number of kinds of resources they can control, and the extent to which they can shape prevailing ideologies, whether social, religious, or political. This control, in turn, confers the power of decisionmaking.

In South Asia, women in general, and poor women in particular, are relatively powerless, with little or no control over resources and little decisionmaking power. Often, even the limited resources at their disposal — such as a little land, a nearby forest, and their own bodies, labor, and skills — are not within their control, and the decisions made by others affect their lives every day.

This does not mean that women are, or have always been, totally powerless; for centuries they have tried to exercise their power within the family (Nelson 1974; Stacey and Price 1981). They also have taken control of the resources to which society has allowed them access, and even *seized* control of resources when they could — the Chipko movement in northern India and the Green Belt movement in Kenya, for example (Misra 1978; Rodda 1991). They have always attempted, from their traditional position as workers, mothers, and wives, not only to influence their immediate environment, but also to expand their space. However, the prevailing patriarchal ideology, which promotes the values of submission, sacrifice, obedience, and silent suffering, often undermines even these attempts by women to assert themselves or demand some share of resources (Hawkesworth 1990; Schuler and Kadirgamar-Rajasingham 1992).

The process of challenging existing power relations, and of gaining greater control over the sources of power, may be termed *empowerment*. This broad definition is refined by feminist scholars and activists within the context of their own regions. For instance:

> The term empowerment refers to a range of activities from individual self-assertion to collective resistance, protest and mobilization that challenge basic power relations. For individuals and groups where class, caste, ethnicity and gender determine their access to resources and power, their empowerment begins when they not only recognize the systemic forces that oppress them, but act to change existing power relationships. Empowerment, therefore, is a process aimed at changing the nature and direction of systemic forces which marginalize women and other disadvantaged sections in a given context (Sharma 1991–1992).

Empowerment is thus both a process and the result of that process. Empowerment is manifested as a redistribution of power, whether between nations, classes, castes, races, genders, or individuals. The goals of women's empowerment are to challenge patriarchal ideology (male domination and women's subordination); to transform the structures and institutions that reinforce and perpetuate gender discrimination and social inequality (the family, caste, class, religion, educational processes and institutions, the media, health practices and systems, laws and civil codes, political processes, development models, and government institutions); and to enable poor women to gain access to, and control of, both material and informational resources. The process of empowerment must thus address all relevant structures and sources of power:

Since the causes of women's inferior status and unequal gender relations are deeply rooted in history, religion, culture, in the psychology of the self, in laws and legal systems, and in political institutions and social attitudes, if the status and material conditions of women's lives is to change at all, the solutions must penetrate just as deeply (Schuler and Kadirgamar-Rajasingham 1992).

Theories that identify any one system or structure as the source of power — for instance, the assertion that economic structures are the basis of powerlessness and inequality — imply that improvement in one dimension would result in a redistribution of power. However, activists working in situations where women are economically strong know that equal status does not necessarily result. If anything, ample evidence exists that strengthening women's economic status, though positive in many ways, does not always reduce their other burdens or eradicate other forms of oppression; in fact, it has often led to intensifying pressures (Brydon and Chant 1989; Gupte and Borkar 1987; Sen and Grown 1985). Similarly, it is evident that improvements in physical status and access to basic resources, like water, fuel, fodder, health care, and education, do not automatically lead to fundamental changes in women's position. If that were so, middle-class women, with higher education, well-paid jobs, and adequate nourishment and health care, would not continue to be victims of wife beating or bride burning.

There is widespread confusion and some degree of anxiety about whether women's empowerment leads to the disempowerment of men. It is obvious that poor men are almost as powerless as poor women in terms of access to and control over resources. This is exactly why most poor men tend to support women's empowerment processes that enable women to bring much-needed resources into their families and communities, or that challenge power structures that have oppressed and exploited the poor of both genders.

Resistance, however, occurs when women compete with men for power in the public sphere, or when they question the power, rights, and privileges of men within the family — in other words, when women challenge patriarchal family relations (Batliwala 1994). This is, in fact, a test of how far the empowerment process has reached into women's lives; as one activist put it, "the family is the last frontier of change in gender relations.... You know [empowerment] has occurred when it crosses the threshold of the home" (Kannabiran 1993).

The process of women's empowerment must challenge patriarchal relations, and thus inevitably leads to changes in men's traditional control over women, particularly over the women of their households. Men in communities where such changes have already occurred no longer have control over women's bodies, sexuality, or mobility; they cannot abdicate responsibility for housework and child care, nor physically abuse or violate women with impunity; they cannot (as is the case in South Asia at present) abandon or divorce their wives without providing maintenance, or commit bigamy or polygamy, or make unilateral decisions that affect the whole family. Clearly, then, women's empowerment does mean the loss of the privileged position that patriarchy allotted to men.

A point often missed, however, is that women's empowerment also liberates and empowers men, both in material and in psychological terms. First, women greatly strengthen the impact of political movements dominated by men — not just by their numbers, but by providing new energy, insights, leadership, and strategies. Second, as we saw earlier, the struggles of women's groups for access to material resources and knowledge directly benefit the men and children of their families and their communities, by opening the door to new ideas and a better quality of life. But most important are the psychological gains for men when women become equal partners. Men are freed from the roles of oppressor and exploiter, and from gender stereotyping, which limits the potential for self-expression and personal development in men as much as in women. Furthermore, experiences worldwide show that men discover an emotional satisfaction in sharing responsibility and decisionmaking; they find that they have lost not merely traditional privileges, but also traditional burdens. As one South Asian NGO spokeswoman expressed it:

> Women's empowerment should lead to the liberation of men from false value systems and ideologies of oppression. It should lead to a situation where each one can become a whole being, regardless of gender, and use their fullest potential to construct a more humane society for all (Akhtar 1992).

The Process of Empowerment

In order to challenge their subordination, *women must first recognize the ideology that legitimizes male domination and understand how it perpetuates their oppression.* This recognition requires reversal of the values and attitudes, indeed the entire worldview, that most women have internalized since earliest childhood. Women have been led to participate in their own oppression through a complex web of religious sanctions, social and cultural taboos and superstitions, hierarchies among women in the family (see Adams and Castle in this volume), behavioral training, seclusion, veiling, curtailment of physical mobility, discrimination in food and other family resources, and control of their sexuality (including concepts like the "good" and "bad" woman). Most poor women have never been allowed to think for themselves or to make their own choices except in unusual circumstances, when a male decision maker has been absent or has abdicated his role. Because questioning is not allowed, the majority of women grow up believing that this is the just and "natural" order.

Hence, the demand for change does not usually begin spontaneously from the condition of subjugation. Rather, empowerment must be externally induced, by forces working with an altered consciousness and an awareness that the existing social order is *unjust* and *unnatural*. They seek to change other women's consciousness: altering their self-image and their beliefs about their rights and capabilities; creating awareness of how gender discrimination, like other socioeconomic and political factors, is one of the forces acting on them; challenging the sense of inferiority that has been imprinted on them since birth; and recognizing the true value of their labor and contributions to the family, society, and economy. Women must be convinced of their innate right to equality, dignity, and justice.

The external agents of change necessary for empowerment may take many forms. The anti-arrack[5] agitation of 1992–1993 in Nellore District of Andhra Pradesh State in southern India, for instance, in which thousands of women participated, was triggered by a lesson in an adult literacy primer depicting the plight of a landless woman whose husband drank away his meager wages at the local liquor shop. The agitation has created a major political and economic crisis for the state government, which earns huge revenues through licensing of liquor outlets and excise duties on liquor (see Box 1; also, Anveshi 1993; Joseph 1993).

A key role of the external activist lies in giving women access to a new body of ideas and information that not only changes their consciousness and self-image, but also encourages action. This means a dynamic educational process. Historically, the poor in much of South Asia, and especially poor women, were beyond the pale of formal education, and so developed learning systems of their own. Valuable oral and practical traditions evolved to transfer empirical knowledge and livelihood skills from generation to generation: about agriculture, plant and animal life, forest lore, weaving, dying, building craft, fishing, handicrafts, folk medicine, and a myriad of other subjects. This body of traditional knowledge and skills was, however, developed within specific ideological and social frameworks. Such knowledge and practices are often suffused with taboos, superstitions, and biases against women. For example, menstruating women are prohib-

ited from touching books, and women and men of certain castes are forbidden to touch religious books.

Through empowerment, women gain access to new worlds of knowledge and can begin to make new, informed choices in both their personal and their public lives. However, such radical changes are not sustainable if limited to a few individual women, because traditional power structures will seek to isolate and ostracize them. Society is forced to change only when large numbers of women are mobilized to press for change. The empowerment process must organize women into collectives, breaking out from individual isolation and creating a united forum through which women can challenge their subordination. With the support of the collective and the activist agent, women can re-examine their lives critically, recognize the structures and sources of power and subordination, discover their strengths, and initiate action.

The process of empowerment is thus a spiral, changing consciousness, identifying areas to target for change, planning strategies, acting for change, and analyzing action and outcomes, which leads in turn to higher levels of consciousness and more finely honed and better executed strategies. The empowerment spiral affects everyone involved: the individual, the activist agent, the collective, and the community. Thus, empowerment cannot be a top-down or one-way process.

Armed with a new consciousness and growing collective strength, women begin to assert their right to control resources (including their own bodies) and to participate equally in decisions within the family, community, and village. Their priorities may often be surprising, even baffling, to the outsider. In the aftermath of the 1991 Bangladesh cyclone, one of the first demands made by women in a badly affected area was the rebuilding of the schoolhouse and the providing of schoolbooks to their children; this was in stark contrast to the demands of the local men, who talked only about houses, seeds, poultry, and loans (Akhtar 1992). In another project in southern India, one of the first issues taken up by the

Women's Mobilizing: Anti-Liquor Agitation by Indian Women

"Even a cow must be fed if you want milk. Otherwise it will kick you. We have kicked! We will do anything to stop saara [country liquor] sales here" (Villager, Totla Cheruvupalli, Andhra Pradesh).

The anti-liquor movement that began in the southern Indian state of Andhra Pradesh in 1992 is unusual among popular uprisings. Initiated and led entirely by poor rural women in a few villages of one district (Nellore), the movement spread rapidly throughout the state. It has no centralized leadership or base in any political party, but is led entirely by groups of women in each village. It has no unified strategy; rather, women use whatever tactics they find most appropriate. The movement has been enormously successful, even overcoming the state government's interest in revenues from taxes on arrack (a crude liquor).

The movement was triggered by the Akshara Deepam (Light of Literacy) campaign, launched by the government and several volunteer organizations in Nellore District. The campaign not only brought women literacy programs, but also raised their consciousness about their status and potential to act. One of the chapters in the literacy primer described the plight of a poor woman whose husband drank away his wages at the local liquor shop. Ignited by this story, which mirrored their own reality all too well, the women readers asked: How is it that liquor supplies arrive in a village at least twice a day, but there are always shortages of food in the government-controlled ration shops, kerosene for lighting, drinking water, medicines at the health center, learning materials for schoolchildren, and myriad other basic essentials?

A decade earlier, the party in power in the state launched the Varuna Vahini (Liquor Flood) policy, through which the state's liquor excise revenues increased from 1.5 billion rupees in 1981–82 to 6.4 billion rupees in 1991–1992. The state government's development outlay for 1991–1992 was 17 billion rupees. Many local employers and landlords pay part of men's wages in coupons that can be used at the local liquor shop, further boosting liquor sales — and ensuring that in most poor households, men's earnings fatten the liquor lobby and state government, while their families

struggle for daily food and survival. Regular harassment and physical abuse by drunken men drives some women to suicide.

The anti-liquor movement began with a few women picketing liquor shops and forcing their closure. News spread through the village grapevine and the media, and soon the whole of Nellore District, then the entire state of Andhra Pradesh, was taken up in the cause. Women used a wide variety of tactics with substantial symbolic import: In one village, for example, the women cooked the daily meal, took it wrapped in leaves to the liquor shop, and demanded that the owner eat all their offerings. "You have been taking the food from our bellies all these years, so here, eat! Eat until it kills you, the way you have been killing us!" The terrified proprietor closed shop and ran, and has not reopened since.

With less arrack being consumed, there is more money for food and other essentials, less physical and emotional abuse of women, and far less violence in general. For the most part, men have reacted surprisingly passively to the whole movement, perhaps because women directed their outrage and attacks at the liquor suppliers, rather than at their men.

The greatest victory of the movement is that no politician or party has been able to derail it, nor has the state government been able to suppress it. It cannot, after all, be characterized as antigovernment or seditious, since it is upholding one of the directive principles of the Indian constitution. However, the state is trying to repress the movement in more devious ways. Officials have floated a rumor that if liquor sales are not resumed, the price of rice will be increased. Attempts are also afoot to sabotage the literacy program that gave rise to the movement. Further, since legal sales have been effectively stopped, liquor contractors and local officials are promoting underground sales by smuggling liquor into villages in milk cans and vegetable baskets.

Though women in the anti-liquor movement have not directly challenged the state, they have managed to weaken it by attacking the nexus between the state and the liquor lobby. Poor women have mobilized and struck a blow for themselves and their families.

Source: Joseph 1993.

emerging Mahila Sangha (women's collective) of one village was the demand for a separate *smashana* (cremation ground); being scheduled castes, they said, they were not allowed to use the upper-caste area. In both cases, external activists were surprised by the women's priorities, which were quite different from those issues the activists considered most pressing.

Traditionally, women have made choices — if, indeed, they can be called choices — only within tight social constraints. For example, a woman can pay a dowry and marry off her daughter, or run the risk that the daughter will remain unmarried and be a burden to the family; a woman can bear many children, especially sons, to prove her fertility, or face rejection by her husband and in-laws. Because of the acute poverty and overwhelming work burden of poor women, most activists face a recurring dilemma: Should they respond to women's immediate problems by setting up services that will meet their practical needs and alleviate their condition? Or should they take the longer route of raising consciousness about the underlying structural factors that cause the problems, and organize women to demand resources and services from the state? Or should they enable women to organize and manage their own services with resources from the state and themselves?

A New Understanding of Power

Empowerment should also generate new notions of power. Present-day notions of power have evolved in hierarchical, male-dominated societies and are based on divisive, destructive, and oppressive values. The point is not for women to take power and use it in the same exploitative and corrupt way. Rather, women's empowerment processes must evolve a new understanding of power, and experiment with ways of democratizing and sharing power — building new mechanisms for collective responsibility, decisionmaking, and accountability.

Similarly, once women have gained control over resources, they should not use them in the same shortsighted and ecologically destructive manner as male-dominated capitalist societies. Women's empowerment will have to lead women — and the "new men" — to address global concerns and issues, including the environment; war, violence, and militarism; ethnic, linguistic, religious, or racial fanaticism; and population.

Such radical transformations in society obviously cannot be achieved through the struggles of village or neighborhood women's collectives. Just as individual challenges can be easily crushed, so can the struggles of small, local collectives of women be negated by far more powerful and entrenched socioeconomic and political forces. In the final analysis, to transform society, women's empowerment must become a political force, that is, an organized mass movement that challenges and transforms existing power structures. Empowerment should ultimately lead to the formation of mass organizations of poor women, at the regional, national, and international levels. Only then can the poor women of the world hope to bring about the fulfillment of their practical and strategic needs, and change both the "condition" and the "position" of women. They can form strategic alliances with other organizations of the poor — such as trade unions, and farmers and tenant farmers groups — and thus involve men in the change process as well. Most important, these federations must remain wholly autonomous and maintain a suprapolitical stance to prevent the cooptation and dilution of the empowerment process by pervasive patriarchal forces. This does not mean that women leaders who emerge through grassroots empowerment cannot participate in political processes like elections; on the contrary, they can, and have done so. However, they should run as candidates of existing parties, not as representatives of autonomous women's federations. This way, the latter can play a vigilant role and call to account its own members if they betray women's aspirations and needs in their performance of other roles.[6]

In a study of selected South Asian NGOs (nongovernmental organizations) engaged in women's empowerment, I was able to gather and review project reports and other published and unpublished material, discuss the empowerment question with project leaders and field workers, and visit with field organizers. Three major approaches to women's empowerment were identifiable: integrated development programs, economic development, and consciousness-raising and organizing among women. These are not mutually exclusive categories, but they help to distinguish among the differing interpretations of the causes of women's powerlessness and, hence, among the different interventions thought to lead to empowerment.

The integrated development approach ascribes women's powerlessness to their greater poverty and lower access to health care, education, and survival resources. Strategies are focused on providing services and enhancing economic status; some NGOs also emphasize awareness building. This approach improves women's condition mainly by helping them meet their survival and livelihood needs.

The economic development approach places women's economic vulnerability at the center of their powerlessness, and posits that economic empowerment has a positive impact on other aspects of women's existence. Its strategies are built around strengthening women's position as workers and income earners by mobilizing, organizing or unionizing, and providing access to support services. Though this approach undoubtedly improves women's economic position *and* condition, it is not clear that this change necessarily empowers them in other dimensions of their lives.

The consciousness-raising and organizing approach is based on a more complex understanding of gender relations and women's status. This method ascribes powerlessness to the ideology and practice of patriarchy and socioeconomic inequality in *all* the systems and structures of society. Strategies focus more on organizing women to recognize and challenge both gender- and class-based discrimination in all aspects of their lives, in both the public and the private spheres. Women are mobilized to struggle for greater access to resources, rather than passively

provided with schemes and services. This approach is successful in enabling women to address their position and strategic needs, but may not be as effective in meeting immediate needs. A more detailed analysis of the goals, strategies, and dilemmas of each of these approaches is contained in Box 2 (on next page).

Lessons for a Women's Empowerment Strategy

No one magic formula or fail-safe design exists for empowerment. Nonetheless, experience clearly shows that empowerment strategies must intervene at the level of women's "condition" while also transforming their "position," thus simultaneously addressing both practical and strategic needs. Within the conceptual framework developed in the first part of this chapter, several elements appear essential. They are designed to challenge patriarchal ideology, and to enable poor women to gain greater access to and control over both material and informational resources. Although these elements are set out below in a particular sequence, they may be reversed or interchanged, or several may be undertaken concurrently, depending on the context.

An organization concerned with bringing about women's empowerment must begin by locating the geopolitical region (urban or rural) in which it wants to work, and identifying the poorest and most oppressed women in that area. Activists then have to be selected and trained. Intensive preparatory training is critical; it must impart to activists an awareness of the structures and sources of power, especially gender, and it must equip them with skills needed to mobilize, while learning from, the women whose consciousness they plan to raise. In general, female activists are preferable, since they are in a better position to initiate the empowerment process with other women, notwithstanding differences in class, caste, or educational background.

In the field, the activists encourage women to set aside a separate time and space for themselves — as disempowered women rather than as passive recipients of welfare or beneficiaries of programs

BOX 2

Empowerment: Three Approaches

Three experimental approaches to empowering women have been undertaken in South Asia: integrated development, economic empowerment, and consciousness-raising. While these approaches differ from each other in concept, most organizations working on the ground take a mix of approaches. Common to all three is the importance placed on group formation to build solidarity among women.

The *integrated development* approach views women's development as key to the advancement of family and community. It therefore provides a package of interventions to alleviate poverty, meet basic survival needs, reduce gender discrimination, and help women gain self-esteem. This approach proceeds either by forming women's collectives that engage in development activities and tackle social problems such as dowry, child marriage, and male alcoholism (Proshika in Bangladesh; RDRS in Rajasthan, India), or by employing an "entry point" strategy, using a specific activity, such as a literacy class or health program, to mobilize women into groups (Gonoshastya Kendra in Bangladesh, United Mission to Nepal, Redd Barna in Nepal).

The *economic empowerment* approach attributes women's subordination to lack of economic power. It focuses on improving women's control over material resources and strengthening women's economic security. Groups are formed using two methods: organizing women around savings and credit, income generation, or skill training activities (Grameen Bank in

Bangladesh, Program of Credit for Rural Women in Nepal); or by occupation or location (SEWA in India, Proshika). These groups may work in a range of areas, including savings and credit, training and skills development, new technologies or marketing, as well as provide such ancillary supports as child care, health services, literacy programs, and legal education and aid.

The *consciousness raising* approach asserts that women's empowerment requires awareness of the complex factors causing women's subordination. This approach organizes women into collectives that tackle the sources of subordination (ASTHA, Deccan Development Society, Mahila Samakhya, WOP in India; Nijera Kori in Bangladesh). Education is central and is defined as a process of learning that leads to a new consciousness, self-worth, societal and gender analysis, and access to skills and information. In this approach, the groups themselves determine their priorities. Women's knowledge of their own bodies and ability to control reproduction are also considered vital. The long-term goal is for the women's groups to be independent of the initiating NGO. This approach uses no particular service "entry point" and attempts to be open-ended and nondirective. It gives considerable emphasis to fielding "change agents," who are trained to catalyze women's thinking without determining the directions in which a particular group may go.

— collectively to question their situation and develop critical thinking. These forums should enable women to evolve from an aggregate of individuals into a cohesive collective, wherein they can look at themselves and their environment in new ways, develop a positive self-image, recognize their strengths, and explode sexist mis-

conceptions. The activists also help women collectively to claim access to new information and knowledge, and to begin to develop a critical understanding of the ideology of gender, the systems and institutions through which it is perpetuated and reinforced, and the structures of power governing their lives. This is the process that expands women's awareness beyond their "condition" to their "position."

With a growing consciousness and collective strength, women's groups prioritize the problems they would like to tackle. They begin to confront oppressive practices and situations both inside and outside the home, and gradually to alter their own attitudes and behavior; this often includes changing their treatment of their girl children and asserting their reproductive and sexual rights. In the course of both individual and collective struggles for change, women also build their skills of collective decisionmaking, action, and accountability and they may forge new strategies and methods, such as forming alliances with other groups of exploited and oppressed people, or involving sympathetic men of their own communities. With the help of training and counsel provided by the NGO or activists working with them, they also acquire real skills — vocational and managerial know-how, literacy and arithmetic competence, basic data collection techniques for conducting their own surveys — that enhance their autonomy and power.

These women's collectives then begin to seek access to resources and public services independently, demanding accountability from service providers, lobbying for changes in laws and programs that are inaccessible or inappropriate, and negotiating with public institutions such as banks and government departments. Collectively they may also set up and manage alternative services and programs, such as their own child care centers, savings banks, or schools. Finally, village- or neighborhood-level women's collectives may form associations at the local, regional, national, and global levels, through which poor women can more effectively challenge higher-level power structures and further empower themselves for the well-being of society as a whole.

Conclusion

Grassroots experiments in empowerment have made considerable headway since the mid-1980s, but it is clear — at least in South Asia — that they have a long way to go. One obvious reason is the absence of a democratic environment. An empowerment process of the kind outlined here is impossible without democratic space for dissent, struggle, and change. Theocratic, military, or other kinds of authoritarian states, based on ideologies of dominance and gender subordination, simply will not allow radical women's empowerment movements to survive. Perhaps for this reason, many approaches to empowerment in South Asia tend to avoid overtly political activities; activists provide women with opportunities and services, and encourage a certain level of awareness, but avoid more serious challenges to the dominant ideology or power structures.

A second, more pervasive, obstacle is a fragmented understanding of the concept and process of empowerment itself, with an accompanying lack of clarity about the nature of power, patriarchy, and gender. Male domination and gender discrimination tend to be oversimplified, equated with conspicuously oppressive practices like child marriage, dowry demands, wife beating, bigamy and polygamy, and denial of women's rights to equal food, employment, education, or physical mobility. The resultant approach focuses on women's practical rather than strategic needs. The organizing and consciousness-raising approach has come somewhat closer to a holistic strategy of empowerment, but still needs to solve many methodological problems before the complexities of the social construction of gender — and the ways in which family, class, caste, religion, and other factors perpetuating women's subordination — can be changed.

Notes

1 This chapter is based on the author's study of empowerment programs in three South Asian countries, entitled "Women's Empowerment in South Asia: Concepts and Practices" (forthcoming), sponsored by the Freedom from Hunger Campaign and Asia South Pacific Bureau of Adult Education).

2 This has come through clearly in my interactions in South Asia with nongovernmental organizations (NGOs), international aid agency representatives, academics, women's activists, government bureaucrats, and others.

3 Development Alternatives with Women for a New Era, a South-driven network of feminist scholars and women's groups, formed in 1984 in Bangalore, India.

4 The promotion of religious obscurantism in India, with its accompanying redefinition of Hinduism, is a case in point. We in the subcontinent are experiencing the revival and spread of a whole ideology, which culminated in the destruction of the Babri Mosque on December 6, 1992.

5 Arrack is a form of country liquor.

6 In India, members of a peasant and landless women's federation in southern Maharashtra, and of an urban slum women's federation (with chapters in 10 major cities) have successfully contested and won elections to municipal and local government bodies with different party platforms. The federations thereafter exercised the right to monitor their performance vis-à-vis the agenda for women's advancement, thus continually pressuring the concerned political parties to take up such issues.

References

Akhtar, F. (UBINIG, an NGO engaged in empowerment of rural women, Dhaka). 1992. Personal communication.

Anveshi. 1993. *Reworking gender relations, redefining politics: Nellore village women against arrack.* Hyderabad.

Batliwala, S. 1994 (forthcoming). *Women's empowerment in South Asia: Concepts and practices.* New Delhi: Food and Agricultural Organization/Asia South Pacific Bureau of Adult Education (FAO/ASPBAE).

Brydon, L., and S. Chant. 1989. *Women in the Third World: Gender issues in rural and urban areas.* New Brunswick, N.J.: Rutgers University Press.

Forgacs, D. (ed.). 1988. *An Antonio Gramsci reader: Selected writings, 1916–1935.* New York: Schocken Books.

Freire, P. 1973. *Pedagogy of the oppressed.* New York: Seabury Press.

Gupte, M., and A. Borkar, 1987. *Women's work, maternity and access to health care: Socioeconomic study of villages in Pune District.* Bombay: Foundation for Research in Community Health.

Hawkesworth, M. E. 1990. *Beyond oppression: Feminist theory and political strategy.* New York: Continuum.

Joseph, A. 1993. Brewing trouble. *The Hindu,* March 7.

Kannabiran, K. (a feminist activist of ASMITA, a women's resource center in Hyderabad, India). 1993. Personal communication.

Misra, A. 1978. *Chipko movement: Uttarakhand women's bid to save forest wealth.* New Delhi: People's Action.

Molyneux, M. 1985. Mobilization without emancipation? Women's interests, the state, and revolution in Nicaragua. *Feminist Studies* 11:2.

Moser, C. 1989. Gender planning in the Third World: Meeting practical and strategic needs. *World Development* 17:1799-1825.

Nelson, C. 1974. Public and private and politics: Women in the Middle Eastern world. *American Ethnologist* 1(3):551-563.

Rodda, A. 1991. *Women and the environment.* London: Zed Books.

Schuler, M., and S. Kadirgamar-Rajasingham. 1992. *Legal literacy: A tool for women's empowerment.* New York: UNIFEM.

Sen, G., and C. Grown. 1985. *Development alternatives with women for a new era: Development crises and alternative visions.* London: Earthscan.

Sharma, K. 1991–1992. Grassroots organizations and women's empowerment: Some issues in the contemporary debate. *Samya Shakti* 6:28–43.

Stacey, M., and M. Price. 1981. *Women, power, and politics.* London and New York: Tavistock Publications.

Walters, S. 1991. Her words on his lips: Gender and popular education in South Africa. *ASPBAE Courier* 52:17.

Young, K. 1988. *Gender and development: A relational approach.* Oxford: Oxford University Press.

10

Women's Burdens: Easing the Structural Constraints

Sonalde Desai

Increasing women's education, improving their income-earning opportunities, and breaking down sociocultural barriers to their health-seeking behavior are necessary but not sufficient means to achieve better health for individuals and families. These individual-level changes are unlikely to lead to desired gains without concomitant improvements in women's physical and social environment that enable women to function more effectively in their multiple roles. Needed is an enabling physical and social environment, including improved infrastructure for basic needs (water, sanitation, and fuel) and women's empowerment in familial relationships.

Health policies and programs emphasize the role of women as health providers in the family and community, while "women in development" policies encourage women to expand their economic activities. Both approaches require increased time commitments from women who are already overburdened. Neither alone takes into account or helps to change inequalities in gender responsibilities for child care and household maintenance, nor does either improve basic infrastructural constraints. Three major responsibilities that fall on women — collecting water, gathering

fuel, and parenting — are reviewed here as examples of enabling conditions that are essential to the empowerment of women and achievement of health for women as well as their families.

Overburdening Mothers

Social science and public health research has revealed the importance of mothers' education and employment for child health and survival. Among the maternal factors influencing children's health, considerable attention has been devoted to characteristics such as education, employment, and maternal position within the household (see Mahmud and Johnston in this volume). An extensive literature on women's education suggests that educated mothers are more likely than less-educated women to adopt safe hygienic practices, thereby reducing children's exposure to gastrointestinal diseases (Caldwell et al. 1990). Additionally, children of educated mothers are more likely than those of less-educated women to receive appropriate and timely medical treatment. Consequently, improvement of female education is one of the primary health recommendations of the 1993 *World Development Report* (World Bank 1993).

The interaction between child health and maternal employment is more complex and less clear. Some have found that employment outside the home reduces time spent in child care or, where the child accompanies the mother, may expose the child to health risks (Basu and Basu 1991). Research on intrahousehold resource allocation has concluded that maternal employment increases a mother's bargaining power within the household and thus results in improvement in child health by increasing resources devoted to children (Acharya and Bennett 1983; Mencher 1988; Thomas 1992).

Drawing on such findings, policy makers have focused on mothers as agents of change. As Bruce and Dwyer have noted (1988), "the invisible women of the economic theorist become the all-powerful mothers of the health and welfare advocates." Primary health care programs that promote community participation rely predominantly on women (Leslie, Lycette, and Buvinic 1988), and many child health programs require intensive time involvement by mothers. Although women already work very long hours, and typically longer hours per day than men (see Table 1), such policies often assume that women's "natural" ability and willingness to undertake more work are limitless (Kabeer 1992). While health policies rely on women's willingness to undertake more work, other social forces have also made increasing inroads into women's time. Policies and programs to incorporate women into development income-generating activities, like health programs, require substantial time and effort by women, often for marginal improvement in income (Buvinic 1983; Heyzer 1992). Further, they tend to ignore the broader context of women's social relations and living conditions (Goetz 1991). (See Box 1.)

Many, if not most, of the women who are the clientele of these policies must spend a substantial portion of each day in domestic activities necessary for family survival. Fuel and water collection

---

BOX 1

Why Holistic Approaches Are Needed

Lillian Nkuzo, a community health worker in South Africa describes her work:

In order to tell you about the Women's Health Project, I should first describe the conditions in Cala. Women in this area live under very oppressive conditions. They are responsible for their children and families, as men generally work away from their homes for a long time. They plant crops in the fields, collect water and fuel such as firewood or cow dung, employ men who can shear the sheep, and then sell the wool (although they have to keep the money until their husbands come home on holiday). They only get money from their husbands once a month, and sometimes nothing comes. Lack of water is the main disadvantage in the area, because sometimes the women have to walk six kilometers to and from the water supply, and can carry only 20 liters of water, which does not provide enough for the family for a day.

Poverty is overwhelming in the whole area. Women buy food from shops on credit every month, as the land is no longer productive because of the drought.

Some people live far from the available health centers, and there is no transport available to assist them even during an emergency, because there are no roads. This situation is really upsetting when a woman is in labor and suffering great pain. She has to be taken to a health center on foot for distances as long as 20 to 30 kilometers, to where transport is available. This commonly results in the death of the newborn, or even the mother. It is awful when accidents occur, and because people do not know about first aid, people sometimes bleed to death. I always advise women to attend first aid and home nursing courses so that they can deal with such incidents.

Source: Klugman 1993.

| | | T A B L E 1 | | | | | | |

Results from Time-Use Studies in Developing Countries

Country Study	Home Production Time		Market Production Time		Total Work Time		Female/Male Ratio
	Males	Females	Males	Females	Males	Females	
Asia							
Bangladesh (rural) Caldwell et al. 1980	0.34	6.20	7.31	4.17	7.65	10.37	1.35
Bangladesh (urban) Caldwell et al. 1980	0.71	5.40	4.20	1.77	4.91	7.17	1.46
Bangladesh (rural) Cain et al. 1979	1.29	6.68	7.04	1.61	8.33	8.29	0.99
Nepal (rural) Nag et al. 1978	2.10	4.76	8.06	7.42	10.16	12.18	1.20
Nepal (rural) Acharya and Bennett 1982	1.74	4.67	6.33	6.15	8.07	10.82	1.59
Philippines Laguna (rural) King and Evanson 1983	1.30	7.42	6.85	2.51	8.15	9.93	1.22
Laguna (rural) Popkin 1983	1.03	7.20	7.30	5.20	8.33	12.40	1.49
Laguna (rural) Folbre 1983	0.49	7.50	8.38	0.89	8.87	8.39	0.95
Indonesia Java Hart 1980	0.80	5.20	7.90	5.90	8.70	11.1	1.28
Java Nag et al. 1980	0.60	4.72	7.80	5.88	8.40	10.6	1.26
Africa							
Botswana (rural) Mueller 1984	1.02	3.94	3.68	2.06	4.70	6.00	1.28
Tanzania (rural) Kamuzora 1980	1.32+	3.89+	10.75	9.98	12.07	13.87	1.15
Central African Republic (rural) FAO 1983	0.22+	3.64+	5.28	4.30	5.50	7.94	1.44
Ivory Coast (rural) FAO 1983	0.75+	5.02+	3.18	1.78	3.93	6.80	1.73
Burkina Faso (rural) McSweeney and Freedman 1980	0.28	5.46	7.27	4.31	7.55	9.50	1.26
South America							
Peru (rural) Johnson 1975	0.96	4.50	4.01	3.62	4.97	8.12	1.63

* Average hours per day. + Excludes child care time.
Source: Calculated from Leslie, Lycette, and Buvinic 1988.

are among the most common and best documented. For example, a study conducted in the hills of Uttar Pradesh in India revealed that women spend as much as five hours per day searching for firewood. Studies in the Sahel show women spending between three and four hours per day walking up to 10 kilometers to collect firewood. (For a review of some of these studies, see Agarwal 1986.) In semiarid parts of southern India, time budget studies show that women spend nearly four hours per day fetching water for family consumption and washing utensils and clothes (Desai and Jain 1992).

Analysts all too often assume that changes in individual behavior can overcome the impact of unfavorable changes of public policy — for example, the removal of public subsidies for food grains. It is sometimes argued that when faced with higher food prices and declining incomes, poor households can shift their consumption habits to maintain their levels of nutrition (Behrman 1988). This type of analysis fails to recognize that some of these changes (such as substitution of millet for rice) may impose considerable time demands on women, not only to cook the food, but also to collect the firewood required for longer cooking time.

As mothers, grandmothers, and sisters, women shoulder almost all responsibilities for child care, regardless of their involvement in economically productive work and household maintenance. In rural southern India, women who are not engaged in outside economic activities spend about seven and a half hours per day in domestic activities, and women who spend seven or more hours per day in market work continue to spend nearly seven hours per day in domestic activities, excluding child care (Desai and Jain 1992). As a result, relatively little time is available to these women for child care. In fact, studies show that some rural women spend no more than one hour per day in direct child care (Ware 1984). This has serious implications for child nutrition and care during illness. Children under two require a considerable amount of food, but can consume relatively little at a single time. Ideally, they

should be fed many times a day, and depending upon the diet, each feeding takes about 20 minutes. Given the domestic and economic demands on women, mothers may not be able to devote this time to feeding children, and as a result, children may be malnourished *even when adequate food is available* (see Box 2).

The multiple demands on women's time also affect their access to health care and their ability to follow prescribed treatments. Oral rehydration therapy is particularly demanding of women's time because it requires constant feeding of very small amounts of solution over a long period. A study conducted in Honduras, for example, documented that in some situations, mothers administer very little of the solution to children (Kendell, Foote, and Martorell 1984). A related problem is that the solution may not meet mothers' felt needs because it does not actually stop diarrhea (Bolton et al. 1989).

Domestic activities, in conjunction with economic activities and child care, force women and girls to reduce time in rest, leisure, and education (Jain and Chand 1982). Research shows that domestic duties routinely interfere with girls' school enrollment (Lloyd and Gage-Brandon 1992) and that high activity levels, combined with low nutritional intake, place women at considerable health risk (Batliwala 1985).

Gender Relations and Paternal Responsibility

We have already noted the generally unequal burden of domestic maintenance and child care responsibilities allocated to women as compared with men. We know of no significant programs to encourage greater male involvement. In fact, a policy focus on mothers' contributions could, if anything, reinforce existing gender inequalities and may even encourage men to abdicate their paternal responsibilities.[1] For a variety of complex reasons, an increasing number of families in both the developed and the developing worlds rely solely on women; this is particularly evident in Latin America and southern Africa. The pathways through which households end up relying

Taking Care of Our Children: The Experiences of SEWA Union

SEWA (Self Employed Women's Association) is a membership-based trade union in India with 50,000 poor self-employed women as paying members. Founded in 1972, SEWA has worked to empower women by addressing the multiple roles of a woman's life, including union organization, credit, artisan and home-based production, milk production, land development and water harvesting, and health services. SEWA focuses in particular on problems and priorities identified by the women themselves.

One SEWA effort is a village-based program to meet the child care needs of working women. Poor women need the security that comes with full employment and regular income. However, their time is often constrained by their role as caretaker, especially for children under age three. Despite the fact that many factories are required by law to provide a crèche on their premises, most do not; in most villages, government child care programs are rarely available. To address this need, SEWA,

in conjunction with 3,000 of its members, developed Shaishav (meaning childhood in Gujarati), a village-based crèche program. The objectives of this program are to provide comprehensive child care services (health, nutrition, and child development activities) for infants and children to age three, to enable workers to work and earn in the fields and tobacco factories, and to support workers in their struggle for full employment.

There are many important benefits of the crèche services: women can go to work more relaxed, knowing their children are being properly cared for; and monthly family income increases because women no longer have to forfeit their wages. The benefits for the children include improved health and nutrition, assistance in obtaining immunizations, better hygiene, and more schooling of older siblings as they are freed from taking care of their younger siblings.

Source: Chatterjee, M. and J. Macwan 1992.

primarily on women's economic contributions are diverse. The causes include divorce in the United States (Sweet and Bumpass 1990); single parenthood in developed countries, Latin America, and some southern African countries, such as Botswana (Lloyd and Desai 1992; United Nations 1990); polygamy or paternal migration in Sub-Saharan Africa (Lloyd 1993); and widowhood in South Asia (Dreze 1990). Table 2 (on next page) illustrates the likelihood that children in selected developing countries will live with their mother only or away from their mother. Children in Asia and North Africa spend only a small proportion of their time living in mother-only families, but the proportion in Sub-Saharan Africa and Latin America is much higher — for

example, in Botswana and Colombia, 26 percent and 13 percent, respectively. These national averages mask significant differences between regions and across social classes.

By and large, families supported primarily by women are poorer than families supported by both men and women, because they have fewer wage earners, they are subject to discrimination in the labor market and in inheritance patterns, and they may not receive economic support from the fathers (Goldscheider and Waite 1991; Mencher and Okongwu 1993; Weitzman 1985). As a result, children in female-supported households experience poorer health than others both in the United States (Mauldon 1990) and in developing countries (Buvinic et al. 1992; Desai 1992b).

Private Responsibility versus Public Infrastructure

In light of the factors discussed above, it is clear that policies to encourage and strengthen individual health behavior must be comple-mented by policies that create enabling condi-tions under which responsible individual action can be undertaken — namely, appropriate infra-structure (for instance, water and sanitation), access to basic needs (such as food and fuel),

| T A B L E | 2 |

Proportion of Time Potentially Spent Living Apart from Mother or Living with Mother Only by Country through Age 15

Country	Away from Mother	With Mother Only	Total
Sub-Saharan Africa			
Botswana	.28	.26	.54
Burundi	.06	.08	.14
Ghana	.18	.08	.26
Kenya	.07	.10	.17
Liberia	.29	.10	.39
Mali	.12	.02	.14
Senegal	.16	.04	.20
Zimbabwe	.15	.08	.23
Average			.26
Asia and N. Africa			
Indonesia	.04	.04	.08
Morocco	.03	.04	.07
Sri Lanka	.03	.05	.08
Thailand	.07	.05	.12
Tunisia	.01	.02	.03
Average			.08
Latin America and Caribbean			
Brazil	.04	.09	.13
Colombia	.06	.13	.19
Dominican Republic	.13	.14	.27
Ecuador	.04	.07	.11
Peru	.04	.09	.13
Trinidad and Tobago	.06	.17	.23
Average			.18

Source: Lloyd and Desai 1992.

supportive institutions (for example, changes in gender relations), and accessible and affordable social services. Elimination of diarrheal diseases in children requires more than promotion of oral rehydration therapy through mothers' nurturing work. It requires, equally, provision of clean drinking water and hygienic sanitation to prevent infection, investments in parents' skills (such as education, especially of girls and women), and shared parental responsibility for the care of children. Similarly, childhood malnutrition should be addressed, not simply through growth monitoring and food supplementation performed by mothers, but also through broader policies, such as food subsidies for the poor, improved economic livelihoods, more equable distribution of parental responsibilities, and investments in parental skills.

Nonetheless, oral rehydration therapy has frequently been favored over improvements in water and sanitation, and targeted nutritional supplementation has been advocated over more generalized food subsidies (United Nations 1990). A search of the POPLINE bibliographic data base revealed, for example, that of the 1,985 entries on diarrhea, 38 percent mention oral rehydration therapy and 22 percent mention education, but only 5 percent mention water supply, 8 percent mention sanitation, and a mere 2 percent mention income. A similar emphasis on individual behavior rather than on an enabling environment was revealed in bibliographic searches on child survival and health. Thus, the focus seems to be on the individual characteristics of the diseased, as well as individual responses to disease, rather than the social conditions that lead to disease (Kent 1991).

It has long been known that disease prevention, particularly prevention of gastrointestinal diseases, is linked to the quantity as well as quality of water supply and to good sanitation (Briscoe 1984, 1987; Mosley and Chen 1984). In fact, the World Bank estimates that the effect of providing access to safe water and adequate sanitation to all who currently lack it would result in two million fewer deaths from diarrhea each year among children under five years of age; 200 million fewer episodes of diarrhea annually; 300 million fewer cases of roundworm infection; 150 million fewer cases of schistosomiasis; and two million fewer cases of guinea worm infection (World Bank 1992). Similarly, the World Health Organization has estimated that improved availability and quality of water would lead to a 16 to 37 percent improvement in morbidity from diarrhea; and improved disposal of excreta would reduce morbidity by 22 percent (Esrey, Feachem, and Hughes 1985). The decade beginning in 1980 was designated as the International Drinking Water and Sanitation Decade. In 1990, partly because of the economic crises of the 1980s and a move toward privatization, nearly 855 million people were still without access to safe drinking water. Nearly 1.7 billion people worldwide do not have access to sanitation services (World Bank 1992).

Public policies can also reduce, rather than improve, poor people's access to fuel. In India, for example, privatization of common property resources in some areas drastically restricts access to forest lands (Guha 1983; 1985). Lack of access to cooking fuel also jeopardizes health by reducing the ability of poor families to regularly boil their drinking water, by compromising the full cooking of food, and by reducing the frequency of cooking. Studies in Bangladesh and the Sahel, for example, have also documented a decline in the number of times food is prepared per day, which may increase the risk of bacterial contamination of food in the absence of access to refrigeration (Agarwal 1986). In the Sahel, two possible dietary effects of fuelwood shortage have been noted: the diet of millet is rarely supplemented by meat, partly because large amounts of firewood are required for cooking meat, and many families seem to be shifting from millet to rice because rice takes a shorter time to cook (Hoskins 1982).

Public Policy

Public health research and practice too often have failed to confront the conflictive aspects of health — namely, the redistribution of power and resources in society required to meet basic needs for all (Chen 1991). Figure 1 compares factors known to enhance health and survival with health policies recommended by international agencies.

Government priorities regarding infrastructural investment are guided by a variety of factors, not the least of which is gender bias due to the absence of women, particularly rural women, at every level of the decision-making process. Failure to invest in water technology provides a classic example of gender bias. Closer proximity to protected water sources, improved water-carrying methods, and running water in the home are high priorities for most poor women. But national and field-level project managers and planners, as well as the decision makers in many international agencies, are men who may not perceive or value the importance of improved household access to water. Even within the community such bias exists. A Kenyan study documented that, although access to water was a high priority among rural women, it was typically considered a low priority by the village leaders, all of whom were men (Elmendorf 1982).

Another source of bias is reliance on narrowly defined economic cost-benefit analyses by the international donor community and governments. For example, some economic analyses have suggested that it may be more cost-effective to provide chemotherapy for tuberculosis than to attempt universal immunization, and that BCG vaccine is cost-effective only when the risk of infection is extremely high (World Bank 1993).[2] Another example are debates about the relative efficacy of investments in water and sanitation projects compared with investments in oral rehydration therapy for the control of diarrheal diseases. Financial calculations show that whereas water and sanitation provision involve substantial investment, oral rehydration therapy can be provided at a fraction of the cost. As a result, donor agencies typically have given priority to the latter over the former (Okun 1987). Such analyses fail to recognize that oral rehydration therapy is simply an immediate response to an acute problem — diarrhea — whereas water and sanitation invest-

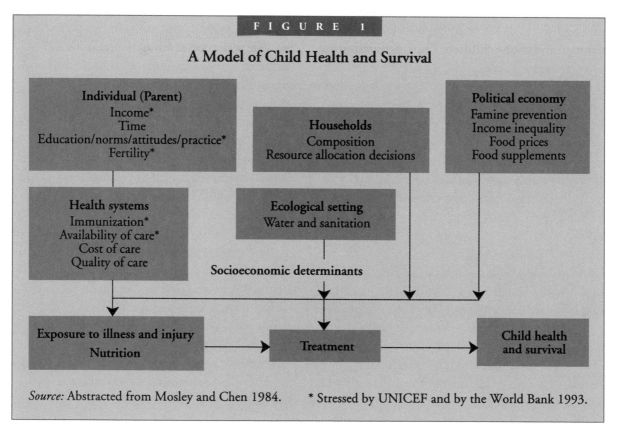

FIGURE 1

A Model of Child Health and Survival

Individual (Parent)
Income*
Time
Education/norms/attitudes/practice*
Fertility*

Households
Composition
Resource allocation decisions

Political economy
Famine prevention
Income inequality
Food prices
Food supplements

Health systems
Immunization*
Availability of care*
Cost of care
Quality of care

Ecological setting
Water and sanitation

Socioeconomic determinants

Exposure to illness and injury
Nutrition

Treatment

Child health
and survival

Source: Abstracted from Mosley and Chen 1984.   * Stressed by UNICEF and by the World Bank 1993.

ments are essential to prevent diarrheal disease to start with.

Nonetheless, the 1993 *World Development Report* (World Bank 1993) advises against public investments in water and sanitation projects based solely on "cost-effective" considerations. It argues that households should pay the costs of water and sanitation services because of productivity and amenity benefits. Under these conditions, substantial health gains are seen as an added bonus achieved at zero cost. Government investments in water and sanitation projects are discouraged on the grounds that "such subsidies compromise the demand-driven approach to services (that is, provision of services that people want and are willing to pay for); lack of accountability and inefficiency are inevitable consequences" (World Bank 1993:93).

This reliance on individual households to pay for improved water supply ignores both gender and class biases in the "willingness to pay" criterion. Household-level decisions about whether to pay for improved water supply may be made by the male household head, while the greatest burden of water collection is typically borne by women and young children. Thus, privatizing the costs of water and sanitation systems and arguing that individual families can decide whether they want to pay might exacerbate, not alleviate, the gender imbalance of burdens within the household.

Additionally, some studies have documented a strong class bias in existing water and sanitation systems (World Bank 1992). At present, most systems are biased in favor of urban consumers and, within this sector, in favor of the more affluent. For example, in Lima, poor people pay as much as $3 for a cubic meter of contaminated water collected by bucket from a private vendor, while the middle class pay $0.30 per cubic meter for treated water provided through taps in their house by the publicly subsidized water company. The 1992 *World Development Report* (World Bank 1992) cites this as an example of a bloated public service utility company, and recommends

reduction in public subsidies. It does not ask why, in spite of their willingness to pay $3 per cubic meter for water, the poor remain without an improved source of water and whether this removal of public subsidies would improve their situation. Complete privatization and market competition is rarely possible with respect to utilities, even in industrial countries. Privatization may lead to a reliance on private monopolies that may exacerbate existing inequalities in access to water and sanitation. Finally, there may be disjunction between private and public good: if a household chooses not to invest in sanitation services, the effects will be experienced by the wider community through environmental contamination.

It may be impossible to achieve high-quality water and sanitation systems for all in many countries. The costs of water supply and sanitation services vary by technology, population density, the hydrological and geological environment, and design standards; costs can range from $15 to $200 per person per year. Design standards of highest quality may not be necessary, however. For example, it may be difficult to provide waterborne sewage systems for all households but it may be possible to develop alternatives such as pour-flush latrines.

Conclusion

It is apparent that efforts to improve child health through the time, skills, and labor of mothers are insufficient. Without concomitant investments in water and sanitation systems, groundwater supply, and the institutions that govern common property resources, as well as the gender division of labor, instrumental approaches not only may increase the costs to women but, in so doing, may reduce the likelihood of success. This brief discussion of infrastructure investments and economic policies that jeopardize basic needs underscores the need to move beyond short-term interventions to long-term development processes that enable women and men to care for their own health and that of their children.

Notes

1 Some studies from the United States have concluded that increased female labor force participation and income may be associated with higher divorce rates and male withdrawal from family commitments (Furstenberg 1988; Farley 1988). Similar research has not yet been done in diverse socioeconomic contexts.

2 Estimates of the efficacy of BCG vaccine in preventing tuberculosis vary from zero to 80 percent (Fine 1988), and there is no consensus on what leads to high efficacy. But there is widespread consensus that BCG is efficacious — as high as 80–95 percent — in reducing the incidence of such serious forms of tuberculosis as miliary tuberculosis and tuberculous meningitis (National Research Council 1993; Schwoebel, Hubert, and Grosset 1992).

References

Acharya, M., and L. Bennett. 1983. Women and the subsistence sector: Economic participation and household decision-making in Nepal. Staff Working Paper No. 526. Washington, D.C.: World Bank.

Agarwal, B. 1986. *Cold hearths and barren slopes: The woodfuel crisis in the Third World*. New Delhi: Allied Publishers.

————. 1991. Engendering the environment debate: Lessons from the Indian subcontinent. Distinguished Speaker Series No. 8. Center for Advanced Study of International Development.

Basu, A. M., and K. Basu. 1991. Women's economic roles and child survival: The case of India. *Health Transition Review* 1:83–103.

Batliwala, S. 1985. Women in poverty: The energy, health and nutrition syndrome. In D. Jain and N. Banerjee (eds.), *Tyranny of the household: Investigative essays on women's work*. New Delhi: Shakti Books.

Behrman, J. R. 1988. The impact of economic adjustment programs. In D. E. Bell and M. E. Rich (eds.), *Health, nutrition and economic crises: Approaches to policy in the Third World*. Dover, Mass.: Auburn House.

Bolton, P., et al. 1989. Health technologies and women of the Third World. In R. S. Gallin, M. Aronoff, and A. Ferguson (eds.), *The women and international development annual*, vol. 1. Boulder, Colo.: Westview Press.

Briscoe, J. 1984. Water supply and health in developing countries: Selective primary health care revisited. *American Journal of Public Health* 74:1009–1013.

————. 1987. A role for the water supply and sanitation in the child survival revolution? *Bulletin of the Pan American Health Organization* 21:93–105.

Bruce, J, and Dwyer, D. (eds.). 1988. Introduction in *A home divided: Women and income in the Third World*. Stanford, Calif.: Stanford University Press.

Buvinic, M. 1983. Women's issues in third world poverty: A policy analysis. In M. Buvinic, M. A. Lycette, and W. P. McGreevey (eds.), *Women and poverty in the Third World*. Baltimore, Md.: Johns Hopkins University Press.

Buvinic, M., et al. 1992. The fortunes of adolescent mothers and their children: The transmission of poverty in Santiago, Chile. *Population and Development Review* 18:269–297.

Caldwell, J., et al. 1990. *What we know about health transition: The cultural, social and behavioural determinants of health*. Canberra: Australian National University Printing Service.

Chatterjee, M., and J. Macwan. 1992. Taking care of our children. The experiences of SEWA Union. Working Paper No. 1. SEWA Paper Series, December. Ahmedabad, India: SEWA Academy.

Chen, L. 1991. Summary of the health transition workshop at Harvard University. *Health Transition Review* 1:115–122.

Cornia, G. A., R. Jolly, and F. Stewart. 1987. *Adjustment with a human face: Protecting the vulnerable and promoting growth, vols. 1 and 2*. Oxford: Clarendon Press.

Desai, S. 1992a. The impact of family size on children's nutritional status: Insights from a comparative perspective. Research Division Working Paper No. 46. New York: Population Council.

————. 1992b. Children at risk: The role of family structure in Latin America and West Africa. *Population and Development Review* 18:689–717.

Desai, S., and D. Jain. 1992. Maternal employment and changes in family dynamics: The social context of women's work in rural South India. Research Division Working Paper No. 39. New York: Population Council.

Desai, S., et al. 1992. Maternal employment and changes in family dynamics: The social context of women's work in rural south India. Research Division Working Paper No. 39. New York: Population Council.

Dreze, J. 1990. Widows in rural India: Development economics program. Paper No. 26. London School of Economics.

Elmendorf, M. 1982. *Women, water and waste: Beyond access*. Washington, D.C.: WASH Project.

Esrey, S. A., R. G. Feachem, and J. M. Hughes. 1985. Interventions for the control of diarrhoeal diseases among young children. *Bulletin of the World Health Organization* 63:757–772.

Ewbank, D. C., and J. N. Gribble, (eds.). 1993. *Effects of health programs on child mortality in Sub-Saharan Africa*. Washington, D.C.: National Academy Press.

Farley, R. 1988. After the starting line: Blacks and women in an uphill race. *Demography* 25:477–495.

Fine, P. E. M. 1988. BCG vaccine against tuberculosis and leprosy. *British Medical Bulletin* 44(3):691–703.

Folbre, N. 1983. Of patriarchy born: the political economy of fertility decisions. *Feminist Studies* 9(2):261-284.

Furstenberg, F., Jr. 1988. Good dads-bad dads: Two faces of fatherhood. In A. Cherlin (ed.), *The changing American family and public policy*. Washington, D.C.: Urban Institute Press.

Goetz, A. M. 1991. Feminism and the claim to know: Contradictions in feminist approaches to women in development. In R. Grant and K. Newland (eds.), *Gender and international relations*. Bloomington: Indiana University Press.

Goldscheider, F. K., and L. J. Waite. 1991. *New families no families? The transformation of the American home*. Berkeley: University of California Press.

Griffin, C. 1992. *Health care in Asia: A comparative study of cost and financing*. Washington, D.C.: World Bank.

Guha, R. 1983. Forestry in British and post-British India: A historical analysis. *Economic and Political Weekly*, October 29.

———. 1985. Scientific forestry and social change in Uttarkhand. *Economic and Political Weekly* 20(45–47).

Halstead, S. B., J. A. Walsh, and K. Warren, (eds.). 1985. *Good health at low cost*. New York: Rockefeller Foundation.

Heyzer, N. 1992. Gender, economic growth and poverty. *Development* 1:50–53.

Hill, K., and A. R. Pebley. 1989. Child mortality in the developing world. *Population and Development Review* 15:657–687.

Hoskins, M. 1982. Women in forestry for local community development: A programming guide. Paper prepared for the Office of Women in Development, U.S. Agency for International Development, Washington, D.C.

Jain, D., and M. Chand. 1982. *Report on a time allocation study—its methodological implications*. New Delhi: Institute of Social Studies Trust.

Jodha, N. S. 1986. Common property resources and rural poor. *Economic and Political Weekly*, July 5.

Kabeer, N. 1992. Triple roles, gender roles, social relations: The political sub-text of gender training. Working Paper No. 313. Dhaka: Bangladesh Institute of Development Studies.

Kamuzora, C. L. 1984. High fertility and the demand for labor in peasant economies: The case of Bukoba District, Tanzania. *Development and Change* 15(1):105-124.

Kendell, C., D. Foote, and R. Martorell. 1984. Ethnomedicine and oral rehydration therapy: A case study of ethnomedical investigation and program planning. *Social Science and Medicine* 19:253–260.

Kent, G. 1991. *The politics of children's survival*. New York: Praeger.

Klugman, B. 1993. *With our own hands: Women write about development and health*. Johannesburg: Department of Community Health, University of the Witwatersrand.

Leslie, J., M. Lycette, and M. Buvinic. 1988. Weathering economic crisis: The crucial role of women in health. In D. E. Bell and M. E. Rich (eds.), *Health, nutrition and economic crises: Approaches to policy in the Third World*. Dover, Mass.: Auburn House.

Lloyd, C. B. 1993. Family and gender issues for population policy. Research Division Working Paper No. 48. New York: Population Council.

Lloyd, C., and S. Desai. 1992. Children's living arrangements in developing countries. *Population Research and Policy Review* 11:193–216.

Lloyd, C. and A. Gage-Brandon. 1992. Does sib size matter? The implications of family size for children's education in Ghana. Research Division Working Paper No. 45. Population Council.

Mata, L. 1988. A public health approach to the food–malnutrition–economic recession complex. In D. E. Bell and M. E. Rich (eds.), *Health, nutrition and economic crises: Approaches to policy in the Third World*. Dover, Mass.: Auburn House.

Mauldon, J. 1990. The effect of marital disruption on children's health. *Demography* 27:431-446.

Mencher, J. 1988. Women's work and poverty: Women's contribution to household maintenance in South India. In D. Dwyer and J. Bruce (eds.), *A home divided: Women and income in the Third World*. Stanford, Calif.: Stanford University Press.

Mencher, J., and A. Okongwu. 1993. *Where did all the men go? Female headed/female supported households in cross-cultural perspective*. Boulder, Colo.: Westview Press.

Mosley, W. H., and L. C. Chen. 1984. An analytical framework for the study of child survival in developing countries. *Population and Development Review* 10 (Supplement):25–45.

National Research Council. 1993. *Effects of Health Programs on Child Mortality in Sub-Saharan Africa*. Washington, D.C.: National Academy Press.

Okun, D. 1987. *The value of water supply and sanitation in development: An assessment of health-related interventions.* Technical Report No. 43. Washington, D.C.: WASH.

Palloni, A. 1981. Mortality in Latin America: Emerging patterns. *Population and Development Review* 7:623–649.

Schwoebel, V., B. Hubert, and J. Grosset. 1992. Impact of BCG on tuberculous meningitis in France in 1990. *Lancet* 340:611.

Shepard, D. S. and E. R. Benjamin. 1990. User fees and health financing in developing countries: Mobilizing financial resources for health. In D. E. Bell and M. E. Rich (eds.), *Health, nutrition and economic crises: Approaches to policy in the Third World.* Dover, Mass.: Auburn House.

Shiva, V. 1988. *Staying alive: Women, ecology and survival.* London: Zed Books.

Sweet, J., and L.L. Bumpass. 1990. *American families and households.* New York: Russell Sage Foundation.

Thomas, D. 1992. The distribution of income and expenditure within the household. Paper presented at the International Food Policy Research Institute–World Bank Conference on Intrahousehold Resource Allocation: Plicy Issues and Research Methods, 12-14 February, in Washington, D.C.

United Nations. 1990. *Patterns of first marriage: Timing and prevalence.* New York.

Victora, C. G., et al. 1993. International differences in clinical patterns of diarrhoeal deaths: A comparison of children from Brazil, Senegal, Bangladesh, and India. *Journal of Diarrhoeal Disease Research* 11:25–29.

Ware, H. 1984. Effects of maternal education, women's roles, and child care on child mortality. *Population and Development Review* 10 (Supplement):191–214.

Weitzman, L. 1985. *The divorce revolution.* New York: Free Press.

Wibowo, D., and C. Tisdell. 1993. Health, safe water and sanitation: A cross-sectional health production function for Central Java, Indonesia. *Bulletin of the World Health Organization* 71:237–245.

World Bank. 1992. *World development report 1992.* New York: Oxford University Press.

———. 1993. *World development report 1993.* New York: Oxford University Press.

11

Women's Status, Empowerment, and Reproductive Outcomes

Simeen Mahmud and Anne M. Johnston

The literature on women's status and fertility has evolved since the 1970s from a narrow focus on specific indicators, such as women's education, to a broader concern with women's autonomy and decision-making power. During the late 1970s and early 1980s, the negative correlation between women's education and fertility was substantiated by considerable empirical evidence, and captured the attention of policymakers. Researchers then attempted to understand the links between fertility and women's access to gainful employment, but found no simple correlation. By the mid-1980s, researchers and advocates recognized that women's status depends on many factors and has multiple dimensions; they recognized, as well, that status is related in complex ways to demographic behavior.

Some of these complexities are examined in the literature of the 1990s, which shifts the focus somewhat away from statistical correlations between women's status and fertility. Instead, analysts have begun to examine the interconnections among the exercise of human rights (such as the right to work, to acquire an education, and to enjoy freedom of movement), women's perception of their own well-being and self-efficacy, and a broad range of reproductive decisions (see Anand in this volume). Such studies have assessed the role of women's autonomy in decisionmaking, and have considered the resources needed to alter or circumvent restrictions on this autonomy at many cultural and institutional levels. Research, policy debate, and action programs are beginning to recognize the centrality of gender-based power relationships in influencing the decision-making processes by which reproduction is determined.

In this chapter, we assess research on the impact of women's education and work on reproduction, review some of the key conceptual questions involved in delineating women's status and autonomy, and describe the possible implications of women's status for reproductive decisionmaking at the individual or couple level. Finally, we reflect on the policy implications of moving beyond earlier, more instrumental treatments of women's education and employment, to concepts of women's autonomy and empowerment that acknowledge and support women as subjects and actors in reproductive decisionmaking.

Empirical Evidence

We review briefly below the findings on female education and reproduction and on women's work and reproduction as the basis for assessing the implications of women's status for reproductive decisionmaking.

Women's Education and Reproduction

Many studies provide evidence of a strong correlation between the educational level of the woman and a couple's fertility, while the educational level of the man correlates less well (Cleland and Rodriguez 1988; Cochrane 1979). World Fertility Survey data also indicate strong associations between women's education and marriage age, desired family size, and contraceptive use in developing countries (United Nations 1987). Data for 30 countries show an average total fertility rate of 6.9 children per woman among those with no education, three children more than among women with seven or more years of schooling.

Researchers hypothesize that more education works indirectly to reduce fertility in a number of ways: by delaying marriage and increasing the chance that a woman will never marry; by reducing desired family size by stimulating aspirations for a higher standard of living and increased investments in fewer children; by preparing women for employment, especially in the formal sector; and by exposing women to new knowledge, attitudes, and practices regarding contraceptive use (Le Vine et al. 1991). Caldwell suggests that education prepares women to respond to more opportunities, challenges traditional values, and weakens the authority of the old over the young, as well as of men over women (Caldwell 1982). Women's education is also the most influential variable in the improvement of child health and reduction of infant deaths (Caldwell 1986a,b).

Although much of the attention to the relationship between women's education and fertility is focused on the impacts of education on the costs and benefits of children to their parents, some studies have attempted to assess how education may influence women's personal attitudes and their roles in reproductive decisionmaking. Cochrane, Leslie, and O'Hara (1982) found, for instance, that education not only delayed the wife's age at marriage, but also increased husband-wife communication and knowledge, and improved attitudes and access to birth control, all of which were negatively related to fertility.

The importance of individual attitudinal changes, both in their own right and in combination with other factors has been frequently emphasized in analyses of the channels through which formal education operates (Cochrane, Leslie, and O'Hara 1982; Le Vine 1982). Several plausible models of the impact of schooling on the attitudes and later behavior of girls have been set out (Le Vine 1982; Le Vine et al. 1991). These include the cognitive growth model, which assumes that "schooling endows the girl with an expanded awareness of means-end relationships in her environment and the capacity to see it in novel contexts as she encounters them"; the self-development model, which posits that schooling "bolsters the self-esteem, sense of personal efficacy, and belief in internal control" of persons in a "position of subordination and compliance"; and the identification, model which hypothesizes that girls are exposed to a new kind of interaction with the adult teacher, which they later imitate as mothers (Le Vine 1982). All of these models describe the impact of education on child care, parenting, and, to a lesser extent, fertility behavior.

Some of the hypotheses in these models are borne out by empirical studies. In discussing the complex mechanism through which improved maternal education raises child survival in rural Punjab, Das Gupta (1990) concludes that education raises maternal skills and self-confidence, increases maternal exposure to information, and alters the way in which others respond to women. Caldwell (1979), examining child mortality differentials by mother's education for Yoruba women in western Nigeria, finds that women who have been to school feel more responsible for the health and welfare of their children than do those with no formal education. They are better able to ensure that their mother-in-law, their husband, or a health worker will behave in ways that are favorable to child survival; for instance, they may succeed in persuading their husbands to contribute a larger share of family resources for children and to demand smaller labor contributions from children.

So far as attitudes toward contraception are concerned, although it is well established that a woman's education is a primary determinant of her contraceptive knowledge and use, and of family size, it is less clear whether it is only formal education that makes a difference (Dixon-Mueller 1993). Most studies assess the easily quantifiable years of schooling, but do not address such other forms of training as adult literacy programs, informal education, and exposure to extension services, which are more difficult to measure.[1]

It is possible that the effective use of birth control, and the adoption of behavioral and investment strategies to maximize the survival and well-being of fewer children depend on the woman's attitude toward, experience of, and knowledge about family planning and health services, *irrespective of whether she has ever attended formal school.* A variety of sources besides formal schooling — such as peer and support networks, women's credit and savings groups, informal education, and other women's programs — may be even more important. For example, in an examination of regional differences in mortality levels in India, the level and nature of political awareness was found to explain differential access to, demand for, and utilization of health services, after income differences were controlled for (Nag 1989). Results of research still under way in this area could provide useful pointers to the connections between programs for women's empowerment and reproductive decisionmaking.

Women's Work and Reproduction

Research on the effects of women's employment has had two foci: implications for women's autonomy, and the extent of incompatibility between women's roles as mothers and as income earners. Employment outside the home has the potential to reduce women's dependence on others; provide alternative sources of social identity and support; increase women's desire to delay marriage; motivate women to terminate unsatisfactory relationships; and space or limit births (Dixon-Mueller 1978; Safilios-Rothschild 1982). While economic activity generally (though not

always) provides women with a resource base, its influence on women's reproductive decision-making is determined largely by the underlying institutional structures that govern the value of women's labor in any society and the conditions under which women engage in economic activity. The relationship between gainful employment and greater reproductive and sexual choices is dependent on a myriad of factors, such as type of occupation, income, motivation, whether the woman works for someone or is self-employed, duration and continuity of work, and whether the work is full- or part-time.

Empirical observations suggest that the impact of women's nondomestic work on fertility differs by type and magnitude of remuneration, workplace, type of activity, and occupation; but there has been little consistency in either the strength or the direction of the observed relationship (Youssef 1982). Investigations of the association relate fertility to the gender division of labor in society, the demand for female labor, and the economic opportunities available to women (Youssef 1982). Where pressure for economic survival forces women to take up market employment, women not only continue to bear the burden of domestic work, but also suffer the consequences of gender-based inequities in the labor market, such as lower wages, less regular employment, and a higher level of underemployment than men. In such situations women's employment may do little, if anything, to strengthen their capabilities to implement their reproductive preferences (Bruce and Dwyer 1988).

Although some evidence exists for a negative association between women's employment and fertility, other studies demonstrate no relation between the two. Studies of maternal role incompatibility[2] conclude that it is the "household's opportunity structure," through which it accumulates status and resources, rather than role conflicts between "mothering" and "working," that determines the relationship between women's work and fertility (Mason and Palam 1985). The lack of clarity regarding the existence and direction of the relationship may be due not only to the nature of the employment and women's broader circumstances, but also to methodological inconsistency and simplistic analytic approaches (Wainerman 1981). Available evidence is insufficient to determine whether women who enter the labor force bear fewer children than others or whether women with fewer children tend to have higher levels of labor force participation (Wainerman 1983).

In some contexts, independent earning by poor women does appear to affect traditional gender relations within the household, enhancing women's participation and voice in decisions. For example, research shows that compared with women who depend entirely on their husband's incomes, poor rural South Asian women who are involved in credit programs supported by government or nongovernmental organizations hold a better position relative to men in the household; the women studied appear to exercise a degree of autonomy, as evidenced particularly by their higher use of birth control and significantly greater physical mobility (Amin and Pebley 1990; Mahmud 1993; Nelson 1979). Outside earning provides women with a critical support mechanism in crises, an enhanced capability to deal with threats, and a higher value in the family as perceived by themselves and others (Bruce and Dwyer 1988). Autonomy is further enhanced if cooperative work settings are available that allow participation in decisionmaking, provide credit and marketing facilities, and improve access to job-related services such as health and child care.

The greatest benefits accrue when women not only earn income, but also directly control that income and achieve economic security as a result. Research in a number of developing countries that assesses women's control over earnings, not just their employment, concludes that control over income is a better predictor of demand for children and subsequent fertility (Kritz and Makinwa-Adebusoye 1993). In Bangladesh, for example, poor rural women with greater control over their own incomes and greater access to

husband's incomes were found to limit births through modern contraceptives more frequently than women who depend entirely on their husband's earnings (Mahmud 1993). In the African context, survey data on currently married women in Nigeria reveal that women's control over their earnings has a strong negative effect on the demand for children (Kritz and Makinwa-Adebusoye 1993). Further research is needed to develop better measures of women's access to income and control over resources at the household level, and to identify the impact on women's decision-making capabilities (see Bruce and Dwyer 1988).

With respect to the impact of maternal employment on child welfare, the importance of the institutional context is even more evident. A growing number of studies reveal a significantly greater allocation of women's incomes than men's to subsistence consumption, including food, and a positive correlation between children's nutritional status and mother's income and subsistence food inputs (Bruce and Dwyer 1988). In contrast, there are situations where maternal employment has been associated with higher infant or child mortality and undernutrition (Basu and Basu 1991).

Research in South India shows that the impact of women's income-earning work on child welfare is mediated by pervasive poverty, women's excessive total work burdens, and lack of access to basic infrastructure (Desai and Jain 1992). Irrespective of the extent of their participation in income earning, the domestic work burdens of rural women in poor regions restrict the time available for child care. The choice between caring for children and engaging in employment hardly exists for women who are completely dominated by the physical demands of their domestic tasks, the imperative to earn income, or both. These findings indicate the need, in future research, to incorporate the larger economic and institutional context in investigations of the relationship between women's employment and reproductive outcomes (see Desai in this volume).

Conceptualizing Women's Status and Autonomy

Increasing understanding of the complexity of women's status has led to the development of alternative concepts such as female autonomy, women's rights, and men's situational advantage. (See Box 1.) Mason's (1984) review of these diverse concepts indicates that most focus on gender inequality. Three dimensions of gender inequality high-lighted most commonly are inequality in prestige, inequality in power, and inequality in access to or control over resources. Because there is more than one dimension and location in which it is possible for men and women to be unequal, women may be "powerful" in one dimension, such as routine household affairs, while completely powerless in another, such as control over productive resources, including their own labor. In addition, gender inequality may vary by location, such as the social unit (family, neighborhood, community, state), and by stage in the life cycle (see Adams and Castle in this volume).

Drawing conclusions from anthropological studies in developing countries, Epstein (1982) defines a woman's role as "the way she is expected to behave in certain situations," and her status as "the esteem in which she is held by different individuals and groups who come in contact with her." If we follow this definition, then status is clearly the esteem that adheres to particular roles and positions within a social hierarchy, and high status does not automatically provide autonomy from the behavioral requirements of the associated role. A particularly difficult dimension of defining or measuring women's status thus has to do with competing sources of "status" and the

---

B O X 1

The Consequences of Forced Marriage in a South African Community

Martha Ndlovu, a community health worker in South Africa, describes the social situation of girls in her community, especially marriage:

"At our home, girls are traditionally forced to get married. When you reach fourteen, you leave school and get married. Older people would say that if you kept attending school and did not get married, you would become stupid and end up as a prostitute, because you were surrounded by so many boys.

"I do not believe that all unmarried women become prostitutes; even married women can be prostitutes. The only thing that I hate about marriage is women's oppression within it. In our area, most of the women are clearly frustrated by early marriage.

"In the early 1970's, my father forced my elder sister to get married. My sister was fourteen at the time, and she disagreed with him because she felt she was too young. But my father kept insisting and threatened to throw my sister out of the house if she disobeyed him. He went to a man who paid R200 as *lobola* [bride price] and then let this man come and collect my sister. My father just frittered that money away.

"My sister was very unhappy in her marriage, but there was nothing she could do about the situation. She did not love the man, and he kept beating her because they could not live together. My sister became lean and ill. She had a heart attack and had to take constant medication. She has not been allowed to go to school, and has to look after four children. Generally, married women are not allowed to make any decisions or say anything which contradicts their husbands. They cannot use contraception of any kind because they should 'give birth until the babies are finished inside the stomach.' It does not matter whether you give birth ten or fourteen times."

Source: Klugman 1993.

value attached to them. For example, in a society that values female seclusion, women who are employed outside the home could gain status through income or the nature of the work, but they could lose status by giving up socially valued seclusion (Youssef 1982). Status and autonomy are both affected not only by attitudes and customs, but also by legal traditions (see Box 2). Nonetheless, improvements in status do not necessarily lead to increases in autonomy.

Dyson and Moore (1983) define equality of autonomy between men and women as "equal decision-making ability with regard to personal affairs." The gap between status and autonomy is evident in the fact that, although women may rise to higher status levels either as producers, as reproducers of labor, as mothers-in-law, or in other social roles, their subordination to men is not necessarily reduced (Safilios-Rothschild 1982). Thus, understanding of the power relations between men and women is essential if women's capability to participate in decisions affecting reproduction is to be enhanced. Furthermore, reproductive decisionmaking, while very much a personal concern for women, is also significantly influenced by family and often community concerns (see Box 2). At no time is this more evident than when a woman is being initiated into fertility behavior and child care responsibilities — namely, as a young bride.

The pathways of influence from women's increased autonomy to their fertility and child care behavior may be both indirect and direct. Empowering experiences that change women's perceptions of self-worth and well-being affect women's dependence on men and their ability to make decisions. These impacts flow back into the hierarchical social structure through women's existing relationships with men and "powerful" women. They also exert influence indirectly to reduce gender inequalities in prestige, control over resources, and decision-making power. Such changes in turn affect fertility and child care behavior by enhancing women's ability to take their own needs for health and well-being into account.

Important impacts may also emerge through the formation in different social locations (house-

hold, community, state, market) of new relationships that enhance self-esteem and self-efficacy, through access to independent information and peer support, and through physical mobility. Such relationships foster women's ability to weigh their own well-being relative to family size preferences, the health needs of their children, birth control preferences, and employment alternatives. Since empowerment is a dynamic process, the effects on reproductive behavior are continuous, responding to external forces and life cycle events as they unfold (see Batliwala in this volume).

Reflections on Policy

This analysis suggests that approaches that treat women's education and employment as instruments to reduce fertility are inadequate. What is needed are strategies for women's empowerment that lead to their increased autonomy and decision-making power, providing them with an alternative power base that is independent of the domination of men. Three crucial questions, among others, must be addressed in assessments of the empowering potential of employment. First, the conditions of work not only must include satisfactory and healthy work environments, protection against unemployment in cases of pregnancy or marriage, and access to appropriate services, such as child care; they also must ensure a reduction in women's total work burden, particularly their obligation to fulfill such basic responsibilities as obtaining water and fuel (see Desai in this volume). Second, women must have not only access to income, but also control over it. Third, employment will be more empowering to the extent that it provides women access to non-kin support, including women's groups, independent sources of information, and contacts with outsiders. Empirical support for this argument is provided by the experience of several nongovernmental organizations, particularly in India and Bangladesh, that have mobilized poor women through informal groups (Batliwala, this volume; Chen 1983).

Even in societies where the balance of power and control over productive resources are highly skewed toward men, women may gain access to power from such processes as conscientization through gender awareness, economic change, or mobilization for economic, social, or psychological support. These empowerment strategies may require new institutional arrangements directed to the needs of specific populations. While formal education may assist women to behave in more "modern ways" with regard to new technology (for instance, to use birth control, oral rehydration therapy, child vaccination, or more nutritious foods), the social barriers to educating girls are still quite strong in many situations. A more informal and contextually relevant type of education could focus better on women's practical and strategic needs, and empower them to bring about social changes affecting their well-being (see Batliwala in this volume).

Available evidence suggests that the most effective strategies are likely to be those that support women to organize peer groups *and* mobilize community resources and public services, including women's health services. Such approaches enable women to overcome negative perceptions of well-being and self-worth. Sen (1990) has argued that such negative perceptions and women's resignation to the "legitimacy of the established order" are important factors in the perpetuation of imbalances of power between women and men. Considerable evidence shows that these can be altered through conscious social policy (Papanek 1990; Sen 1990) and programs that treat women as subjects who can and ought to shape their own destinies. Adoption of such strategies would move population policies far beyond their past treatment of women as instruments.

Finally, if women are to implement their reproductive preferences, then it is essential that their empowerment occur not only within their personal spheres, but also in the broader spheres of the community and the state. As Dixon-Mueller (1993) has pointed out, the promotion of policies that encourage contraceptive use and smaller families are futile if not accompanied by the eradication of legal, social, and economic constraints on women.

Notes

1 It is important to note that the Convention on the Elimination of Discrimination against Women promotes equal access to these modes of training, all types of institutions, choice of curricula, financial aid, and scholarships. These areas warrant further investigation as indicators of knowledge exposure in relation to reproductive decisionmaking.

2 Maternal role incompatibility refers to the hypothesis that women's employment reduces fertility where contraception is widely available and where the roles of worker and mother are most incompatible — that is, where the job is away from home.

References

Amin, S., and A. R. Pebley. 1990. Gender inequality within households: The impact of a women's development program in 36 Bangladeshi villages. Paper presented at the Annual Meeting of the Population Association of America, May 3–5, in Toronto.

Armstrong, A., et al. 1993. Uncovering reality: Excavating women's rights in African family law. *International Journal of Law and the Family* 7:314-369.

Basu, A. M., and K. Basu. 1991. Women's economic roles and child survival: The case of India. *Health Transition Review* 1:83-103.

Batliwala, S. 1993. The Mahila Samakhya strategy for women's mobilization and empowerment. Unpublished manuscript.

Boserup, E. 1970. *Women's role in economic development.* New York: St. Martin's Press.

Bruce, J., and D. Dwyer. 1988. Introduction. In D. Dwyer and J. Bruce (eds.), *A home divided: Women and income in the Third World.* Stanford, Calif.: Stanford University Press.

Cain, M. 1981. Risk and insurance: Perspectives on fertility and agrarian change in Bangladesh and India. *Population and Development Review* 7:435-474.

Cain, M., and S. Nahar. 1979. Class, patriarchy and women's work in Bangladesh. *Population and Development Review* 5:405-438.

Caldwell, J. 1976. Towards a restatement of demographic transition theory. *Population and Development Review* 2:321-366.

————. 1979. Education as a factor in mortality decline: An examination of Nigerian data. *Population Studies* 33(3):395-413.

————. 1982. Education and fertility: An expanded examination of the evidence. In G. P. Kelly and C. M. Elliot (eds.), *Women's education in the Third World: Comparative Perspectives.* Albany, N.Y.: SUNY Press.

————. 1986a. The role of mortality decline in theories of social and demographic transition. In United Nations Department of International Economic and Social Affairs (ed.), *Consequences of mortality trends and differentials.* New York.

————. 1986b. Routes to low mortality in poor countries. *Population and Development Review* 12(2): 171–220.

Chen, M.A. 1983. *A quiet revolution: Women in transition in rural Bangladesh.* Cambridge, Mass.: Shenkman Publishing Co.

Cleland, J., and G. Rodriguez. 1988. The effect of parental education on marital fertility in developing countries. *Population Studies* 42(3):419-442.

Cleland, J. C., and C. Scott. 1987. *World fertility survey.* Oxford: Oxford University Press.

Cochrane, S. H. 1979. *Fertility and education: What do we really know?* Baltimore, Md.: Johns Hopkins University Press.

Cochrane, S. H., J. Leslie, and D. J. O'Hara. 1982. Parental education and child health: Intracountry evidence. *Health Policy and Education.* 2(3–4): 213–250.

Das Gupta, M. 1990. Death clustering, mother's education and the determinants of child mortality in rural Punjab, India. *Population Studies* 44(3):489-505.

————. 1993. What motivates fertility decline? Paper presented at the conference on Population Reconsidered: Empowerment, Health, and Human Rights, December 6-10, in Harare, Zimbabwe.

Desai, S., and D. Jain. 1992. Maternal employment and changes in family dynamics: The social context of women's work in rural South India. Paper presented at the Annual Meeting of the Population Association of America, in Denver, Colorado.

Dixon-Mueller, R. 1978. *Rural women at work: Strategies for development in South Asia.* Baltimore, Md.: John Hopkins University Press.

————. 1993. *Population policies and women's rights.* Westport, Conn. and London: Praeger.

Dyson, T., and M. Moore. 1983. On kinship structure, female autonomy, and demographic behavior. *Population and Development Review* 9(1):35-60.

Epstein, T. S. 1982. A social anthropological approach to women's roles and status in developing countries: The domestic cycle. In R. Anker, M. Buvinic, and N.H. Youssef (eds.), *Women's roles and population trends in the Third World.* London and Sydney: Croom Helm.

Klugman, B. 1993. *With our own hands: Women write about development and health.* Johannesburg: Department of Community Health, University of the Witwatersrand.

Kritz, M. M., and P. Makinwa-Adebusoye. 1993. Women's resource control and demand for children in Africa. Paper prepared for the International Union for the Scientific Study of Population Committee on Gender and Population, in Dakar, Senegal.

Le Vine, R. A. 1982. Influences of women's schooling on maternal behavior in the Third World. In G. P. Kelly and C. M. Elliot (eds.), *Women's education in the Third World: Comparative perspectives.* Albany, N.Y.: SUNY Press.

Le Vine, R. A., et al. 1991. Schooling and survival: The impact of maternal education on health and reproduction in the Third World. Working Paper No. 3. Harvard School of Public Health.

Mahmud, S. 1993. Female power: A key variable in understanding the relationship between women's work and fertility. Dhaka: Bangladesh Institute of Development Studies. Unpublished manuscript.

Mason, K. O. 1984. *The status of women: A review of its relationships to fertility and mortality.* New York: The Rockefeller Foundation.

Mason, K. O., and V. T. Palam. 1985. Female employment and fertility in peninsular Malaysia: The maternal role incompatibility hypothesis reconsidered. *Demography* 18:549-575.

Nag, M. 1989. Political awareness as a factor in accessibility of health services: A case study of rural Kerala and West Bengal. Working Paper No. 3. New York: The Population Council.

Nelson, N. 1979. *Why has development neglected rural women: A review of south Asian literature.* Oxford: Pergamon Press.

Papanek, H. 1990. To each less than she needs, from each more than she can do: Allocations, entitlements, and values. In I. Tinker (ed.), *Persistent inequalities: Women and world development.* New York and Oxford: Oxford University Press.

Safilios-Rothschild, C. 1982. Female power, autonomy and demographic change in the Third World. In R. Anker, M. Buvinic, and N. H. Youssef (eds.), *Women's roles and population trends in the Third World.* London and Sydney: Croom Helm.

Sen, A. K. 1990. Gender and cooperative conflicts. In I. Tinker (ed.), *Persistent inequalities: Women and world development.* New York and Oxford: Oxford University Press.

Singhunetra-Renard, A. 1993. Complex relationship between production and reproduction. Paper presented at the Conference on Population Policy Reconsidered: Empowerment, Health, and Human Rights, December 6-10, in Harare, Zimbabwe.

Wainerman, C. H. 1981. *Female work and fertility in Argentina: Ideational orientations and actual behavior,* vol. 3. Geneva: International Union for the Scientific Study of Population, International Population Conference.

United Nations. Department of International economics and Social Affairs. 1987. Fertility behavior in the context of development: Evidence from the World Fertility Survey. New York.

———. 1983. The world of values and ideas: Women and work. In C. H. Wainerman, E. Jelin, and M. del C. Feijoo (eds.), *On what women want to do and do.* Mexico: El Colegio de Mexico y PISPAL.

Youssef, N. H. 1982. The interrelationship between the division of labor in the household, women's roles and their impact on fertility. In R. Anker, M. Buvinic, and N. H. Youssef (eds.), *Women's roles and population trends in the Third World.* London and Sydney: Croom Helm.

12

Gender Relations and Household Dynamics

Alayne Adams and Sarah Castle

Empowering women to make reproductive decisions requires understanding the web of intrahousehold relations within which women are caught. While recent research and policy have recognized the role of gender relations in decisionmaking, and their impact on household welfare, much of this analysis remains overly general. Lacking is a systematic assessment of power relations both between and within genders, and their influence on reproductive behavior and outcomes. Also overlooked are ways in which these relations change over the life cycle, and how they constrain or enable different kinds of reproductive decisions. Finally, by focusing excessively on fertility, research and policy have tended to neglect other reproductive decisions central to the health of women and children.

In this chapter we examine reproductive decisionmaking in the light of women's social and economic power, their prestige, their access to material and nonmaterial resources, and their control over these resources both within and beyond the household in rural West Africa. These dimensions of status are analyzed not only in terms of how women differ from men, but also in terms of how they differ from each other in the household, as well as in society at large. Recognizing that "…West African family structure typically places reproductive decisionmaking in the

hands of the husband and the economic burden mainly on the shoulders of the wife" (Caldwell and Caldwell 1987:421), we suggest that the capacity of an individual woman to gain and apply knowledge relevant to reproduction is strongly related to her social and economic power at any particular point in the life cycle.

Although fertility patterns and household forms vary widely in West Africa, and although these patterns depart sharply from classic Eurasian models — characterized by spousal coresidence, maternal childrearing, and some degree of cooperative decisionmaking (Lloyd 1993) — we hold that there are fundamental similarities in the importance of power and control within and beyond the household and in their influence on women's reproductive decisions and outcomes.

Recent Demographic and Health Surveys (Agounké, Assogba, and Anipah 1988; Demographic and Health Survey (DHS) 1988; Ndiaye, Sarr, and Ayad 1987; Traoré, Konate, and Stanton 1987) in West Africa indicate that large proportions of married women have no education, few use modern contraceptives, and many are in polygynous unions. Low median age at marriage and high total fertility rates are also apparent in these countries, with the notable exception of Ghana.[1] However, as Mason (1984) has argued, these conventional indicators of women's status are unidimensional, ignoring the many sources of women's status and the multiplicity of roles that women play simultaneously and throughout the life cycle. Thus, our discussion will focus instead on the nature of women's status as it pertains to their power, prestige, access to and control over resources within and beyond the household. While these variables are less easily measured, they reveal the dynamic constraints on women's reproductive decisions over the life cycle and provide insight on how fertility declines may be facilitated.

We begin with a discussion of some of the existing explanations of the social, cultural, and economic determinants of reproduction in West Africa. After clarifying and refining the concept of the household, we consider the influence of power relations, between and within genders, on the roles assumed by women, and their implications for women's autonomy and control over reproduction. Turning to social and economic relations beyond the household, we suggest how women's access to extrahousehold networks both contributes to and is a consequence of their status in the domestic domain. We conclude by focusing on the changing context and character of women's reproductive decisions over the life cycle.

Refining the Concept of the Household

The absence of a significant fertility decline in West Africa has been attributed to sociocultural and economic forces that preclude a change in the direction of intergenerational wealth flows, an intensification of child-rearing styles, or an increase in female status within the household and the community (Caldwell 1977; Caldwell and Caldwell 1987).[2] One important sociocultural force that sustains and rewards high fertility is the system of patrilineal descent that predominates in West African society. Indeed, given high rates of infant and child mortality in the region, high fertility has frequently been interpreted as an adaptive strategy to perpetuate the lineage.[3]

High fertility is also essential to subsistence farming and household survival in rural areas where a shortage of labor (not land) is a serious constraint to production. Having many offspring,

both biological and fostered, facilitates increased production and diversification of income. Offspring are also valued for their future obligation to provide economic and social security to their parents in old age.

Men and women in West Africa thus have strong motivation to maximize their fertility, and they do so through early and universal female marriage; polygynous unions, which ensure the supply of husbands; pressure on widows of reproductive age to remarry; and widespread antipathy toward or ambivalence about fertility control, especially among men (Lesthaeghe 1989).[4] These behaviors and attitudes, along with women's reproductive decisions and outcomes, are mediated through relationships inside and outside of households.

The household, however, is a problematic unit of analysis. Demographers collecting and using survey or census data generally employ definitions centered on the provision of food from a common granary, the use of a common hearth or cooking pot, or the enumeration of all persons who look to the same household head (United Nations 1980). Cross-sectional analyses of this kind have resulted in the widespread misconception that households are clearly bounded entities with an age- and gender-based hierarchical structure. Overlooked are complex intrahousehold relationships and functions, and important networks of support and obligation that extend beyond household boundaries.

Anthropologists, on the other hand, prefer the term "domestic domain," which relates not only to the preparation of food, but also to processes such as the socialization of children, the transference of property, and the maintenance and reproduction of household values and influence (Bender 1967; Goody 1976). Anthropological inquiry tends to focus on the classification of kinship and household size and profile (whether a stem, joint, or multiple family) in relation to production activities. While useful, this approach does not illuminate what goes on *within* households, and especially how social, economic, and power relationships influence reproductive behavior.

Proponents of the "new household economics" also tend to overlook important disparities among social, economic, and power relations central to the analysis of reproductive decisions and outcomes. They assume instead that all household members are united by a common desire to pool resources and maximize collective benefits (Becker 1976). Alternative models of household economic behavior have been advanced to better capture the variations in individuals' means and motives by conceptualizing theories of bargaining or "cooperative conflict" (Sen 1985, 1990). These theories recognize inequalities between individuals in the same household in terms of their access to economic resources and power, and thus document intrahousehold and extrahousehold economic transactions in a more realistic way. However, their primary focus on economic activity underestimates other important motives influencing individual and household behavior, including reproductive decisionmaking. Responding to monetary-based theories of economic activity, Bruce (1989) emphasizes how intrahousehold transactions and negotiations often involve currencies other than cash — such as labor, time, and information. Even this analysis pays little attention to differentiation within genders.

In this chapter, we integrate and refine demographic, anthropological, and economic conceptions of the household, viewing the household as a dynamic, functional system in which relations between and within genders define the context of decisionmaking. Households are characterized by internal social structures that are constantly changing because of migration, divorce, mortality, and fission. Morover, they have porous external boundaries, and are influenced by a wide system of networks through which important transfers of information and resources occur.

Women's Roles within and beyond the Household[5]

Oppong and Abu (1987) elaborate the multiple roles of women as mothers, wives, domestics, kin, workers, community participants, and individuals, and propose that women's health and reproductive decisions be viewed in terms of the relative satisfaction and resources accruing via each of these roles as they compete, complement, or change over the life cycle. However, the researchers do not recognize the impact of relations between and within genders on women's roles, and therefore overlook the influence these relations have on the power, prestige, and resources women can summon when making reproductive decisions. We first show how the roles described above are structured by "between-gender" relations (power relations involving men and women) and "within-gender" relations (specifically, power relations occurring among women). We then discuss how additional power is accrued from relations beyond the household.

Between-Gender Relations

In West Africa, marriage is not simply a contract between two individuals, but a definitive transfer of rights from one lineage to another. With the payment of brideprice, rights to sexual access, female reproduction, and labor (agricultural and domestic) are passed from the natal to the marital household. Even after the death of the husband, the institution of levirate, whereby a widow is inherited by her late husband's brother, frequently obliges a woman to stay within the marital lineage. Further entrenching the individual and lineage power of men over women is the widespread practice of polygyny (Goody 1976).

Within the marital household, gender relations are defined by segregation of roles between husband and wives, and between men and women more generally. Practices of early arranged marriages and polygyny, the influence and coresidence of kin, and the frequent separation of spouses due to migration discourage conjugal intimacy and the development of a strong husband-wife bond (Oppong and Abu 1987). In these patriarchal societies, men have ultimate authority over material resources in the household, such as land, and over the labor of women and junior household members. Women, having no direct access to land or male labor, must request these resources from their husbands or from other males in the household to whom they are obligated. Indeed, under systems of land tenure widespread in patrilineal societies in West Africa, the fields that a woman works are returned to the control of the marital household on her death or divorce.

Despite the apparent subordination of a woman's social and political power to her husband and his family, she maintains considerable economic independence. Separation of men's and women's financial budgets in West Africa is well documented and appears to persist even among the urban and highly educated (Abu 1983). This separation of spousal budgets helps to perpetuate polygyny by relieving men of financial responsibility for their wives (Abu 1983; Desai 1991). Women's financial independence from men can foster greater autonomy in reproductive matters relating to the health and nutrition of children, but not necessarily in fertility decisions. Men may be indifferent about or hostile to limiting family size, particularly if they bear little economic responsibility for their wives and offspring.

Between-gender relations thus have considerable influence on the biological outcomes of fertility. Through the exchange of bridewealth, men gain absolute rights to intercourse with their wives, have control over children born of such unions, and command their wives' labor to benefit the marital family. Among Fulani communities in rural Mali, bridewealth is sometimes paid after the birth of the couple's first child — in other words, after the woman's fertility has been proved (Castle 1992). Even in the case of divorce, women are valued as wives insofar as they are able to produce and reproduce (see Box 1). As a result of this social and economic emphasis on fecundity, women's self-esteem and perceived self-worth or self-efficacy are substantially determined by their reproductive performance. Whereas the benefits of high fertility accrue to both genders, reproductive failure, infertility, and subfecundity are frequently matters of shame and reproach borne by women alone.

B O X   1

Calculating the Value of a Woman

Hawa Salmana is a 25-year-old Fulani woman who lives in Mali. Like her husband, she has been divorced twice. She is renowned within her marital family for her feisty and forceful behavior. Before her third marriage, she had borne two children. Hawa has a very lucrative business selling kola nuts within the village. After her second divorce, her value was enhanced by her economic prowess and her demonstrated reproductive capabilities. As a result, she was bid for competitively by a number of suitors. Even though traditional bridewealth transactions for divorced women consist of a single monetary payment of 5,000 CFA ($15), her husband offered her family 30,000 CFA ($90) and gave Hawa an additional 5,000 CFA worth of clothes to secure her hand in marriage.

Source: Castle 1992.

Although the level and timing of childbearing can be said to result largely from the social control of men over women both in the household and in the wider community, as we argue next, these "fixed" outcomes can be sidestepped by actions and information associated with relations among women. These relations are, nonetheless, structured largely by the prevailing system of patriarchy that exists in West Africa.

Within-Gender Relations

In view of the separation of men's and women's time, financial budgets, and spheres of influence, it is important to examine how rural women differ from each other with respect to social, economic, and intellectual resources for reproductive decisionmaking. In relations with men, inequalities of power and influence are mainly due to differences in control over material resources, such as ownership of and access to land, labor, and capital. Differences among women relate mainly to inequalities in access to or control over nonmaterial resources, such as time, information, and labor within the domestic domain. Social and political relations among women have a significant impact on reproductive preference and performance, because they govern both access to services and use of information for child health and nutrition, pregnancy, and fertility regulation (Castle 1992). In addition, within-gender power relations influence women's parenting, marriage patterns, and use of time.

In West Africa, parenting patterns may be determined by both biological and social factors (Castle 1992; Isiugo-Abanihe 1985; Page 1989). Indeed, in the case of Sierra Leone, "methods of family formation are predominantly post-natal and socially managed and therefore the customary 'cost-benefit' calculus of biological fertility has little meaning in daily life" (Bledsoe 1990). Social strategies such as child fostering reduce the immediate time and economic costs of high fertility to biological parents and thereby remove an important inducement to fertility reduction. Among the Malian Fulani, the transfer of children is rigorously controlled by the *female* social hierarchy. Older women who have completed their childbearing and who require company or labor have unquestionable rights to claim the children of young female relatives who are obligated to them. The latter are required to give up their biological offspring to be fostered by senior, more socially powerful women, regardless of whether they wish to do so (Castle 1993).

Table 1 presents DHS data on the proportion of children living away from their biological mothers in three West African countries. It is important to note, however, that evidence from a study of Fulani and Dogon communities in rural Mali indicates that conventional survey methodologies, such as those employed by the DHS, may substantially underestimate the proportions of children under five living away from their biological mothers (Castle 1993). While a cross-sectional survey of 334 mothers using a "DHS approach" estimated that 5 percent of children under five live under nonmaternal care, results from a longitudinal study of the same population indicate that nearly one-third of weaned children under five live away from their biological mothers.

Another feature of the West African household that has implications for gender relations between women is the institution of polygyny. As Goody (1976: 51-52) states, "domestic organization is…more complex and domestic relationships more diffuse when many households consist of a plurality of wife/mothers, at least for a part of their cycle of development." With the addition of a co-wife, roles and relations in the household change. The sharing of household chores allows women greater freedom to pursue independent economic activity (Adams 1992). Polygyny may also benefit the reproductive health of women and the health and nutrition of children by facilitating prolonged post-partum sexual abstinence.[6] Cooperation in the polygynous household is of-

---

TABLE 1

Percentage of Children Living Away from Their Biological Mother, by Age

Country	Total	Age		
		0-4	5-9	10-14
Ghana	15.2	4.2	18.2	29.4
Mali	10.5	3.6	13.5	17.8
Senegal	13.6	5.7	16.3	24.0

Source: Lloyd and Desai 1991.

ten counterbalanced by conflict as jealousy develops between co-wives over the attentions of their husband. In some cases, women play out these rivalries within the domain of reproduction, using children as political pawns to further their objectives within the household economy. For example, Bledsoe (1993) describes how, in Sierra Leone, conflicts among co-wives over the educational prospects of their respective children have led to accusations of witchcraft, or to senior women's assigning arduous chores to the children of more junior co-wives. In the same setting, co-wives were noted to decrease their duration of breast-feeding to hasten their return to fecundability, in hopes of "outdoing" rival wives in terms of the number of offspring they produced for their husband (Bledsoe 1987).

Finally, the degree of a woman's autonomy in the household can influence her reproductive decisions and behavior. When a woman's labor is controlled by other family members, she may be constrained by a lack of time or autonomy from fulfilling personal reproductive goals. By contrast, if she is free to engage in individual economic activity, she can gain access to considerable economic and social resources that facilitate her acquisition and use of information to control her fertility and the health of her children. Evidence suggests that, independent of the effects of education and socioeconomic status, as women gain autonomy within and outside the household, they are more likely to innovate or take risks (Miles Doan and Bisharat 1990) — for example, to adopt modern contraceptive methods and seek health care for themselves and their children (Dyson and Moore 1983). Figure 1 traces the female life cycle in West Africa, highlighting the relative balance of individual versus household production, and the degree of social and economic power women wield in the domestic and external environments.

Women's Relationships beyond the Household

In West Africa, roles and relationships beyond the marital household are conditioned by a woman's stage in her reproductive life. Particular importance is given to menarche, first birth, and menopause. At the same time, women gain considerable knowledge, information, and control from interactions in the external world, which in turn affect reproductive decisions taken within the household. Social and economic roles and relations beyond the household may involve other households, as well as the community and market economy.

Role in Other Households

Research in other cultural settings has indicated that a woman's relationships with members of her natal family are important to her sense of security and psychological well-being (Jeffery, Jeffery, and Lyon 1989; Zeitlin, Ghassemi, and Mansour 1990). While studies in Asia have considered marriage distance and its relationship to women's status (Dyson and Moore 1983; Fricke, Axinn, and Thornton 1992), little work has been done on this subject in Africa, nor have the consequences for reproductive decisionmaking been considered. In Mali, where marriage constitutes a work relationship between a woman and her husband's relatives, women are often returned to their natal families when they cannot carry out household duties because of childbirth, child care, or ill health. For example, all Fulani women return to their mother's house in the seventh month of their first pregnancy and remain there for up to a year afterward. Men may also send married women back to their natal families as a coping strategy during periods of stress, risk, and food insecurity.[7] Removed from the influence of their husbands and other senior household members, and supported by natal kin, women may enjoy greater autonomy. It should be noted, however, that the balance between extrahousehold support and commitment, and intrahousehold obligations must be carefully negotiated. If these boundaries are overstepped, tragic consequences for women's reproductive health and well-being may result (see Box 2 on page 168).

Role in the Community

Given the nature of gender relations in most West African societies, women's involvement and leadership in the community are largely confined to the female sphere. Nevertheless, women's relations with the broader community may enhance their knowledge about reproductive matters, including fertility and its control, and give them confidence to apply it. For example, among the Ibo of Nigeria and the Akan of Ghana, women entering marriage must appear before a council of older women who explain to them the rules that

FIGURE 1

Women's Life Cycle in West Africa

AGE	STAGE	DESCRIPTION
0-2	Infancy	Universal breast-feeding of infants is associated with intensive maternal care.
2-6	Young childhood*	The care of young children is assumed by older siblings through the weaning period (about age 2). During this stage, the risk of a child's dying is greater than in infancy.
6-9	Childhood	Young girls begin to be socialized to the household labor economy.
9-13	Pre-adolescence	Pre-adolescent girls assume increased responsibility as productive members of their fathers' families (fetching firewood and water, providing child care).
13-17	Puberty	With the onset of menses, arrangements for marriage are finalized.
16-18+	Marriage 1st birth 2nd birth ▼ to 6-7th birth	On average, the total fertility rate is 6-7 live births per woman. Sahelian childhood mortality (0-5) is 200-250/1000. Therefore, a woman on average can expect to lose 2-3 children during her reproductive career. During this stage, a woman's reproductive and productive duties to her marital family outweigh autonomous activities for personal social and financial gain.
32-40	1st child marries	If a daughter-in-law joins the household, the woman is released from domestic duties allowing for greater involvement in commercial and agricultural activity for personal gain. If her daughter marries into another household, she loses an important source of domestic assistance
45+	Menopause	This stage is marked by increased community and familial sociopolitical power by virtue of a woman's postmenopausal status. She also gains considerable public stature and respect as a diagnostician and healer.
50+	Widowhood	With the death of her husband, the sociopolitical power gained as a mother-in-law is largely lost. The widespread practice of levirate means that widows are inherited by their husband's younger brother, and remain in the marital family. However, in some cases, she may live separately and rely on nearby daughters (and **not** daughters-in-law) for subsistence.
55-60+	Death	

* Research indicates no sex differentials in anthropometric status, feeding practices or mortality risks in West Africa (Garenne et al. 1987; Gbenyo and Locoh 1989). This reflects the perceived importance of female's productive and reproductive roles to household viability, and their contribution to the welfare of male members.

Conflicting Loyalties: Marital Obligations and Natal Affiliations in West Africa

Dikko Allay is a Fulani woman aged 43 who lives with her husband, his parents, and her five surviving children in Mali. In December 1991, she underwent her 10th delivery — a stillborn boy. A few days after the birth, she developed a severe postpartum infection and needed to be hospitalized. Her marital family refused to organize the necessary transport and cash because Dikko had broken customary restrictions on interactions with her natal family.

Dikko loved her biological sister and brother, and to express her affection, she had paid for her sister's dowry (*ginna*). She had also given her sister valuable gold earrings, which according to patrilineal tradition, should have gone to the elder of Dikko's two daughters. In addition, she had given her brother one of two cows which in theory should have gone to one of her three sons. Her husband was furious at her display of disloyalty to his family and children, and told her that she could not expect any help or support from him.

Dikko's natal family also appeared unwilling to help. Her mother said Dikko's husband was responsible for looking after his wife. Dikko's sister volunteered to go with her to the dispensary, but their mother would not let her. Finally, because Dikko would have died, the researcher, together with Dikko's brother and sister, took her on a donkey cart seven kilometers to a hospital. The researcher paid for the treatment, and the brother and sister remained by Dikko's bedside for 10 days and nursed her back to health. During Dikko's stay in the hospital, neither her mother nor any member of her marital family came to visit. Although her doctor told her to refrain from intercourse, she said that she could not refuse her husband sex, which she believed would be a Quranic sin. She returned home after an injection of Depo Provera to protect her from pregnancy for three months.

Source: Castle 1992.

govern their sexual and reproductive lives (Mair 1953). For the most part, entry into the wider community is biologically determined; the onset of menarche signals initiation into age-set affiliations, while the onset of menopause endows women with widely respected social and political power.

Role in the Economy

Owing to the segregation of spousal budgets, most West African women participate in some form of market commerce. However, the gains from participating in the external economy are not simply financial. Skills used in interactions in the marketplace — including bargaining, management, the manipulation of individuals and goods, forward planning, and investment — may be useful in the domestic domain as well. Given

the low levels of formal female education in West Africa, such skills are likely to have important consequences for reproductive decisions. In particular, these skills enhance a woman's bargaining power in sexual relations and decisionmaking relating to the health and well-being of her children.

Reproductive Decisions over the Life Cycle

Women's motivation and capacity to use knowledge about sexuality and reproduction are influenced by their age and stage in their marital and reproductive careers. For example, in the Gambia, Bledsoe et al. (1993), found that women choose contraceptives according to three main criteria, the balance among which varies over the life cycle. The first consideration is the degree of confidentiality that particular contraceptives afford; the second relates to the speed with which fecundity resumes after contraceptive use terminates; the third concerns the likelihood of impaired fertility in the long term.

Life cycle changes sometimes can result in conflicts of interest regarding a woman's current and future reproductive needs and goals. For example, despite Malian women's frequently verbalized preference for boys, research suggests that they benefit immensely from daughters' help with child care, food preparation, and assistance with household tasks (Castle 1992). Thus, although patriarchal and patrilineal systems of marriage and inheritance make women dependent on sons for old age security, daughters often provide greater advantage in the short run. The fostering of young girls as domestic labor, therefore, reflects women's multiple needs and the variety of strategies they pursue to maximize both short- and long-term security.

As Figure 2 describes, women's multiple roles as mothers, wives, domestics, kin, workers, community participants, and individuals vary at different stages of the life cycle, and dictate in large part the degree of interhousehold and intrahousehold activity, influence, and movement that women enjoy. For example, an unmarried daughter has fairly loose ties to the domestic environment because she has yet to assume the roles of wife and mother. Her domestic responsibilities are performed out of respect for her natal kin, not because she has a social obligation to female in-laws. She is therefore able to move freely beyond the household and to fulfill roles as kin, individual and worker. She has, however, little power, prestige, or control over resources. Daughters-in-law, by contrast, carry out domestic and reproductive duties expected of them by their husbands' mothers and perform such activities within, rather than beyond, the household. These young

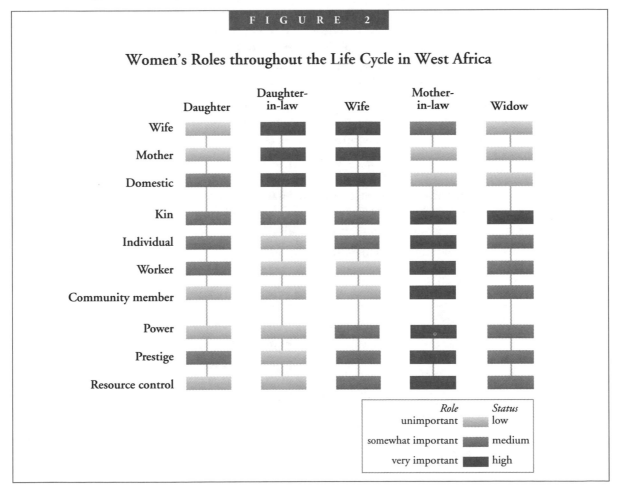

FIGURE 2

Women's Roles throughout the Life Cycle in West Africa

women begin childbearing early to win prestige and approval from their husband and his family, and use the roles of wife and mother to gain status in the eyes of the individuals to whom they are obligated. In the case of the daughter-in-law, therefore, intergender and intragender relations determine the context within which reproductive decisions are made. By contrast, married women who are not subject to the authority of a mother-in-law or co-wife have more power, prestige, and resource control within the household. While they are still subject to the patriarchal authority of their husbands and other male kin, their increased status may result in greater individual autonomy in reproductive matters.

Women whose daughters and daughters-in-law have begun their own reproductive careers are permitted to gain prestige and autonomy through economic activity rather than through childbearing. Indeed, in many West African societies it is considered shameful to continue bearing children after becoming a grandmother. Instead, the availability of children as domestic labor, together with older women's prestige by virtue of their senior status in the household or their position as mother-in-law, frees them for independent activity as kin, individual, worker, and community member. While their biological role as mother is ended, their social control over reproduction is considerable. Prestige and resources gained through independent economic activity, and their social power vis-à-vis younger women, may be wielded to obtain foster children from other households. In the same way, their senior status gives them considerable say in matters concerning pregnancy, child care, and nutrition. Widowed women may have some economic autonomy, but the absence of a male partner compromises their social power.

Conclusion

There are indications that the traditional reproductive regimes described here are changing as a result of external economic and social forces. For example, it is argued that the prolonged faltering of national economies since the 1980s due to structural adjustment, rising costs of imports, declining commodity prices, and increasing food insecurity is contributing to a change in the perceived costs of children (Lesthaeghe 1989). This is especially apparent in countries like Ghana and Nigeria, where increased school fees and high unemployment challenge the social and economic bases of high fertility. Further destabilizing traditional fertility and marriage patterns are changes with respect to land tenure and lineage control, and increases in social stratification due to differential wealth, education, and wages, as well as to migration and urbanization (Lesthaeghe 1989).[8]

Studies among urban educated and migrant populations have indicated change in the midst of continuity. While there is evidence of increased individualism, marital disruption, and a dwindling of the rights and duties of the conjugal family in some spheres of activity (Oppong 1982), the household and lineage remain central to social and economic life. Rather than being abandoned, traditional household structures and relationships are sometimes synchretically adapted and redefined. For example, the preference for modern nuclear units has in many cases led to relegation of polygynous wives to *deuxième bureaux*, or second households, and not to the rejection of polygyny (Fainzang and Journet 1988). As Bruce (1989) contends, economic pressures and social change such as the rise in male migration and marriage disruption are "spinning the family as traditionally defined down to its core — mothers and children."

In this chapter we have argued that intrahousehold dynamics are a critical determinant of women's reproductive decisions and outcomes. In reappraising the concept and definition of the household, we urge that analysis, policies, and programs heed the many competing interests and multiple economies found within and beyond its boundaries. In particular, it is important to consider the complex power relations between and within genders in the household as they are forged and negotiated via bargaining over material and nonmaterial resources.

Consideration of women's reproductive decision-making within the household has two broad policy implications. First, given that the economic and time costs of high fertility do not necessarily fall on biological parents, demand for family planning services may be limited in societies where fixed demographic outcomes such as "completed family size" can be manipulated socially by institutions such as fosterage. The value of children as productive members of the household economy from an early age and their obligation to provide old age security to their parents also discourage men and women from limiting offspring. In this context, coordinated policies and programs to provide social and livelihood security, education, and improved agricultural and domestic technologies may help facilitate change in reproductive expectations and outcomes (see Desai in this volume).

Second, it is imperative that population policies be sensitive to the particular needs and constraints of women at the various stages of their reproductive careers. Not only do reproductive needs and constraints vary over women's life cycle, so too does the complex of power relations within and beyond the household that influence their reproductive options and behavior. These relations determine women's control over resources needed to access reproductive health services and information, and, ultimately, over reproductive outcomes. Broadly based policies and programs are required to strengthen younger women's economic and social power within and beyond the household, and enhance their access to and command over both material and nonmaterial resources.

Notes

1 Ghana has many anomalous characteristics. High levels of education across all age groups, a later age at marriage, and a greater prevalence of contraceptive users (despite small total numbers) in older age groups point to the uniqueness of Ghana vis-à-vis the rest of West Africa. This may well be related to the fact that the Akan and Ashanti, who constitute nearly half the population in Ghana, are matrilineal and thus practice different systems of residence and inheritance than the patrilineal societies found in the rest of the region (Phillips 1953).

2 Analyses of DHS data indicate the start of a fertility transition in Botswana, Kenya, and Zimbabwe; except in Senegal, this trend is absent in West Africa(Agounké, Assogba, and Anipah 1988; DHS 1988; Ndiaye, Sarr, and Ayad 1987; Traoré, Konate, and Stanton 1987). In Senegal, a later age at marriage has been associated with a small decline in fertility, whereas in Botswana, Kenya, and Zimbabwe, increased contraceptive use has resulted in larger and more sustained fertility declines.

3 Evidence suggests, however, that more important than absolute numbers of surviving children is the degree of social control that senior household members wield over them. A survey in the Seno-Mango region of Mali requested Fulani and Dogon women to describe numerically what they considered "a lot" of children. When asked what disadvantages were associated with the number of children they cited, all referred to a lack of social control over many offspring, who might, for example, abandon them to seek employment. Rather than problems with sheer numbers of children, it was the children's potential lack of obedience or loyalty that was perceived as difficult (Castle 1992). Similarly, in a survey of Bambara agriculturists in central Mali, only two of 148 respondents associated household food insecurity with too many mouths to feed (Adams 1992).

4 Balancing these norms and practices are compensatory fertility-controlling practices, which include pressures against premarital fertility, widespread postpartum female sexual abstinence, and a common resort to permanent female abstinence once women become grandmothers (Caldwell 1977). It should be noted, however, that many of these "fixed" cultural practices are sidestepped or negotiated. For example, in Sierra Leone, a prolonged prohibition on intercourse during breastfeeding is overturned by the use of tinned milk, which culturally sanctions an earlier return to sexual relations (Bledsoe 1987).

5 The following discussion of power relations within the household focuses largely on households in which both genders are present and women are not household heads. While there is a growing literature on female-headed households (Bruce 1989; Bruce and Lloyd 1992), relatively little work has been done on the power relations within them. For policy purposes, the growing incidence of female-headed households and their reproductive health needs merits increased attention.

6 Polygyny, however, can also facilitate transmission of reproductive tract infections among the co-wives.

7 In a longitudinal study in central Mali, one Dogon woman who had 18-month-old twins and an additional child under five was returned to her natal village by her mother-in-law because she was too occupied with child care to carry out household duties (Castle 1992). Similarly, among the Bambara, household food insecurity often precipitates the temporary migration of women to their natal villages during the dry season, which relieves

their husbands' families of the burden of feeding them (Adams 1992).

8 According to the World Bank (1992), on average, about 30 percent of the total population in West Africa live in major urban centers; the proportion varies from only 9 percent in Burkina Faso to 40 percent in Côte d'Ivoire. Among the fast-growing population of urban migrants are increasing numbers of young unmarried women, who are often expected to support extended family members in rural areas.

References

Abu, K. 1983. The separateness of spouses: Conjugal resources in an Ashanti town. In C. Oppong (ed.), *Female and male in West Africa*. London: George Allen and Unwin.

Adams, A. M. 1992. Seasonal food insecurity in the Sahel: Nutritional, social and economic risk among Bamana agriculturists in Mali. Ph.D. thesis. Faculty of Medicine, University of London.

Agounké, A., M. Assogba and K. Anipah. 1988. Enquête Démographique et de Santé au Togo. Columbia, Md.: Demographic and Health Surveys, Institute for Resource Development, Westinghouse.

Becker, G. 1976. *The economic approach to human behaviour*. Chicago: University of Chicago Press.

Bender, D. 1967. A redefinement of the concept of household: Families, coresidence and domestic functions. *American Anthropologist* 70(2):493–504.

Bledsoe, C. 1987. Tinned milk and child fosterage: Side-stepping the post-partum sexual taboo. Paper prepared for Rockefeller Conference on the Cultural Roots of African Fertility Regimes, February 25–March 1, in Ife, Nigeria.

———. 1990. Transformations in Sub-Saharan African marriage and fertility. *Annals of the American Academy* 510:115–125.

———. 1993. The politics of polygyny in Mende education and child fosterage transactions. In B. Miller (ed.), *Sex and gender hierarchies*. Cambridge: Cambridge University Press.

Bledsoe, C., et al. 1993. Local cultural interpretations of Western contraceptives in rural Gambia. Paper presented at Program for International Cooperation in Africa Workshop, February 5–6, at Northwestern University, Evanston, Illinois.

Bruce, J. 1989. Homes divided. *World Development* 17(7):979–991.

Bruce, J., and C. Lloyd. 1992. Finding the ties that bind: Beyond headship and household. Working Paper No. 41. New York: Population Council Research Division.

Caldwell, J. C. 1977. The economic rationality of high fertility: An investigation illustrated with Nigerian survey data. *Population Studies* 31(2):189–217.

Caldwell, J. C., and P. Caldwell. 1987. The cultural context of high fertility in Sub-Saharan Africa. *Population and Development Review* 13(3):409–437.

Castle, S. E. 1992. Intrahousehold variation in illness management and child care in rural Mali. Ph.D. thesis. Faculty of Medicine, University of London.

———. 1993. Fostering and the nutritional status of children in rural Mali: The importance of definition, context and research methodology. Unpublished.

Demographic and Health Survey (DHS). 1988. Ghana Statistical Service, Accra. Columbia, Md.: Demographic and Health Surveys, Institute for Resource Development, Westinghouse.

Desai, S. 1991. Children at risk: the role of family structure in Latin America and West Africa. Working Paper No. 28. New York: Population Council Research Division.

Dyson, T., and M. Moore. 1983. On kinship structure, female autonomy and demographic behaviour in India. *Population and Development Review* 9(1):35–60.

Fainzang, S., and O. Journet. 1988. *La femme de mon mari: Anthropologie du mariage polygamique en Afrique et en France*. Paris: L'Harmattan.

Fricke, T. E., W. G. Axinn, and A. Thornton. 1992. Going home again: Interfamilial relations, marriage and women's contact with their natal families in two Nepali communities. Paper presented at the annual meeting of the Population Association of America, April 30–May 2, in Denver, Colorado.

Garenne, M., et al. 1987. *Risques de décès associés à différents etats nutritionnels chez l'enfant d'age préscolaire: Rapport final*. Dakar: ORSTOM, Orana.

Gbenyo, K., and T. Locoh. 1989. Les différences de mortalité entre garçons et filles. In G. Pison, E. van de Walle, and M. Sala-Diakanda (eds.), *Mortalité et Société en Afrique*. Paris: INED and Presses Universitaires de France.

Goody, J. 1976. *Production and reproduction: A comparative study of the domestic domain*. Cambridge: Cambridge University Press.

Isiugo-Abanihe, U. C. 1985. Child fosterage in West Africa. *Population and Development Review* 11(1):53–73.

Jeffery, P., R. Jeffery, and A. Lyon. 1989. *Labour pains and labour power: Women and childbearing in India*. London: Zed.

Lestaeghe, R. J. 1989. Production and reproduction in Sub-Saharan Africa: An overview of organizing principles. In R.J. Lesthaeghe (ed.), *Reproduction and social organization in Sub-Saharan Africa*. Berkeley: University of California Press.

Lloyd, C. 1993. *Family and gender issues for population policy*. Proceedings of the UN Expert Group Meeting on Population and Women. New York: Population Council Research Division.

Lloyd, C., and S. Desai. 1991. Children's living arrangements in developing countries. Working Paper No. 31. New York: Population Council Research Division.

Mair, L. 1953. African marriage and social change. In A. Phillips (ed.), *Survey of African marriage and family life*. Oxford: Oxford University Press.

Mason, K. 1984. *The status of women: A review of its relationships to fertility and mortality*. New York: Rockefeller Foundation.

Miles Doan, R. M., and L. Bisharat. 1990. Female autonomy and children's nutritional status: The extended family residential unit in Amman, Jordan. *Social Science and Medicine* 31(7):783–789.

Ndiaye, S., I. Sarr, and M. Ayad. 1987. Enquête Démographique et de Santé au Sénégal. Columbia, Md.: Demographic and Health Surveys, Institute for Resource Development, Westinghouse.

Oppong, C. 1982. Family structure and women's productive and reproductive roles: Some conceptual and methodological issues. In R. Anker, M. Buvinic, and N. H. Youssef (eds.), *Interactions between women's roles and populations trends in the Third World*, London: Croom Helm.

Oppong, C., and K. Abu. 1987. *Seven roles of women: Impact of education, migration and employment on Ghanaian mothers*. Geneva: International Labour Office.

Page, H. 1989. Childrearing v. childbearing: Co-residence of mother and child in Sub-Saharan Africa. In R. J. Lesthaeghe (ed.), *Reproduction and social organization in Sub-Saharan Africa*. Berkeley: University of California Press.

Phillips, A. 1953. *Survey of African marriage and family life*. Oxford: Oxford University Press.

Sen, A. 1985. Women, technology and sexual divisions in trade and development. United Nations Council on Trade and Development, Working Paper No. 6. New York: United Nations.

_____. 1990. Gender and cooperative conflicts. In I. Tinker (ed.), *Persistent inequalities: Women and world in development*. New York: Oxford University Press.

Traoré, B., M. Konate, and C. Stanton. 1987. Enquête Démographique et de Santé au Mali. Columbia, Md.: Demographic and Health Surveys, Institute for Resource Development, Westinghouse.

United Nations. 1980. *Principles and recommendations for population and housing censuses*. New York: Department of International Economic and Social Affairs.

World Bank. 1992. *World development report: Development and the environment*. Oxford: Oxford University Press.

Zeitlin, M., H. Ghassemi, and M. Mansour. 1990. *Positive deviance in child nutrition—with emphasis on psychosocial and behavioural aspects and implications for development*. Tokyo: United Nations University.

Reproductive and Sexual Health

13

Reproductive and Sexual Health Services: Expanding Access and Enhancing Quality

Iain Aitken and Laura Reichenbach

For the population field, the concept of "reproductive health"[1] has gained increasing significance. There exists a growing recognition that reproductive health approaches to population have the potential of both expanding the constituencies that support population policies and enhancing the performance of family planning programs. Many innovative reproductive health programs have been launched by nongovernmental organizations (NGOs), especially women's groups, and some governments are attempting to offer a wider array of high-quality reproductive health services. Important questions remain to be addressed if access is to be expanded and quality enhanced. What constitutes the core of reproductive health services? How important are reproductive health problems? Do we have effective interventions against them? And how best can these services be provided? To begin to answer these questions, this chapter defines and estimates the burden of reproductive health problems; compares and prioritizes reproductive and other health interventions; and analyzes the barriers to expanding access and enhancing quality.

Data presented will demonstrate that reproductive health problems place very heavy burdens on women and children. Low-cost yet effective interventions to ameliorate most of these problems exist. When compared with other health interventions through cost-effectiveness analyses, these interventions are among the "best buys" in terms of health returns for each dollar invested (World Bank 1993). Reproductive health services, therefore, deserve high priority in virtually all societies. Nonetheless, in expanding access to these services and enhancing their quality, substantial challenges need to be overcome. We examine three of these: how to improve technical and social support for health workers, how to strengthen functional linkages in reproductive health programs, and how to integrate reproductive health and related services so as to attain program efficiency and effectiveness in diverse communities around the world.

Definition

Reproductive and sexual health as a concept encompasses a set of health problems or diseases associated with the physical and social risks of human sexuality and reproduction. Germain and Ordway (1989) define a reproductive health approach that enables women and men, including adolescents, everywhere to regulate their own fertility safely and effectively by conceiving when they desire, terminating unwanted pregnancies, and carrying wanted pregnancies to term; to remain free of disease, disability, or death associated with reproduction or sexuality; and to bear and raise healthy children. This approach does not demarcate which reproductive health problems are more important than others. Rather, it refers to clusters of health problems that impede healthy sexual and reproductive functioning, and vary according to the health circumstances of diverse populations.

Protection against disease and illness in fulfilling basic human functions of sexuality and reproduction is not simply a medical or technical challenge, but has major social, political, and developmental aspects. Especially relevant are the two-way relationships of reproductive health to human rights and empowerment, discussed elsewhere in this volume. Avoidance of premature death and unnecessary illness due to sexuality and reproduction deserves consideration as a basic human right. Good reproductive health enables people to pursue socioeconomic opportunities as part of individual and social development. Protecting human rights, both civil-political and sociocultural, and broadening access to material and social resources are vital to shaping the reproductive health of populations. The concept of reproductive and sexual health, therefore, goes beyond simply the prevention or treatment of disease and should be viewed as part of equity-oriented human development.[2]

Reproductive and Sexual Health Burdens

Reproductive and sexual health is concerned with a coherent set of specific health problems, identifiable clusters of client groups, and distinctive program goals and strategies. Everyone — women, men, young people, children, and the elderly — has social and reproductive health needs; some, such as adolescents and commercial sex workers and their clients, face especially high risk.

Table 1 summarizes common reproductive health threats, provides estimates of the mortality and morbidity impact of these problems, and

indicates the types of programs that have been launched to address them. The problems include lack of access to good-quality contraception and safe abortion, hazardous birthing environments, infertility, maternal and child malnutrition and infection, and the Human Immunodeficiency Virus (HIV) and sexually transmitted diseases (STDs).[3] These health problems exert an enormously heavy illness burden on adults, young people, and children, often with long-term physical and social consequences. About 500,000 pregnancy-related deaths occur each year; of these, perhaps one-quarter to one-third are due to the lack of access to safe abortion services (WHO 1993). Pregnancy-related deaths are only the tip of an iceberg; it has been estimated that for every such death, another 100 women suffer significant complications with long-term physical and social sequelae. In other words, as many as 50 million women may suffer serious maternal morbidity each year (Koblinsky, Campbell, and Harlow 1993).

Of the 7 million perinatal deaths among children worldwide, about half are associated with low birth weight (under 2,500 g), due predominantly to maternal protein-calorie malnutrition and anemia, and in some cases to STDs (Elliott et al. 1990; Kramer 1987; Villar and Belizan 1982). The prevalence of low birth weight varies between 10 percent and 20 percent; in some regions, like South Asia, it may exceed 30 percent. Of the 25 million low-birth-weight babies born each year in developing countries (WHO 1992b), a significant proportion are underweight because of chronic nutritional stunting of mothers, an intergenerational transmission of malnutrition (WHO 1992b). Many mothers are at nutritional risk during pregnancy because of their own deprived nutritional growth and development in early childhood and adolescent years. About 60 percent of pregnant women in developing countries suffer from anemia, due mostly to iron deficiency and, in some settings, malaria. Maternal anemia increases mortality risk, both directly and through the hazard of postpartum hemorrhage (WHO 1990).

HIV and STDs constitute another major cluster of reproductive health problems (see Box 1 on next page). The median prevalence rate for syphilis and chlamydia is about 8 percent among women attending family planning clinics in developing countries, compared with 14 percent among commercial sex workers (Wasserheit and Holmes 1992). Women are disproportionately at risk of STD transmission, and they more commonly suffer from STD complications. STD transmission from men to women is estimated to be up to 50 percent more efficient than that from women to men. Untreated STDs can lead to acute pelvic inflammatory disease (PID) in 5-10 percent of women; PID, in turn, can cause ectopic pregnancy, chronic pelvic pain, adverse pregnancy outcomes, and infertility (Brunham and Embree 1992; Weström 1980; Weström, Bengtsson, and Mårdh 1981). Worldwide levels of infertility average 3-5 percent. In parts of Africa, this rate may be double the worldwide average, mostly because of STDs, and the rate

T A B L E   1

Reproductive and Sexual Health Problems, Estimated Impacts, Program Interventions

Health Problem	Estimated Worldwide Annual Impact Mortality	Morbidity	Illustrative Programs
Women and men			
Unwanted pregnancy	–	80 million	Family planning
Unsafe abortion	110,000	25 million	Legal, safe abortions
Infertility	–	60 million couples	Prevent reproductive tract infections
Obstetrical risk	350,000	35 million	Safe motherhood
Maternal anemia	40,000	58 million	Prenatal care
HIV	–	1.9 million	HIV/STD control
AIDS	1 million	1 million	HIV/STD control
Gonorrhea	(a)	20 million	HIV/STD control
Chlamydia	(a)	50 million	HIV/STD control
Syphilis	(a)	4 million	HIV/STD control
Adolescents			
Teen pregnancy		(b)	Sex education, health services, delay marriage
Children			
Birthing risk	1,750,000	(a)	Safe motherhood
Low birth weight	3,500,000	24 million	Nutrition
Perinatal infection	1,400,000	(a)	Immunization, HIV/STD control
High risk and others			
Gender-based violence		(a)	Social/legal

(a) Data not available
(b) Teenage pregnancy as a high risk category should be restricted to those less than 17 years. Worldwide data on this category are not available.

Sources: Fathalla 1992; Mann, Tarantola and Netter 1992; Tinker and Koblinsky 1993; WHO 1992a; WHO 1992b.

reaches as high as 30-40 percent in some severely affected communities (Frank 1983). In addition to the threat of death and disability, infertility can have important social consequences, including ostracism by spouse, family, or community.

The very heavy burdens of reproductive health problems are shown in Figures 1 and 2 (World Bank 1993). These figures present disease burden as DALYs (disability-adjusted life years lost), a measure that combines the loss of healthy life years due to both mortality and morbidity associated with specific diseases.[4] Figure 1 shows the distribution of disease burden by cause for children under five and women ages 15-44 in developing countries. Among children, high-risk delivery and the infection-malnutrition dyad account for nearly three-quarters of the perinatal disease burden. For adult women, reproductive health problems (maternal, STDs, and HIV) constitute 36 percent of the burden of disease. Differences among regions in the burden of reproductive health problems are highlighted in Figure 2. These problems constitute 60 percent of the female adult disease burden in Africa, with about two-thirds due to HIV and STDs.

Cost-Effectiveness of Interventions

The 1993 World Development Report "Investing in Health" presents comprehensive information on the cost-effectiveness of various health

Controlling HIV and Sexually Transmitted Diseases

According to a 1990 estimate by the World Health Organization, there are worldwide more than 250 million new cases of sexually transmitted diseases (STDs) each year. STDs, including Human Immunodeficiency Virus (HIV), usually affect people in the 15–44 age group, and certain STDs, such as syphilis, are major causes of neonatal morbidity and mortality. STDs are of particular concern to women because of greater male-to-female transmission for most STD pathogens, the lack of female-controlled preventive methods, and, in many settings, gender power dynamics that limit women's ability to determine the conditions under which sexual intercourse occurs. Since men are responsible for much STD transmission, disease control measures, to be effective, must be targeted to both sexes.

Because STDs facilitate the transmission of HIV, controlling these infections is most important for AIDS control. The diagnostic, preventive, and therapeutic interventions against STDs have mixed efficacy in terms of availability and cost. For some STDs, such as syphilis, treatment is inexpensive and simple (between one and three injections of penicillin). For others, especially viral agents, therapy can be very difficult. Where technology is available, STD treatment can be very cost-effective, yielding among the highest health returns per dollar invested. Case management of chlamydia and gonorrhea (bacterial infections) can be highly cost-effective, as can treatment of chancroid in areas where it is common.

Although pilot experimental community-based intervention efforts and clinic-based interventions have been field-tested, experiences in launching population-based STD control efforts are limited. The worldwide HIV/AIDS epidemic and the women's health movement have helped to bring attention to HIV and STDs; many innovative programs have been launched. Documenting successful experiences in STD and HIV education and control is likely to be extremely useful in designing public health approaches to STD and HIV control.

Source: World Bank 1993.

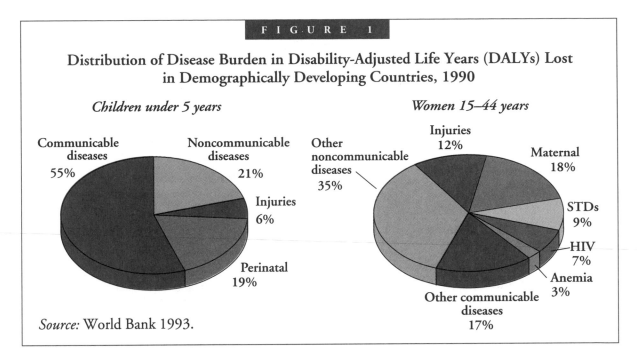

FIGURE 1

Distribution of Disease Burden in Disability-Adjusted Life Years (DALYs) Lost in Demographically Developing Countries, 1990

Children under 5 years

Communicable diseases 55%

Noncommunicable diseases 21%

Injuries 6%

Perinatal 19%

Women 15–44 years

Other noncommunicable diseases 35%

Injuries 12%

Maternal 18%

STDs 9%

HIV 7%

Anemia 3%

Other communicable diseases 17%

Source: World Bank 1993.

interventions (World Bank 1993). Cost-effectiveness is an analytic measure that can help guide decisions about the relative priority to be accorded to a range of health actions. Of various investment options, reproductive health interventions rank among the "best buys" available. In other words, each dollar invested in reproductive

health interventions gives a higher health return than comparable investments against many other diseases. Estimates of cost-effectiveness range from less than $7 per DALY saved for tetanus toxoid immunization and tuberculosis chemotherapy to nearly $5,000 per DALY saved for treatment of cardiovascular disease (Jamison and Mosley 1993;

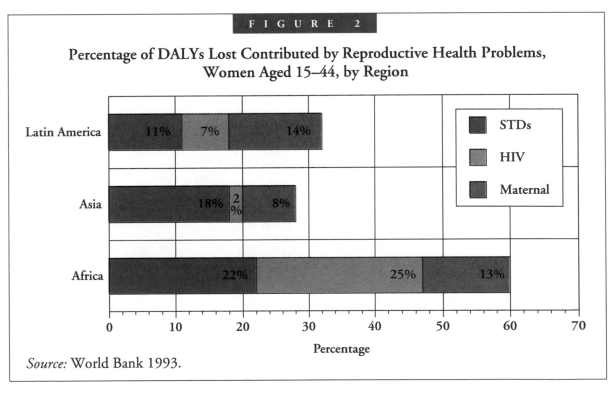

FIGURE 2

Percentage of DALYs Lost Contributed by Reproductive Health Problems, Women Aged 15–44, by Region

Latin America: 11%, 7%, 14%

Asia: 18%, 2%, 8%

Africa: 22%, 25%, 13%

STDs

HIV

Maternal

Percentage

Source: World Bank 1993.

Kutzin 1993; World Bank 1993). Most reproductive health interventions are at the low-cost, high-yield end of this spectrum — at about $30-$60 per DALY saved for such services as improved prenatal and delivery care, contraception, immunizations, and nutritional and micronutrient supplementation. Certain interventions to screen and treat STDs are also extremely cost-effective. Information, education, and communication combined with condom subsidies range from $1 to $50 per DALY saved, and STD treatment ranges from $1 to $55 per DALY saved (Over and Piot 1993).

The favorable cost-effectiveness of many reproductive health interventions is shown in Table 2 (Jamison and Mosley 1993). The highest-cost intervention examined is the secondary treatment or rehabilitation of cardiovascular disease by angioplasty or bypass surgery, estimated at $5,000 per DALY saved. By comparison, the various reproductive health interventions in Table 2 all appear extremely favorable: most would save more than 50 times as many DALYs as the highest-cost intervention; even the most expensive one, palliative treatment of AIDS, is six times as cost-effective as treatment of cardiovascular disease.

The ranking of these health interventions would be expected to vary between countries. In some low-income countries where fertility levels are high and the use of contraceptives is low, birth control services are highly cost-effective because of their influence on health risk factors such as birth spacing and the reduction of unwanted or high-order pregnancies. In other settings, the returns of

T A B L E 2		
Cost-Effectiveness of Reproductive Health Interventions		
Intervention	Cost per DALY Saved($)	Ratio to Highest-Cost Intervention[*]
Women		
Delivery of family planning services	30 – 150	.018
Prenatal and delivery	30 – 250	.028
Iodine injections for pregnant women	25	.005
Promotion of breast-feeding	30	.006
Tetanus case management	100	.02
Women and Children		
Nutrition Supplementation		
Pregnant Woman	25	.005
Preschool Child	70	.0002
Nutrition Rehabilitation	150 – 250	.04
Women, Men, and Children		
HIV/STD screening and referral	1 – 250	.0251
STD treatment	1 – 55	.0056
Palliative treatment of AIDS with medical or surgical interventions	80 – 1250	.133

[*] The highest-cost intervention is taken as secondary prevention or rehabilitation of cardiovascular disease (angioplasty or bypass graft surgery), at a cost per DALY saved of $5,000. Calculation of the numerator involved taking the average of the range.

Source: Jamison and Mosley 1993.

increasing contraceptive use are smaller. The benefit of other direct interventions to improve health, such as expanding prenatal care, immunization, and obstetric services, is very high, especially in populations experiencing high mortality levels (Kutzin 1993). In all societies, safe motherhood and HIV or STD prevention programs would rank among the very highest priorities. Decisions to invest in these reproductive health services, of course, should be based only in part on health benefits; other values, such as choice, freedom, and equity, should also be considered.

It is important to underscore that the net benefit of reproductive health interventions is undoubtedly even greater than the computations suggest because these interventions can have multiple beneficiaries. Existing analyses usually consider only the health benefits that accrue to a single beneficiary, the mother or a child. But improving the health of mothers can generate secondary health benefits for children and other family members, today and into future generations (Kutzin 1993).

Expanding Access and Enhancing Quality

Although some believe access to and quality of services are competitive in terms of resource allocation, we believe that any health system must seek to achieve both simultaneously. Strategies to expand access to services of poor quality, and to enhance quality for only a few, are seriously inadequate. Resources are needed for both, and improvements in either will strengthen and facilitate the other. The allocation of resources between these two aspects of service must be appropriate to diverse situations.

Data on the coverage provided by reproductive health services around the world are scanty. Coverage undoubtedly varies with different service components. Contraception is now being practiced by nearly half of all eligible couples in the world, although at least 100 million women are estimated to have an "unmet need" for contraception (Fathalla in this volume; Dixon-Mueller and Germain 1992). Control of HIV and STDs presumably covers only a limited proportion of eligible clients; young people and women in the general population are particularly underserved. The proportion of deliveries that are attended by trained personnel is inexcusably low in developing countries and provides an indicator of obstetric service coverage (see Figure 3 on next page). In industrialized countries, virtually all births are attended by trained personnel. In Latin America, a very high proportion of births are also professionally attended. Yet more than half of all births are unattended in Asia, and nearly two-thirds are unattended in Africa.

The quality of reproductive health services is widely reported to be poor, yet quality is believed to be a key factor determining how private consumers utilize fee-for-service providers and whether or not public service, even if free, is utilized. Bruce (1989), focusing on family planning services, developed a framework consisting of six elements of service quality: full client choice in method use, adequate information for and counseling of users, technical competence of providers, positive interpersonal relations between providers and clients, mechanisms for follow-up and continuity of care, and an appropriate constellation of services. Quality criteria are less well developed for other reproductive health services, such as sex education and safe motherhood interventions.

Many barriers exist to expanding access to and enhancing the quality of reproductive health services. Physical, social, and economic factors may constrain access; quality depends not only upon necessary logistical support and technical competence, but also on the staff's motivation and dedication. Both access and quality, as well as the factors that affect them, are undergoing rapid change in many parts of the world. In this volume, Anand, Batliwala, Desai, and Zeitlin and colleagues review some of the socioeconomic structural factors that affect access and quality, such as development policies, women's empowerment, and resource allocation; Germain, Nowrojee, and Pyne suggest how approaches to reproductive and sexual health can be expanded to encompass men's responsibility for their own sexual behavior, sexuality, and gender relations;

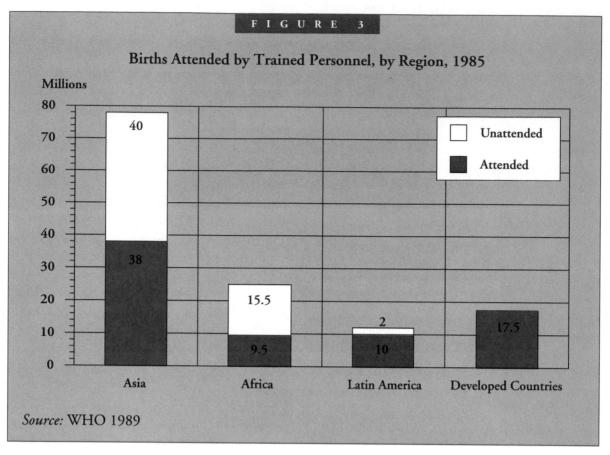

FIGURE 3

Births Attended by Trained Personnel, by Region, 1985

Millions

Legend:
- Unattended
- Attended

Region	Attended	Unattended
Asia	38	40
Africa	9.5	15.5
Latin America	10	2
Developed Countries	17.5	

Source: WHO 1989

Hawkins and Meshesha review means to over-come the obstacles to providing information and services to young people; and several chapters assess the ethical dimensions of expanding access and enhancing the quality of services. In the remainder of this chapter, we will focus on three dimensions of reproductive health services — the critical provider-client interface, the functioning of services as a coherent system, and the integration of reproductive health with other health services — all of which pose challenges and opportunities for improved access and quality.

Provider-Client Interface

In villages and slums around the world, access to and quality of reproductive health services depend upon the availability of a technically competent primary health worker within geographic and economic reach of potential clients. That ultimate interaction between the health worker and client is one of the most critical, neglected dimensions of health services. Three

aspects of the provider-client interaction are especially important — worker density, technical skills, and human qualities.

Field studies have repeatedly demonstrated that service access is possible only with a certain minimal density of health workers in the community that provides the capacity for sustained and repeated provider-client contacts. In a review of client relations in many family planning programs in northern India and Bangladesh, Simmons, Koblinsky, and Phillips (1986) identified worker density as the basic determinant of frequency of contact between family planning workers and villagers. In India in the 1970s, female village workers were expected to serve populations of 10,000 people, usually in several villages. This density of worker coverage is probably too low for effective performance. Because of cultural constraints on their movements, female workers often restricted themselves to the populations closest to their residences, while distant villagers remained underserved. In the Bangladesh government programs of the 1980s, the populations served were smaller, and the rate of client-worker contact was higher than in India. However, it was in the nongovernment program at Matlab, Bangladesh, in which a worker was responsible for only the 1,200 people of her own village, that contact was frequent and family planning utilization high. Nonetheless, of the many factors that have been credited for the "success" of the Matlab program, worker density has been relatively neglected.

If services are to be effective, the health worker must have the requisite technical skills, along with appropriate equipment, drugs, and supplies. Given the scarcity of trained human resources in many developing countries, attempts to increase access and to enhance quality have involved delegation of critical tasks to peripheral workers closest to the clients. Studies have repeatedly demonstrated that the technical reliability of even illiterate community-based distributors of contraceptive pills, oral rehydration packets, and antibiotics can be extremely high (Osborn and Reinke 1981). In fact, there is general agreement that routine, frequently performed tasks, like contraceptive distribution, prenatal care, and supervision of a normal delivery, can be well managed by briefly trained workers. How to delegate less frequently performed, but important life-saving tasks — like manual removal of a placenta or vacuum aspiration of retained products of conception after an incomplete abortion — is a challenge faced by all programs.

At the heart of the health worker's performance, however, is the human dimension. Reproductive health workers must address some of the most intimate aspects of sexuality and life-changing, life-giving, and sometimes life-threatening events. The quality of the relationship between provider and client is thus vital to the quality of care. Attention, therefore, should be given to health workers' own needs. Their attitudes and behaviors are, in many cases, simply the reflection of the ways in which they are treated by their supervisors. Under poor working conditions, it is hardly surprising that many peripheral

health workers work less than half-time and spend most of their time with better-off families — sometimes even developing negative attitudes toward other community members and making insufficient efforts to understand people's various needs and aspirations. In their review of family planning performance in India and Bangladesh, Simmons, Koblinsky, and Phillips (1986) noted that the quality of client relations depended not only on frequency of contact, but also on the attitudes of the health workers. Both of these require that health workers have acceptable living conditions, an appropriate workload, adequate training, realistic work targets, and, most importantly, supportive supervision. These conditions are infrequently met, however, at least partly because health workers in villages or peripheral health centers are often women and have little formal education (see Box 2 on page 187).

Functioning Systems

Once midwives in villages and slums, health workers in health centers, and doctors in hospitals are technically trained, they must be functionally connected. Effective health systems require that the whole be more than the sum of the individual parts. The challenge to develop efficient and effective health systems in which several parts contribute to a functioning whole faces every country, rich and poor alike.[5]

Table 3 (on next page), constructed from various World Health Organization (WHO) technical guidelines (1990, 1993), shows the different types of services required for a well-functioning reproductive health care system at three levels — community, health center, and referral center. The bulk of reproductive health services can and should be community-based, including, for example, sex education, nonclinical contraceptive distribution, prenatal care, low-risk deliveries, and recognition and referral of complications. Referral and support services are also essential and must be provided at more sophisticated facilities. The health center, usually the first professional level, operates as a critical pivot point. This is true especially with reproductive health services, because many women face difficulty in traveling to hospitals as a result of physical and economic barriers as well as social restraints (for example, needing a husband's or other relative's permission to travel) (Thaddeus and Maine 1990). Several critical reproductive health services require hospitalization, but these should not take precedence in resource allocation over the bulk of reproductive health services that can and should be delivered in the community and at health centers.

A functional system is therefore based on systematic assessment of the types of services that should be performed at each level, which tasks can be delegated to the community level, and how the referral systems for emergencies and more technically complicated tasks can be improved. Clear delegation of life-saving skills to community-level and health center staff is the best way currently available to reduce physical, social, and other barriers to reproductive care. A

		TABLE 3	

Reproductive Health Tasks at Different Levels of Care

	Community	Health Center	Referral Center
Contraception	• Promote/educate • Nonclinical methods • Referral for complications	• Promote/educate • Nonclinical and clinical methods • Manage side effects • Refer for surgical methods	• Surgical methods
Reproductive Tract Infections	• Education in STD prevention/management • Referral for treatment	• Diagnose/treat • Serology	
Abortion	• Educate • Referral for safe abortion	• Manage incomplete abortion • Referral • Menstrual regulation	• Manage severe side effects
Prenatal Care	• Educate • Distribute iron, folic acid, and antimalarial pills • Risk assessment • Refer complications	• Risk assessment • Monitor progress • Diagnose • First aid and referral	• Manage severe complications • Blood transfusion for severe anemia
Delivery Care	• Normal delivery • Refer complications	• Monitor labor progress • First aid and referral • Management of third stage • Removal of placenta	• Oxytocic augmentation for prolonged labor • Cesarean section or instrumental delivery • Blood transfusion • Manage postpartum hemorrhage
Postpartum care	• Promote breast-feeding • Educate • Refer breast and genital tract infections • Neonatal eye care	• Diagnose and manage puerperal infection • Refer severe sepsis and fistulae	• Manage or refer severe sepsis and fistulae

Source: World Health Organization 1990, 1993

The Loneliness of a Front-Line Health Worker

Anna is an assistant nurse-midwife (ANM) in Ramnagar, a village of 10,000 in the southern Indian state of Andrah Pradesh. Like the 100,000 other ANMs in India, Anna provides maternal and child health, nutrition, immunization, family planning, communicable disease control services; trains traditional midwives (*dais*); and registers vital events for the people. A low-caste Christian, Anna was posted to Ramnagar eight years ago. She had hoped for a warm welcome, instead, she felt isolated. Her district supervisors were not interested in her work, other than her monthly quota of family planning acceptors. She soon discovered that her lack of medicines and injections left her helpless in the eyes of the villagers.

Anna attempted to train and strengthen *dais* in the village, but few were willing to change their profitable practices. Of the eight

villagers trained as voluntary community health guides, only two continued to practice, and one of these ignored Anna completely, setting up her own private services. Recently, the government appointed another ANM to Ramnagar, the second wife of the leader of a nearby village. Although this additional ANM should have assisted Anna, she instead competed with Anna for clients, competition Anna can ill afford, because she is a widow with three children in school. Even though her government salary is high by village standards, Anna has to supplement her income with private payments for attending deliveries.

Many of Anna's classmates in ANM training face similar social and professional problems.

Source: Prakasamma 1993.

number of standard management protocols for prevention and treatment at the various levels have been developed by the WHO (1990, 1993). Such protocols enable even briefly trained workers to provide technically demanding health services at the community and health center levels. It may be possible to delegate even more complex tasks to nurses and health auxiliaries. Many of the less frequently performed emergency procedures required at a health center share with the routine tasks of monitoring labor and inserting an IUD the need for the common skill of being able to perform and interpret a pelvic examination. Taking the idea of common skills one step further, we can see that someone trained to insert and remove IUDs can also be trained to use a manual vacuum extractor for menstrual regulation or incomplete abortion. This principle has already been demonstrated by auxiliaries in Bangladesh who do manual vacuum aspirations very safely (Bhatia, Faruque, and Chakraborty 1980; Dixon-Mueller 1988).

Community-level services must be made effective and efficient to encourage clients to use these services rather than unnecessarily going into hospitals. At the same time, the delegation of tasks to the lowest level possible within the health system requires access to emergency services at higher levels. Referral linkages thus must be given high priority. Sorting out interactions among various service levels requires careful design and evaluation of pilot projects (Freedman 1987) and a process of consultation that includes people from all levels of the system, including clients, to ensure decisions that are both realistic and feasible, and to enable all necessary actors to take ownership of the system that is ultimately developed (Aitken, Kargbo, and Gba-Kamara 1985).

Integration

The functional quality of reproductive health services is dependent upon interconnections not only between various reproductive health interventions, but also between reproductive and other

Silent Endurance: Women in Rural Egypt

Zahra, who is 19 years old, has been married for seven years and has two living children after five pregnancies. After her last delivery by caesarean section, Zahra did not menstruate. Eager to conceive again, she sought medical advice, only to discover that a hysterectomy had been performed without permission from her or her husband.

Han'a, who is 16 years old, has been married for two years and has one daughter who has been slow to develop. Han'a tested positive for syphilis, and was treated but then reinfected when her husband came home from work in Libya. Han'a knew nothing about STDs, did not realize that her husband could infect her and also never imagined that her daughter's poor health could be connected to her own.

Yasmin, who is 19 years old, was married when she was eleven and has only one living child after four pregnancies. Wanting more children, her husband threatened to divorce her and also refused to allow her to get treatment for a heart condition. When Yasmin became pregnant again, she gave birth prematurely and the baby died.

These three cases illustrate the "silent endurances" required of women in rural Egypt by relatives, social traditions, isolation from information, and health professionals.

Source: Khattab 1992.

health services. In the 1960s and 1970s, the population field invested heavily in vertical family planning programs. In addition, while conceptually strong and rhetorically supported, the linkages of reproductive health with primary or general health services have in practice been infrequently tried and have involved only a narrow range of services. In reproductive health, vertical programs in traditional birth attendant training, contraception, and AIDS control (sometimes even distinct from STD control) have proliferated. The picture, of course, varies enormously between countries.

Several compelling reasons have been offered for why integration is particularly relevant for reproductive health services. Synergy among health components is one. Upgrading the quality of care in contraceptive delivery, for instance, relies heavily on related support services to screen for contraindications, including STDs; to counsel; and to provide follow-up services (see Jain and Bruce in this volume). Consultations for contraceptive services provide an efficient context for dealing with other health concerns, including child health; preventive education;

condom promotion; screening for STDs and HIV/AIDS; and screening and treatment for anemia. A second reason is client demand. Many studies have revealed the extent to which health services have failed to meet women's perceived reproductive health needs and the frustration of many women because services for them and their children are not coordinated (Simmons, Koenig, and Huque 1990). Additional reasons for better integration of reproductive health components are the urgent need to prevent and manage STDs, including HIV and AIDS, and the desirability of introducing a life-cycle approach to coordinating the management of pregnancies, family planning, and child care. Often lack of attention to the coordination of care and to clients' perceived needs and convenience is a major cause of skepticism and underutilization of health services (Simmons, Koenig, and Huque 1990). The time constraints on women's lives (see Desai in this volume), as well as strong medical and cost reasons, require a "supermarket approach," enabling women to attend to their own and their children's needs in the same facility at the same time.

Despite the compelling reasons to integrate services, for four decades, international conferences and policy makers have debated integration — most often between health and family planning and, less often, across the various components of reproductive health services. Several attempts to study the cost-effectiveness of integrating contraception with a few maternal and child health services have been undertaken — in Narangwal and Khanna in India (Taylor et al.

1983; Wyon and Gordon 1971), Danfa in Ghana (University of Ghana Medical School 1979), "Taylor-Berelson" projects in several sites (Taylor and Berelson 1971), and the Matlab health and family planning project in Bangladesh (Simmons and Phillips 1987). The anticipation of improved contraceptive utilization that motivated integration in many of the projects was not always met. It has turned out that good contraceptive utilization depended primarily on a well-planned and

---

BOX 4

Integrating Women's Health into Development: BRAC in Bangladesh

To meet the health needs of the poorest of the rural poor, BRAC, one of the world's largest non-governmental agencies (NGOs), launched an experimental Women's Health and Development Program (WHDP) in 1991. The WHDP objective is to "improve the quality of life of the rural poor by bringing about an improvement in their health and nutritional status...thus reducing the morbidity and mortality burden." The overall strategy is to serve in a comprehensive fashion the health needs of women, children, and adolescents. Health and education are integrated with and reinforced by activities in rural development, credit, income-generation, development of skills, and awareness building.

The current program operates in three regions of Bangladesh serving 1,637 villages and an estimated population of 1.9 million. Approximately 800 workers are assigned to area offices each covering 6–8 villages. Program organizers (POs), both female and male, work with community volunteer ("shasto shehikas"), traditional birth attendants, and the participants themselves to ensure access to a range of critical reproductive health services delivered either by the government program or directly by BRAC, including:

- Contraceptive services at village level provided by female resident "Depot Holders"

who also work on pregnancy identification and pre- and postnatal care.

- Nonformal primary education for girls ages 11–18 using curriculum materials that include nutrition education and hygiene, reproductive health, and nutritional monitoring of children.

- Immunization of children as part of the national Expanded Programme of Immunization (EPI) program involving mobilizing communities for vaccination services provided by the government.

- Growth monitoring of all children through the female adolescent education program that undertakes child weighings and nutritional education.

- Water and sanitation obtained through loans and self-help.

Innovative aspects of the BRAC program are its simultaneous work with government and the private sector, the priority accorded to health problems of women, children, and female adolescents, and integration and reinforcement by other parallel BRAC programs in credit, rural development, and social mobilization.

Source: Adapted from Chowdhury 1993, with permission.

well-implemented contraceptive program, and additional maternal and child health services increased utilization only after that was achieved (Simmons and Phillips 1987).

Studies in Mexico have shown how integration of maternal care and family planning have led to improved client-provider relationships and increased contraceptive utilization (Potter, Mojarro and Nunez 1987). Recently a new generation of small-scale programs has begun to evaluate the operational and cost implications of providing integrated reproductive health services. These experiments have yielded preliminary evidence that the provision of a substantial range of integrated reproductive services can be both effective and affordable (Dos Santos et al. 1992; Eschen and Whittaker 1993; Kay and Kabir 1988). (See box on page 246.) Some experiments integrate several reproductive health service components with other women's development activities. (See Box 4 on page 189.)

Conclusion

In this chapter we have examined the definition, quantified the burden, and assessed the operations of reproductive health services. The burden of reproductive health problems is extremely heavy, but highly cost-effective interventions are available. The challenge everywhere is the joint planning of population and health investments to generate cost-effective packages of good-quality integrated services shaped to the specific needs of diverse clients in different settings and available to all who need them.

Improving the provider-client interface, we believe, must be at the heart of all efforts to meet the next challenge. Services must ensure sufficient density of technically competent health workers within geographic and economic reach of potential clients. The human quality of the provider-client relationship is critical, dependent not only on the personal characteristics of the worker, but also on the support of supervisors and the health care system. That support must be part of a system where the components are interconnected as a functioning whole. In reproductive health,

most service tasks can be performed by briefly trained workers in communities, backed by a health center. Very few services need to be performed in sophisticated and expensive hospitals. Delegation of responsibility and adequate support are the major ingredients of a successfully functioning system.

More difficult are the linkages between reproductive health and primary health or general health services. "Integration" is a buzzword that has revisited the population and health fields for decades. Many, if not most, reproductive health services have been provided through vertical systems — immunization, family planning, HIV and STD control. Horizontal development of integrated health care must be developed if reproductive and sexual health and rights are to be universally achieved.

Notes

1 For brevity and clarity of presentation, the term "reproductive and sexual health" is frequently shortened to simply "reproductive health" in this chapter.

2 The United Nations Development Programme's human development index consists of a composite of health, education, and income indicators (UNDP 1993; see also Anand in this volume). The attainment of reproductive functions — either controlling unwanted fertility or overcoming infertility — is not now, but could easily be, included in assessments of human development.

3 Widespread problems that are less well documented and not covered in this chapter include gender-based violence; gynecologic problems, including cancers; and problems of menopause.

4 For the methodology of computing DALYs, see World Bank (1993), Appendix B.

5 One of the wealthiest health care systems in the world, that of the United States, is currently undergoing reforms to blend diverse elements into an affordable, functioning health care system.

References

Aitken, I. W., T. K. Kargbo, and A. M. Gba-Kamara. 1985. Planning a community-oriented midwifery service for Sierra Leone. *World Health Forum* 6:110-114.

Bhatia, S., A. S. G. Faruque, and J. Chakraborty. 1980. Assessing menstrual regulation performed by paramedics in rural Bangladesh. *Studies in Family Planning* 11:213-218.

Bruce, J. 1989. *Fundamental elements of the quality of care: A simple framework*. New York: Population Council.

Brunham, R. C., and J. E. Embree. 1992. Sexually transmitted diseases: Current and future dimensions of the problem in the third world. In A. Germain et al. (eds.), *Reproductive tract infections: Global impact and priorities for women's reproductive health*. New York: Plenum Press.

Chowdhury, S. 1993. Women's health and development program. Dhaka, Bangladesh: Bangladesh Rural Advancement Committee (BRAC).

Dixon-Mueller, R., and A. Germain. 1992. Stalking the elusive "unmet need" for family planning. *Studies in Family Planning* 23(5):330-335.

Dixon-Mueller, R. 1988. Innovations in reproductive health care: Menstrual regulation policies and programs in Bangladesh. *Studies in Family Planning* 19(3):129-140.

Dos Santos, R. B., E. M. P. Folgosa, and L. Fransen. 1992. Reproductive tract infections in Mozambique: A case study of integrated services. In A. Germain et al. (eds.), *Reproductive tract infections*. New York: Plenum Press.

Elliot, B., et al. 1990. Maternal gonococcal infection as a preventable risk factor for low birth weight. *Journal of Infectious Disease* 161:531-536.

Eschen, A., and M. Whittaker. 1993. Family planning: A base to build on for women's reproductive health services. In M. Koblinsky, J. Timyan, and J. Gay (eds.), *The health of women: A global perspective*. Boulder, Colo.: Westview Press.

Fathalla, M. 1992. Reproductive health in the world: Two decades of progress and the challenge ahead. In J. Ishanna, P. F. A. Van Look, and P .D. Griffin (eds), *Reproductive health: A key to a brighter future*. Special programme of research, development and research training in human reproduction. Geneva: World Health Organization.

Frank, O. 1983. Infertility in sub-Saharan Africa: Estimates and implications. *Population and Development Review* 9(1):137-144.

Freedman, R. 1987. The contribution of social science research to population policy and family planning program effectiveness. *Studies in Family Planning* 18:57-82.

Germain, A., and J. Ordway. 1989. *Population control and women's health: Balancing the scales*. New York: International Women's Health Coalition.

Jamison, D. T., and W. H. Mosley. 1993. Selecting disease control priorities in developing countries. In D.T. Jamison et al. (eds.), *Disease control priorities in developing countries*. New York: Oxford University Press.

Kay, B. J., and S. M. Kabir. 1988. A study of costs and behavioral outcomes of menstrual regulation services in Bangladesh. *Social Science and Medicine* 26:597-604.

Khattab, H. A. S. 1992. *The silent endurance: Social conditions of women's reproductive health in rural Egypt*. G. Potter (ed). Cairo: UNICEF and Population Council.

Koblinsky, M. A., O. M. R. Campbell, and S. D. Harlow. 1993. Mother and more: A broader perspective on women's health. In M. A. Koblinsky, J. Timyan, and J. Gay (eds.), *The health of women: A global perspective*. Boulder, Colo.: Westview Press.

Kramer, M. S. 1987. Determinants of low birth weight: Methodological assessment and meta-analysis. *Bulletin of the World Health Organisation* 65:663-737.

Kutzin, J. 1993. Cost-effectiveness issues in women's health. Background Document for the Women's Health Best Practices Paper, Population, Health and Nutrition Department, World Bank, April 20, in Washington D.C.

Maine, D. 1990. *Safe motherhood programs: Options and issues*. New York: Center for Population and Family Health, School of Public Health, Columbia University.

Mann, J., D. J. M. Tarantola, and T. W. Netter (eds.). 1992. *AIDS in the world: A global report*. Cambridge: Harvard University Press.

Osborn, R. W., and W. A. Reinke (eds.). 1981. *Community-based distribution of contraception: A review of field experience*. Baltimore, Md.: Johns Hopkins Population Center, School of Hygiene and Public Health, The Johns Hopkins University.

Over, M., and P. Piot. 1993. HIV infection and sexually transmitted diseases. In D. T. Jamison et al. (eds.), *Disease control priorities in developing countries*. New York: Oxford University Press.

Prakasamma, M. 1993. Incongruence of Indian rural health policies with village realities: Rethinking rural health policy. Takemi Program Paper, Harvard School of Public Health.

Potter, J. E., O. Mojarro, and L. Nunez. 1987. The influence of health care on contraceptive acceptance in rural Mexico. *Studies in Family Planning* 18:144-156.

Simmons, R., M. A. Koblinsky, and J. F. Phillips. 1986. Client relations in South Asia: Programmatic and societal determinants. *Studies in Family Planning* 17:257-268.

Simmons, R., M. A. Koenig, and A. A. Zahidul Huque. 1990. Maternal-child health and family planning: User perspectives and service constraints in rural Bangladesh. *Studies in Family Planning* 21:187-196.

Simmons, R., and J. F. Phillips. 1987. The integration of family planning with health and development. In R. J. Lapham and G. B. Simmons (eds.), *Organizing for effective family planning programs*. Washington, D.C.: National Academy Press.

Taylor, C. E., et al. 1983. *Child and maternal health services in rural India. The Narangwal experiment: Integrated family planning and health care*, vol. 2. Baltimore, Md.: Johns Hopkins University Press.

Taylor, H. C., and B. B. Berelson. 1971. Comprehensive family planning based on maternal/child health services: A feasibility study for a world program. *Studies in Family Planning* 2:22-54.

Thaddeus, S., and D. Maine. 1990. *Too far to walk: Maternal mortality in context.* New York: Center for Population and Family Health, School of Public Health, Columbia University.

Tinker, A, and M. A. Koblinsky. 1993. Making motherhood safe. World Bank Discussion Paper No. 202. Washington, D.C.: World Bank.

United Nations Development Programme (UNDP). 1993. *Human development report 1993.* New York: Oxford University Press.

University of Ghana Medical School, Department of Community Health. 1979. *The Danfa Comprehensive Rural Health and Family Planning Project, Ghana.* Los Angeles, Calif.: Division of Population, Family and International Health, School of Public Health, UCLA.

Villar, J., and J. M. Belizan. 1982. The relative contribution of prematurity and fetal growth retardation to low birth weight in developing and developed societies. *American Journal of Obstetrics and Gynecology* 143:793-798.

Wasserheit, J. N., and K. K. Holmes. 1992. Reproductive tract infections: Challenges for international health policy, programs, and research. In A. Germain et al. (eds.), *Reproductive tract infections: Global impact and priorities for women's reproductive health.* New York: Plenum Press.

Weström, L. 1980. Incidence, prevalence and trends of acute pelvic inflammatory disease and its consequences in industrialized countries. *American Journal of Obstetrics and Gynecology* 138:880-92.

Weström, L., L. P. H. Bengtsson, and P. A. Mårdh. 1981. Incidence, trends and risks of ectopic pregnancy in a population of women. *British Medical Journal* 282:15-18.

World Bank. 1993. *World development report 1993:* Investing in health. New York: Oxford University Press.

World Health Organisation (WHO). 1989. *Coverage of maternity care: A tabulation of available information,* 2nd ed. Geneva: Division of Family Health.

———. 1990. *The prevention and management of postpartum haemorrhage.* Geneva.

———. 1992a. *The prevalence of aenemia in women: A tabulation of available information.* Geneva.

———. 1992b. *Low birth weight: A tabulation of available information.* Geneva.

———. 1993. *The prevention and management of unsafe abortion.* Geneva.

———. 1994 (forthcoming). *Care of mother and baby at the health centre.* Geneva.

Wyon, J. B., and J. E. Gordon. 1971. *The Khanna study: Population problems in the rural Punjab.* Cambridge: Harvard University Press.

14

A Reproductive Health Approach to the Objectives and Assessment of Family Planning Programs

Anrudh Jain and Judith Bruce

Population policies and family planning programs are at a crossroads. On the one hand, population policy increasingly has come to be equated narrowly with fertility reduction through family planning programs. On the other hand, many are advocating reproductive health and rights approaches to population policy that would broaden both the objectives and the array of services provided. Broadening family planning programs poses several dilemmas, however, regarding program definition, the complexity of program operations, and the evaluation of services.

In this chapter, we reexamine the scope and objectives of population policies and family planning programs in view of the demands for a reproductive health approach. We also examine the evaluation issues raised by a shift in the goals of family planning programs from reducing both wanted and unwanted fertility to reducing only unwanted and unplanned childbearing and closely associated reproductive morbidity. We review the relevance and utility of current family planning program indicators and evaluation frameworks. Then we propose a new methodology to assess how well programs help women to achieve their reproductive intentions safely and effec-

tively. To begin, we propose a new vision and strategy for services. Neither family planning programs nor reproductive health services can be responsible for achieving population policy objectives. Rather, we also propose, broader social and economic policies must become responsible for reducing desired family size.

What Should a Reproductive Health Approach Entail?

Two approaches might be used to promote provision of reproductive health services through family planning programs. The first would be to justify it as a means to reduce fertility. The second is to redefine the rationale, objectives, and scope of population policies and family planning programs. There is no empirical evidence to support the first alternative. We discuss below how the second can be achieved.

Population Policies and Family Planning Programs

Population policies in developing countries have been guided primarily by two rationales: a concern for reducing aggregate population growth, and an individual's right to control his or her fertility. Most formal population policy statements in developing countries specify the goals of a population policy in terms of a reduction in the population growth rates. In the absence of mass international migration and high mortality, this can occur only through fertility reduction. While such population policies usually also specify the means to modify fertility, they rarely specify the means to reduce mortality and to influence the movement of people.

This narrow specification of population policy derives from intense concern among various groups, in both developed and developing countries, about rapid population growth. A reduction in population growth in developing countries has been asserted to be advantageous for the planet and for the social and economic development of the countries concerned. While this argument has had political appeal, a globalized concern about rapid population growth does not necessarily provide useful guidance for action by national governments, communities and families, or individuals. Moreover, a search for the solution to the global population problem should be concerned not only with the optimal size of population, but also with improving human welfare and achieving a more equitable balance between people and resources.

Most population policies, as currently operationalized, depend upon family planning programs as the primary means to reduce fertility. Although levels of contraceptive use and fertility are highly correlated, age at marriage, abortion, and postpartum infecundability associated with breast-feeding and abstinence also determine fertility. In addition, a variety of socioeconomic factors powerfully affect individuals' and couples' desire for children and their ability to implement these desires. These factors include levels of infant and child mortality, female education, employment and livelihood opportunities for women, and women's empowerment in general. Policies and measures to influence these pivotal factors are typically addressed (if at all) in a country's multi-faceted development policies and programs. Population policies do not, as currently operationalized,

have any influence over the design of these broader development and health programs or control over the resources for their implementation.

When fertility fails to decline at a desired pace, planners search for potential interventions in the only population policy implementation arm they know — the family planning program. At times the result has been to impose more stringent performance targets on service providers and managers, to add incentives for clients, and, in some instances, to use coercion. Such actions are justified by many as a means to achieve the "common good." At the same time, no special effort is made to create conditions conducive to fertility decline by changing the powerful social and economic determinants of fertility at the individual level.

Lacking other visible concerns and employing no policy instruments save the promotion of contraceptive services, population policy is thus viewed solely as a fertility reduction policy and is identified with family planning programs.[1]

Reproductive Health and Its Place in Population Policy

Should we redefine population policies and family planning programs to include reproductive health? There would seem to be very little scope to include reproductive health in the mandate of current family planning programs as described above. If, on the other hand, population policy is redefined to include concern with the reduction of morbidity and mortality, then reproductive health has a legitimate place in that policy, whether reproductive health services are offered in their own vertical program or are integrated with the provision of fertility regulation or other health services. Similarly, the broadest interpretation of population policy — which is not so different from a thoughtful development and human welfare policy — would naturally embrace reproductive health as an important goal.

Our Vision and Strategy

Our long-term vision is one in which population policy is very similar to development policies attentive to reducing class, ethnic, and gender disparities. Such policies, whether labeled population policies or development policies, would pay attention to both the quantity of available goods and their distribution in relation to people. Good social and economic development policy and just population policy would become indistinguishable. Family planning would be subsumed within reproductive health, which in turn would be subsumed within health. This goal, despite being highly desirable, is unlikely to be pragmatic in the near future, because governments and international agencies are functionally organized around various sectors — each with its own sphere of activity and budget. Therefore, we propose a transitional strategy for the next 10–15 years, the "1994 strategy." It focuses primarily on fertility reduction and would encompass actions to accomplish the following goals:

■ promote policies and legal frameworks to create conditions conducive to voluntary fertility decline — for example, give priority attention to girls' education, increase women's access to and control of valued resources, reduce childhood mortality and morbidity, and distribute cost-benefits of children[2] more equitably between parents;

■ redefine family planning programs to emphasize helping individuals to achieve their reproductive intentions *in a healthful manner*; and

■ increase attention to those aspects of reproductive health that interact directly with the avoidance of unwanted and unplanned childbearing.

The proposed strategy implies a balanced, comprehensive, and humane approach to the reduction of fertility and population growth rates that optimizes the synergistic effects across development, health, and family planning sectors. Our proposal is based on the assumptions that it is legitimate, indeed important, for public policy to address population size and growth,[3] and that public funds will continue to be invested in the population sector. The issue is how to allocate

these funds to optimize human welfare as well as to reduce population growth rates. The means used to achieve population goals must therefore be just in and of themselves. Assurance that the means, in fact, will be just, depends substantially on whether a distinction is made between family planning programs that function as voluntary contraceptive service programs, and family planning programs that function as arms or centerpieces of fertility reduction programs.

The first element in the proposed strategy emphasizes an examination of development and health policies and legal frameworks to ensure that their impact on factors influencing individuals' desired family size is consistent with the overall fertility reduction objectives of population policy. Funds allocated to population would include support for professionals to identify implementation strategies, budgetary goals, and points of advocacy to bring about changes in a broad range of development policies and programs in order to accelerate voluntary fertility decline.

In the second element of the 1994 strategy, we intentionally have added the phrase "in a healthful manner." We thus propose that the primary objective of family planning programs be modified from societal fertility reduction to an explicit concern with assisting individuals to meet personal reproductive goals. This approach would allow family planning programs to pursue voluntary fertility reduction while giving attention to neglected aspects of reproductive health that are of immediate consequence to reaching personal fertility objectives. At the aggregate level, this means that instead of remaining responsible for reducing the rate of population growth or total (wanted and unwanted) fertility, family planning programs should become responsible for reducing unplanned and unwanted childbearing and related morbidity and mortality. Broader social and economic policies must then become responsible for reducing the level of wanted fertility.

We propose that family planning programs pay attention to those aspects of reproductive health that interact directly with the avoidance of unwanted fertility in a healthful manner. This implies that in addition to making various contraceptives available, they should make services available for safe abortion; diagnosis and treatment of pre-existing conditions that would make the use of a particular contraceptive method unhealthful, such as reproductive tract infections; and diagnosis and treatment of unhealthful effects of contraceptive use. Which of these services gets priority in a particular setting would depend upon the local conditions and the felt needs of clients.[4]

Current Measures of the Efficacy of Family Planning Programs

Voluntary family planning programs try to influence fertility behavior by providing accessible and affordable services for fertility regulation, information about contraceptive methods (and in some countries, safe abortion), and promotional activities and motivational messages about the benefits of small families and birth spacing to attract new users.[5] The first two types of activities are designed to facilitate contraceptive use and abortion among those who wish to regulate their fertility behavior or those who may be ambivalent about it. Activities of the third type are designed to influence family size norms; however, since reproductive goals are influenced mainly by social, economic, and cultural conditions, the potential impact of these motivational activities on the reduction in women's desired family size is dubious.

In the past, most of the efforts to measure the efficacy of family planning programs have derived from a demographic perspective. Likewise, the common theme in designing input and output indicators has been a desire to measure the impact of family planning programs on fertility. Before discussing the implications of the proposed shift in the objectives of these programs, we review the indicators and the evaluation frameworks typically used to measure the efficacy of family planning programs in terms of their current objectives.

Current Indicators

The development and use of indicators have been guided both by the interest in fertility reduction and by the availability of data. The input indicators used to describe family planning programs include type and density of workers and clinics, availability of and accessibility to contraceptive services, program effort, and, more recently, quality of care. Among these, only quality of care focuses upon service giving; the others emphasize policy commitment or quantity and distribution of services, and do not observe or describe service giving. (See Jain, Bruce, and Kumar 1992 for comparisons of these input indicators.)

Indicators used to judge the performance of family planning programs include the annual rate of population growth, crude birthrate (CBR), and total fertility rate (TFR). The data to estimate the annual population growth rate are usually available from decennial censuses. The CBR usually is estimated from registration systems of births and deaths, which are deficient in most developing countries. Efforts to estimate the CBR from cross-sectional surveys have not been very successful. However, the data to estimate the TFR have become more widely available for a number of countries as a result of international investments in cross-sectional survey projects — World Fertility Surveys, and Demographic and Health Surveys. In the absence of accurate and timely estimates of these indicators, various other indicators have been developed and used as proxies to measure the output of these programs, including contraceptive acceptance rate, continuation rate, births averted, couple years of protection (CYP), and contraceptive prevalence rate (CPR). Acceptance and continuation rates and births averted were more commonly used in the mid-1960s, at the initial stages of family planning programs. At present, continuation rates are used primarily in clinical studies of new contraceptive methods.

The CPR is commonly estimated from the data collected in cross-sectional surveys of women of reproductive age. In comparison, CYP is based on the distribution of supplies (pills, condoms, foaming tablets), the number of IUD insertions, and the number of sterilizations performed

(Wishik and Chen 1973). It is the easiest indicator to calculate because it depends only on supply information and does not require any contact with the assumed users.

The value of CYP can grossly overestimate the number of active users or the protection provided by the use of contraception, because it does not take into account the wastage in the distribution system and nonuse of a method or duration of its use. Different values of CYP can reflect differences in the catchment areas of various service facilities because it does not take into account the number of individuals who can be served through these facilities. This is not the case with the CPR, because its denominator includes all individuals who can be served by a family planning program. Neither CYP nor the CPR reflects the irregularity of use by individuals, differential effectiveness of various contraceptives in preventing pregnancies, or individuals' experiences with different methods over time. Neither makes any adjustment for overlap of contraceptive use with postpartum amenorrhea, postpartum abstinence, or noncontraceptive sterility. (See Shelton 1991 for additional pitfalls of CYP.)

CYP compares apples and oranges. It gives a false sense of comparability among various service delivery programs and methods that are explicitly designed to meet the needs of different individuals. For example, the conversion factors used in estimating CYP imply that one sterilization, in terms of CYP accumulated, is equivalent to five IUDs inserted or 162 cycles of pills or 1,250 condoms distributed. Permanent methods, however, cannot be used for spacing purposes and therefore are not comparable to reversible methods. Similarly, social marketing and sterilization projects, even though they are considered the most cost-effective programs (about $2 per CYP) cannot replace community-based distribution projects and clinics that provide multiple methods and information. Studies using current measures have found these programs to be the least cost-effective — $13–14 per CYP (Huber and Harvey 1989). Service delivery programs that provide continuity of care are thus likely to be penalized in comparison with programs that move more supplies through the system.

Some, but not all, of the pitfalls of CYP can be corrected by improving data collection methods and using situation-specific conversion factors, as originally recommended by Wishik and Chen (1973), to estimate CYP. However, the collection of data from clients required to estimate situation-specific conversion factors would reduce the simplicity and utility of CYP. Moreover, the experience from India indicates that even if one improves the methodology to estimate an index equivalent to the CPR from the distribution figure, the outcomes could include an overestimation of contraceptive use, inconsistencies between contraceptive use and fertility, and, above all, an overemphasis on sterilization and a highly skewed method mix. (See Department of Family Welfare 1989:51 for methodology; Visaria, Visaria, and Jain 1992 for incongruence between distribution and client-based estimates of the CPR.) If the job performance of program managers or of field-workers is evaluated in terms of CYP accumulated (or an equivalent number of sterilizations performed, as in India), there is great risk of an increasingly inappropriate emphasis on sterilization.

An increase in CYP and the CPR often has been used to infer program effectiveness in terms of fertility decline. There is no empirical evidence to confirm the relationship between CYP and fertility. Cross-country comparisons, however, have revealed a quite robust relationship between the CPR and fertility (see, for example, Mauldin and Ross 1991). However, owing to such factors as irregularity of use, overlap of contraceptive use with postpartum amenorrhea, age at marriage, and use of abortion, an increase in a country's CPR over time is not always consistent with the observed fertility reduction (see, for example, Adamchak and Mbizvo 1990 for Zimbabwe). Similarly, the relationship between the CPR and fertility in cross-areal comparisons within a country do not always correspond to the strength of these relationships observed in cross-country comparisons (see, for example, Jain 1985 for India).

Current Evaluation Frameworks

Efforts to evaluate the impact of family planning programs have focused on addressing the following questions: Do these programs reduce fertility? If yes, by how much? Is the program a causal or a contributing factor in fertility decline? The vast literature on this subject is guided by supply-demand frameworks, though the definitions of these two terms vary from one analysis to another. (See, for example, Chandrasekaran and Hermalin 1975; Phillips and Ross 1992; and Ross and Lloyd 1992.)

Evaluation designs commonly used include cross-country comparisons and comparisons within countries. These analyses try to address one basic question: What would have happened to fertility had there been no family planning program in an area or a country? An experimental design comes closest to answering this question, but rarely do circumstances permit this approach. The Matlab experiment in Bangladesh is the example most often cited in recent years. It demonstrated that delivery of services adapted to local conditions and a client-centered approach can increase contraceptive use even in conditions of extreme poverty, which had been assumed to foster high fertility norms (Phillips et al. 1988).

At times, the performance of family planning programs is judged by the pace and the magnitude of decline in population growth and fertility. A slow decrease in the population growth, birth, or total fertility rate in a country should be interpreted as a failure of the entire development planning process, including the family planning program; instead it usually is interpreted as a family planning failure. A lack of decline in the population growth rate, however, may reflect the effect of in-migration or, more likely, the effect of a mortality decline that is greater than or equivalent to fertility decline. Similarly, a lack of fertility decline in a country may reflect high fertility norms or preference for sons, among other factors. Identifying the slow pace of fertility decline in a country as evidence of the failure of its family planning program, therefore, implicitly assumes that

these programs are organized not only to help individuals meet their current reproductive goals, but also to change these goals. The pace of fertility decline is often confused with an objective judgment about the effectiveness of its family planning program; this thinking is tautological. For example, until recently, the program in Kenya had been interpreted as a failure, but as soon as national surveys started showing an increase in the CPR and a decline in the TFR, the program was deemed a success.

The use of time trends in a single country to infer causality is problematic because we cannot determine with certainty what would have happened in the absence of this intervention. Cross-country comparisons try to get around this problem. These studies use a statistical technique — multiple regression analysis — to try to control for the effect of confounding socioeconomic factors and to estimate the "net" effect of family planning programs on fertility decline over a specified time period (see, for example, Bongaarts, Mauldin, and Phillips 1990; Boulier 1985; Cutright 1983; Lapham and Mauldin 1984; Mauldin and Ross 1991).

These cross-country analyses are likely to overestimate the net contribution of family planning programs to "voluntary" fertility decline, however, because they rely on the program effort indicator to measure the strength of family planning programs (see Lapham and Mauldin 1984). The overestimation of the program impact can arise for three reasons: a bias introduced in the collection of data used to estimate the program effort, the lack of specification of the boundaries of "family planning" programs, and the lack of a distinction between the "voluntary" and "involuntary" elements of the program.

First, the high correlation often observed between program effort and the CPR or TFR at one point in time or over a period of time is likely to reflect, in part, the fact that the experts who provided information on a country's program inputs were also aware of the levels and trends in the CPR and TFR, which would influence their assessments of inputs.[6]

Second, the definition of program boundaries can also influence conclusions about the effect of family planning programs on fertility decline. Of the 30 measures included in the program effort index, 10 refer to items outside the scope of a program oriented to providing services and information. Some of these 10 measures (such as import laws and legal regulations) can be considered determinants of program services, and a few others (such as policy on age at marriage) are unrelated to the provision of services and information. For all developing countries together, these 10 measures account for 32 percent of the program effort score.

Third, without establishing the degree of voluntarism, attempts to estimate net effects are likely to overestimate the contribution of family planning programs to voluntary fertility decline. This point is illustrated by considering the analyses undertaken by Bongaarts, Mauldin, and Phillips (1990), and Bongaarts (1992). The program effort index used by these and other researchers in cross-country analyses does not include elements that can distinguish between the voluntary and involuntary nature of a country's effort to reduce fertility. The pressures on clients to accept a particular method or to conform to a given fertility level in China, India, and Indonesia, for example, are substantially different than in Egypt and Kenya. The TFR in China declined from the pretransition level of 6.3 births to 2.5 in the late 1980s, in India from 6.0 to 4.3, and in Indonesia from 5.7 to 3.0. Inclusion of China in the UN statistical system itself created a favorable impression about the effectiveness of family planning programs. Excluding China, the TFR in developing countries declined by one birth between 1960–65 and 1980–85, from 6.0 to 5.0; including China, the decline was 1.9 births, from 6.1 to 4.2.

The total decline of 1.4 births per woman attributed to family planning programs in all developing countries (Bongaarts 1992) consists of 0.7 attributed to the program in China, 0.2 in India, and 0.1 in Indonesia, and 0.4 to programs in other developing countries. The impact attrib-utable to voluntary programs, however, would be less than that attributable to all programs. The magnitude of the difference between the two would depend upon the assumptions about what would have happened in these countries in the absence of pressures on clients to accept a particular method or to conform to a given fertility level. If, for example, we assume that the voluntary component of the programs constituted about 50 percent and 70 percent of the total effort in China and India, respectively, and 100 percent in all other developing countries, then the impact attributable to the voluntary program would be around 1.0 birth, instead of 1.4 births attributable to the total program.

Implications of a Shift in Program Objectives for Measuring Efficacy

The second element of the 1994 strategy proposes that the primary objective of family planning programs be redefined to help individuals achieve their reproductive goals in a healthful manner. Instead of remaining responsible solely for reducing population growth or total (wanted and unwanted) fertility, these programs would become responsible for reducing unplanned and unwanted childbearing and the associated morbidity and mortality. This shift in emphasis has important implications for service provision and evaluation.

The proposed shift in the primary objective of family planning programs implies certain criteria for measuring the efficacy of these programs. The evaluation framework must follow and evaluate the clients' behavior rather than the service delivery point or a given method. It must not penalize the services that foster or effectively support switching among methods or service points; in other words, it must accommodate the variability of clients' paths to a desired outcome. It must acknowledge the desirability of voluntary, freely chosen use of fertility regulation. It should allow for the disaggregation of clients into significant subgroups whose needs are distinct. The framework must include in its universe only those women who express a need for fertility regulation,[7] rather than assume that all women of reproductive age are equally in need of contraception or implicitly create an incentive to serve some groups at the expense of others. The framework must permit comparisons of efficacy between programs or service points. Finally, the reproductive health impact of the program should be explicitly incorporated in the framework, not only in terms of mortality, but also in terms of morbidity encountered by women in their attempts to regulate their fertility.

Developing an index that would meet all these criteria is fairly straightforward at the individual level. Suppose a woman does not want to have another child for a given number of years. The program can be termed successful if it helps or empowers her to avoid childbearing for that period in a healthful manner.[8] The program is a failure if she has an unwanted or unplanned pregnancy or dies or suffers severe morbidity (that is, requires treatment) while trying to avoid unwanted or unplanned childbearing during the period of observation.

Transforming this principle to measure the impact of a program at the aggregate level is a bit tricky. Some of the available indicators can be modified to incorporate some, but not all, aspects of this principle. For example, the CPR, as currently estimated from cross-sectional surveys, implicitly assumes that all women of reproductive age are equally in need of contraception. Although the CPR can be estimated separately for different subgroups of clients (on the basis of their reproductive intentions), it cannot be linked explicitly with the achievement of stated reproductive goals of individual clients. Similarly, the TFR can be divided into unwanted and wanted fertility, and program success can be measured in terms of the decline in unwanted fertility. However, the information collected retrospectively about the wantedness of a child already born is usually biased (Bongaarts 1990). Women understandably are reluctant to report that a child already born was unplanned or unwanted.

A better link between reproductive intentions and subsequent behavior can be established when the information is collected for the same women (users and nonusers) through a panel study or through a follow-up survey[9] of those who initiate contraception from a service facility. If one wants to evaluate the effectiveness of a program (meaning the multiple service delivery avenues available in a given area) in terms of the revised objective, then a sample of users and nonusers of reproductive age needs to be included in the panel study, and the required information needs to be collected prospectively: women are asked first about what their reproductive intentions are, and this information is linked with their subsequent fertility behavior. We have to address three issues: the indicator of unwanted childbearing, the definition and indicator of unhealthful manner, and data collection.

Proposal for a New Measure

The HARI index — an acronym for Helping Individuals Achieve their Reproductive Intentions, proposed by Jain (1992), incorporates individuals' reproductive intentions but not the morbidity associated with reproduction.[10] In terms of morbidity, the question is whether to compute a separate reproductive health index or have one index for both. In either case, we have to start with two components: the proportion of clients who achieved their reproductive intentions during the observation period, and the proportion of clients who experienced morbidity while trying to do so. This can be done easily, assuming that the classification and measurement of morbidity is handled by an explicit, locally determined process. A separate reproductive health index can be defined in terms of 100 minus the percentage of women who experience severe morbidity while trying to avoid an unplanned or unwanted pregnancy. A joint reproductive intention and health index can be defined by a modified HARI index as being equal to 100 minus the percentage of women who have an unplanned or unwanted pregnancy, or experience severe morbidity related to reproduction, during a specified period of observation. In programs that also provide services for safe abortion, the HARI index can be modified further and estimated by 100 minus the percentage of women who have an unplanned or unwanted birth, or experience severe morbidity related to reproduction, during a specified period.

The modified HARI index meets almost all of the criteria for an efficacy indicator mentioned above. It is client-centered, allowing clients to define the need to be met, with their wishes dominant over the efficacy perspectives that are driven by an interest in program or method performance. Implicit in this line of reasoning is the assumption that the clients are making voluntary statements. However, we must acknowledge that their "voluntarism" is inherently limited to the extent that women may be under considerable pressure from sex partners, the community, or family elders, or cannot negotiate contraceptive protection at the time of intercourse. The measure does not insist that a client continue with a specific or even any method, or that she receive services from a single service point; rather, it counts a client who avoids unwanted pregnancy as a "success," regardless of the number of other services and strategies she has used as means to avoid unwanted pregnancy. On the other hand, "failures" are attributed to the program for failing to empower the client sufficiently to meet her reproductive intentions, whether or not she is connected to a given service point.

Three issues need further clarification. What happens if a woman wants to have a child but cannot? What happens if a woman dies in childbirth? What happens if a woman changes her reproductive intention during the period of observation? The first two issues can be incorporated in the HARI index if the program is explicitly responsible for addressing them. These services may be integrated with contraceptive services in some countries, but if the resources are not controlled by the family planning program, the efficacy measure need not incorporate these two dimensions. The chance that a woman's reproductive intentions will change is likely to increase with the period of observation. If women are contacted periodically (for instance, every

year), these changes can be detected and incorporated in the index. On the other hand, if the reported change in intention from not wanting to wanting follows a pregnancy, we have to assume that the client is rationalizing, and we classify that pregnancy as a failure of the program.

The HARI index will be equal to 100 if the program is completely successful in helping individuals achieve their reproductive intentions in a healthful manner;[11] it will be equal to 0 if the program is a complete failure with respect to both unwanted pregnancy and unnecessary morbidity. It implies, but does not measure directly, the logical intervening steps — choice of technology, adequate information exchange, and so forth.

Insofar as the HARI index is derived from a population-based sample, it is automatically weighted to reflect the correct balance of clients' needs. But a program manager might want to look more closely at emerging constituencies or to identify groups for whom the program is performing below par. The utility of the index is enhanced if clients' experiences are disaggregated according to reproductive intentions. For example, women who wish to space have different needs and are potentially more challenging to serve (and in some settings demographically more important to serve) than women who wish to limit. With the HARI index disaggregated by clients' intentions, we can measure how effective a given program is with regard to serving women who wish to continue childbearing, who wish to space, and who wish to limit.

The index's value is enhanced when measurement is complemented by an analysis of types of failures; these classifications and their weights can provide the attentive manager with vital information for adjusting program operations. As an illustration, the calculation of the HARI index, combined with such case studies (see Figure 1 on next page) could distinguish between failures due to inadequacies of methods (that is, when continuous or compliant use of a method nonetheless leads to a pregnancy), failures due to poor quality of the information exchange (such as when a client uses a method inappropriate to her health

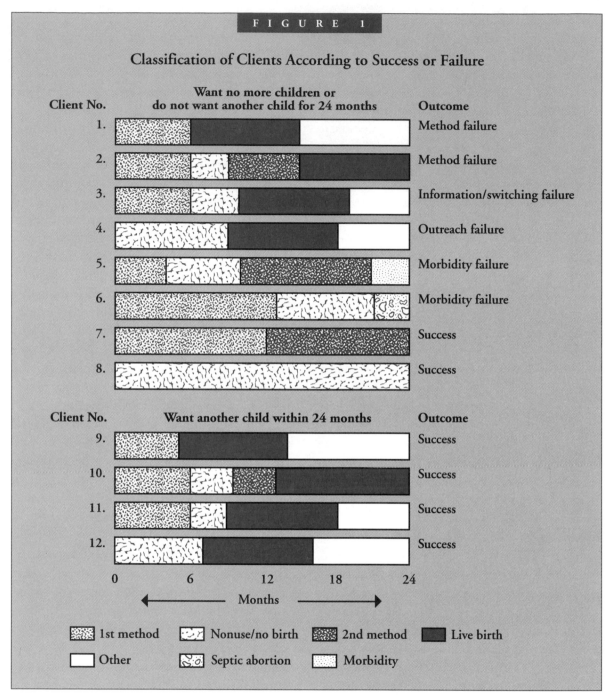

FIGURE 1

Classification of Clients According to Success or Failure

Client No.	Want no more children or do not want another child for 24 months	Outcome
1.		Method failure
2.		Method failure
3.		Information/switching failure
4.		Outreach failure
5.		Morbidity failure
6.		Morbidity failure
7.		Success
8.		Success

Client No.	Want another child within 24 months	Outcome
9.		Success
10.		Success
11.		Success
12.		Success

0   6   12   18   24

◀ Months ▶

1st method   Nonuse/no birth   2nd method   Live birth

Other   Septic abortion   Morbidity

status or the nature of her sexual relationship, or when a client is not informed about the possibility of switching methods or sources of supply), and failures due to inadequacies in outreach efforts (when a potential client does not get enough or appropriate information or access to a service facility).

To make the reproductive health link, we might add morbidity failure, when a client indicates that she has suffered undue morbidity while trying to avoid unwanted childbearing. This morbidity can occur at different points in the service process; it can be a problem inadequately addressed when a woman initially seeks contraception or safe abortion, or a problem that occurs during her use of a method, including morbidities arising from poor technique or improper or septic procedures. Morbidity also can be due to septic abortion, even if abortion is legal and safe services are widely available, because the woman was desperate to avoid the unwanted birth, but did not know where to go for safe services.

Illustrative Case Studies

Numerous pathways exist for an individual to achieve her reproductive goals, not all of which can be enumerated. However, as an illustration, in Figure 1 we summarize the experiences of 12 clients who were successful or experienced different types of failures. We consider 24 months of experience for each client, the reproductive intentions at the beginning of the period, and subsequent fertility and morbidity experiences. We assume that abortion is legal and available; therefore, failure is indicated by an unwanted pregnancy leading to an unwanted birth, an unwanted pregnancy terminated by a septic abortion, or an experience of morbidity. These clients first are classified into two groups: one group consists of eight women who want no more children or do not want another child for at least two years; the second group consists of four women who want another child within the next two years.

The experiences of clients 1–4 are classified as failures because they had unwanted births while trying to avoid them (1 and 2 as method failure, 3 as information failure, and 4 as outreach failure). Method failures can be reduced by better counseling on method use, by the availability of more effective contraceptive methods, and by the availability of safe abortion to deal with the not insignificant risk of method failure. Information failures can be reduced if, at the time method use is initiated, adequate information is provided about the possibility of switching if the method turns out to be unsuitable or unhealthful. Outreach failures can be reduced through special efforts to contact women at home and provide them with information about various service outlets and methods offered by the program.

The experiences of clients 5 and 6 are classified as failures because they experienced significant morbidity either while using a method or while terminating an unwanted pregnancy. These ex-

periences would have been classified as successes if unwanted births were the indicator of failure.

The experiences of clients 7 and 8 are classified as successes because they were able to delay their childbearing for the intended period under various circumstances, including the nonuse of contraception. Clients 9–12 also are classified as successes, because these women had a planned and wanted birth within the period of observation. If the reproductive intentions at the beginning of the observation period had not been ascertained (as is the case with cross-sectional or typical follow-up and panel surveys), these experiences would have been classified as failures (9 and 10 as method failure, 11 as information or switching failure, and 12 as outreach failure).[12]

Utilization of the HARI Index

What difference will the HARI index make to measuring the efficacy of family planning programs? To illustrate the utility of this index, we have used the information available from a follow-up survey of IUD initiators in Taiwan and panel studies conducted in the Philippines, Sri Lanka, Taiwan, and the United States. (Refer to Desai 1991 for the Philippines; De Silva 1992 for Sri Lanka; Freedman, Hermalin, and Chang 1975 for Taiwan 1967–70; Hermalin et al. for Taiwan 1967–74; Freedman and Takeshita 1969 for Taiwan follow-up survey; and Westoff and Ryder 1977 for the United States.) None of these studies, however, was conducted for this purpose. The information on reproductive intentions was collected from answers to questions about wanting or not wanting any more children. No information was collected at the initial contact about the timing of the next wanted birth, and none was collected retrospectively about whether clients suffered undue morbidity. Finally, from the available information, we cannot distinguish between the types of failure for Sri Lanka and the United States. For these reasons, failures include only those women who had a birth during the observation period even though they said at the beginning of the period that they did not want any more children. This classification scheme *overestimates* the value of the HARI index and success in our terms, because women having unplanned births or experiencing morbidity associated with the use of contraception and abortion are included in the success category.

In Figure 2, we compare the value of the HARI index with four other indicators of program evaluation estimated from a follow-up survey in Taiwan. The utility of following women and incorporating their reproductive intentions in measuring the efficacy of a program is clear. The conclusion about the program's effectiveness would be different if the focus was on the performance of a particular method rather than on the *total* experience of women. At one extreme, only 28 percent of women continued to use the same IUD for about 30 months; at the other extreme, 93 percent achieved their reproductive intentions during a period of three years. (Thus, the focus on the women's experience

rather than on a method provides a considerably improved picture of the program's degree of success.) Notwithstanding that the HARI index is a bit overestimated for the reasons mentioned above, an indicator based on the total experiences of women obviously captures reality better than that based on the performance of a particular method.

The values of the HARI index based on panel studies in Sri Lanka, the United States, and Taiwan (1967–70) are 93–94 (see Figure 3). Once the period of observation in Taiwan is increased from three to seven years, the value of the index declines from 93 to 88. This suggests that the failure rate may increase with the duration of exposure. The HARI index is lower for the Philippines (50), which probably reflects the known deficiencies in that country's program.

A further analysis of the data from the Philippines and Taiwan indicates that the outreach failure in the Philippines is 33 percent of all

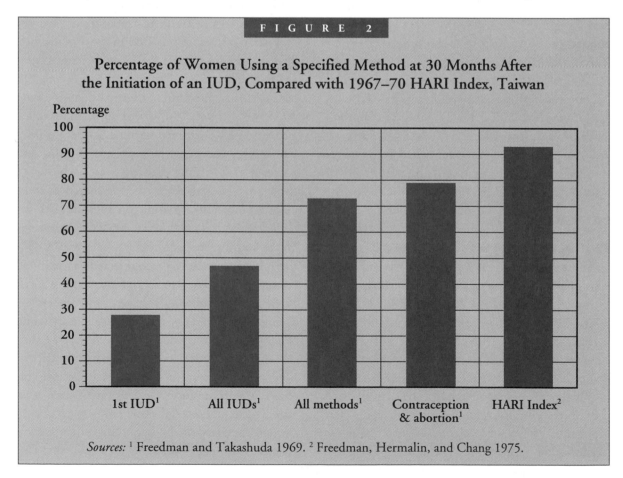

FIGURE 2

Percentage of Women Using a Specified Method at 30 Months After the Initiation of an IUD, Compared with 1967–70 HARI Index, Taiwan

Sources: [1] Freedman and Takashuda 1969. [2] Freedman, Hermalin, and Chang 1975.

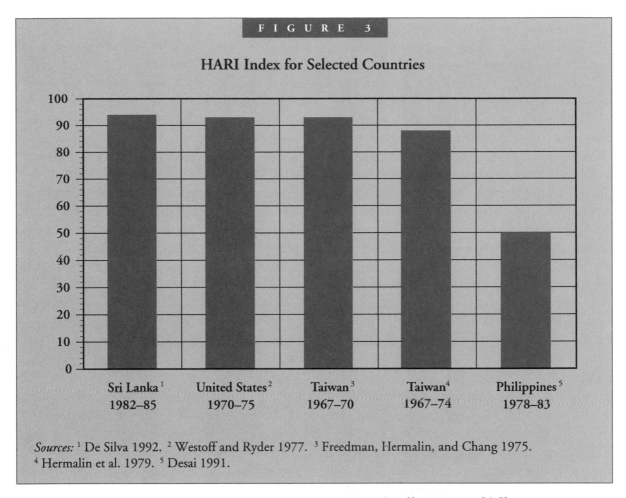

FIGURE 3

HARI Index for Selected Countries

| | Sri Lanka[1] 1982–85 | United States[2] 1970–75 | Taiwan[3] 1967–70 | Taiwan[4] 1967–74 | Philippines[5] 1978–83 |

Sources: [1] De Silva 1992. [2] Westoff and Ryder 1977. [3] Freedman, Hermalin, and Chang 1975. [4] Hermalin et al. 1979. [5] Desai 1991.

women, in comparison with 6 percent in Taiwan. The switching and method failures in the Philippines are 9 percent and 8 percent, respectively. In comparison, the two failures together in Taiwan come to 2 percent of all women. The differences between these two countries in the extent to which women successfully achieve their desired fertility levels in part reflects that abortion is legal and widely available in Taiwan, but not in the Philippines. Nevertheless, these comparisons indicate that the program in the Philippines needs to focus on how to provide services and information that will enable more women who wish to avoid pregnancy to do so, by offering adequate contraceptive choices and helping women sustain use more effectively.

In addition to measuring the efficacy of a service delivery program at the national or subnational level, the HARI index can be used to compare the performance of various service delivery points, to compare the effectiveness of different interventions at the same outlet, and to estimate the overall effectiveness of all services provided by one outlet. The use of the HARI index may not be advisable, however, to evaluate the performance of some types of programs, especially social marketing and commercial programs. In these programs, since the client is sharing the cost of commodities, the sales figures over a period of time would start reflecting their use. The rate of growth in the sales figures itself would be an indicator of success or failure of a social marketing program. Conversion of the sales figures to CYP or some other index would add very little to the comparison of cost-effectiveness of various social marketing programs. It is, however, important to understand clients' needs and behavior, even in these programs. The required information can be collected through specialized marketing surveys, as is usually done in evaluating the performance of marketing programs of other commodities.

Conclusion

With greater or lesser clarity and emphasis, two themes or rationales — an individual's right to regulate his or her fertility behavior, and a nation's interest in reducing its population growth rate — have guided the evolution of population policies and family planning programs in developing countries since the mid-1960s (see Dixon-Mueller 1993, for a detailed discussion and historical account of these two themes). The dilemmas posed by these themes are that the means adopted to reduce the rate of population growth are not always consistent with individuals' rights and welfare, and that there is skepticism that efforts guided by concern for individuals' rights and welfare will not solve the aggregate problem. Indeed, the explicitness of the conflict in some cases has seemed to increase while, paradoxically, a growing proportion of individuals are seeking to regulate their fertility voluntarily.

In our view, the population movement needs to delink family planning programs from the societal fertility reduction objective. This linkage has adversely affected the quality of contraceptive services and, in some circumstances, has led to dependence upon undesirable means to induce fertility decline, including community-wide incentives, quotas, and coercion. Instead, the design of family planning programs should be guided by the individual's right to regulate her or his fertility safely and effectively.

The indicators and evaluation frameworks used to measure the efficacy of family planning programs have been guided by an overriding interest in fertility reduction, rather than improvement of individuals' welfare. No single indicator can resolve all the problems associated with current efforts to measure the efficacy of family planning programs. We have argued that the efficacy measure needs to be linked with the stated objectives of these programs. The evaluation approach we have suggested is based on a proposed shift in these programs' objectives. In our view, efforts to measure the efficacy of family planning programs need to move beyond estimating their "net contribution to fertility de-

cline." Instead, these efforts should focus on measuring the efficacy of these programs in terms of the degree to which they are successful in assisting individuals to achieve their reproductive intentions in a healthful manner.

The available data are not adequate to incorporate this shift and to use the proposed efficacy indicator and evaluation framework. Naturally some experimentation is required in data collection and measurement of morbidity before we can define an index that can be used in cross-cultural comparisons. We believe that the highest priority needs to be assigned to defining indicators of morbidity associated with the avoidance of unwanted or unplanned childbearing and use of contraception, and to designing panel studies in a few selected countries to collect data from individuals that can link their reproductive intentions with their subsequent fertility and morbidity experiences.

It is not appropriate for us to present a detailed design of such studies. One possibility is to do so in collaboration with an ongoing cross-sectional survey, like the Demographic and Health Surveys, or clinic-based situation analyses. We suggest that in these panel and follow-up studies, women, at the time of initial contact, be asked about their reproductive intentions — namely, whether and when they want to have their next child. (For those pregnant at the time of interview, this information would refer to the next pregnancy.) The response can be recorded in the exact number of months reported by a woman or in discrete categories, such as never, not for five years, not for two years, and within two years. Other responses, such as that the woman is uncertain or it is "up to God," can be classified as if the individual wants a child within two years. At the initial contact, questions also could be raised about the reproductive health services women are seeking, whether they have any health problems they believe are related to their use of contraception or that interfere with their use of contraception or limit their range of choices, and whether they have had any significant reproductive health problems. In subsequent interviews, questions can be asked regarding clients' experience of any pregnancy, its timing, its outcome, and circumstances under which the pregnancy occurred. At these interviews, questions also should be asked relating to the women's experience of any "substantial" discomfort, infections, or need to switch methods for clear medical reasons, as opposed to personal preference. (Difficulties or delays in switching methods that are unsuitable owing to health effects should be considered a negative.)

These types of data from a number of countries are required to appropriately measure the efficacy of family planning programs in terms of the revised objectives. We also propose that new alliances be created between contraceptive and reproductive health services. Countries interested in fertility reduction, in addition, need to create alliances between population and development policies.

Acknowledgements

The authors gratefully acknowledge the valuable research assistance provided by Shelly Friedland and helpful suggestions made on an earlier version by John Bongaarts, Adrienne Germain, Albert I. Hermalin, and Beverly Winikoff.

Notes

1   According to the Population Policy Data Bank maintained by the United Nations Population Division, out of 131 developing countries, 74 considered their fertility level to be too high, 9 perceived it to be too low, and 48 perceived it to be satisfactory. These three groups account for, respectively, 85, 1, and 14 percent of the people living in developing countries. Of the 74 developing countries that considered their fertility to be too high, 64 have policies to reduce their fertility rate and provide direct support to family planning programs. (These 64 countries contain 82 percent of the population of developing countries.) An additional 39 countries also provide direct support to family planning programs, but for improving health. The remaining 28 countries do not provide direct support to family planning programs (United Nations 1987-90, 1992).

2   A vast literature on the determinants of fertility indicates that the costs of rearing children and the benefits derived from them are not shared equally by mothers and fathers. Moreover, parents have large families for reasons such as old age security, to provide extra help in domestic and field work, and to support other siblings — in other

words, to enhance their own welfare. Thus, a shift toward an improvement in the welfare of children and a more equitable sharing of the costs and benefits of children between men and women would create conditions conducive to fertility decline. We do not deal with this issue.

3   This assumption is necessary, because in the absence of a clearly perceived population problem, there is no need for a separate population policy or a population sector, and we can move directly to the long-term vision stated above.

4   It can be argued that family planning programs also should offer services for identification and treatment of infertility, which would enable some women to achieve their reproductive goals. We have excluded these services from our list because the incidence of primary sterility in most societies is very low — about 3 percent (Bongaarts and Potter 1983) — and the cost of such services is very high. Prevention of sexually transmitted and other infections or traumas that result in infertility will thus be more effective for larger numbers of people. In certain settings with elevated rates of infertility, it may make sense to include these services. Our proposal also implies that other reproductive health services — for example, those advocated by Germain, Nowrojee and Pyne, and Aitken in this volume — should be provided through the health sector.

5   Can cash or other kinds of incentives and disincentives for the use of contraception or avoidance of a birth be included in a voluntary program? These activities may be very effective in reducing fertility without either influencing family size norms or necessarily helping individuals meet their existing goals.

6   One analysis carried out by Jain (1989) also suffered from this bias. This analysis showed a very high effect of availability on contraceptive use. The author acknowledged the bias in a footnote, but carried on the analysis anyway.

7   Reproductive intentions of individuals, in the presence of means to regulate fertility, strongly influence their subsequent use of contraception and abortion, as well as their fertility. (See for example, Freedman, Jain, and Sun 1970 and Freedman et al. 1971 for Taiwan; and Westoff and Ryder 1977 for the United States.)

8   The concept of "healthful manner" needs to be developed further for measurement purposes. The word "healthful" was added to generate an interest among service providers and to address those reproductive health needs that are closely related to contraceptive use and fertility regulation. "Unhealthful" contraception would be that which results in mortality (easily defined) and morbidity (less easily defined). Not only is defining morbidity in different locations a challenge, but so is measuring it.

9 A panel study can be set up by taking a subsample of the respondents included in a cross-sectional survey (for example, the Demographic and Health Surveys) and reinterviewing them after one, two, and three years. A follow-up survey can be used to evaluate the efficacy of services provided through a service facility.

10 The Index is a modification of the concept of extended use-effectiveness proposed by Tietze and Lewit (1968), with one major difference: the extended use-effectiveness concept attributes pregnancies that occur among spacers after the initiation of a contraceptive method to program failure, whereas the HARI index does not. Moreover, the extended use-effectiveness concept does not incorporate women who do not initiate contraceptive use, whereas the HARI index can incorporate non-users through a panel study. The HARI index may be confused with the concept of unmet need, defined as women who want to delay or stop childbearing, but are not using contraception. The extent of unmet need is not an indicator of program performance; instead it is used to justify program expansion. The HARI index, in comparison, by linking reproductive intentions with subsequent fertility behavior, can be used to measure the impact of service delivery on meeting the unmet need. In the absence of panel or follow-up studies, we cannot judge the accuracy of statements about reproductive intentions or the impact of services on eliminating unmet need.

11 The value of this index also will be high in settings in which a large majority of women do not want to regulate their fertility — that is, are not in need of fertility regulation methods.

12 Should women who want to have a child but did not have one during the period of observation be treated as a failure of the program? We recommend that these women be treated as failures only if they were unable to have a child because of infertility and the program is responsible but unable to help them.

References

Adamchak, D. J., and M. T. Mbizvo. 1990. The relationship between fertility and contraceptive prevalence in Zimbabwe. *International Family Planning Perspectives* 16(3):103–106.

Bongaarts, J. 1990. The measurement of wanted fertility. *Population and Development Review* 16(3):487–506.

———. 1992. The fertility impact of family planning programs. Paper presented at the International Planned Parenthood Federation Congress on Meeting Challenges: Promoting Choices, October, in New Delhi.

Bongaarts, J., W. P. Mauldin, and J. F. Phillips. 1990. The demographic impact of family planning programs. *Studies in Family Planning* 21(6):299–310.

Bongaarts, J., and R. G. Potter. 1983. *Fertility, biology, and behavior: An analysis of the proximate determinants.* New York: Academic Press.

Boulier, B. 1985. Family planning programs and contraceptive availability: Their effects on contraceptive use and fertility. In N. Birdsall (ed.), *The effects of family planning programs on fertility in the developing world,* Staff Working Paper No. 677. Washington, D.C.: World Bank.

Chandrasekaran, C., and A. I. Hermalin (eds.). 1975. *Measuring the effect of family planning programs on fertility.* Paris: Organization for Economic Cooperation and Development.

Cutright, P. 1983. The ingredients of recent fertility decline in developing countries. *International Family Planning Perspectives* 9(4):101–109.

Department of Family Welfare. 1989. *Family welfare programmes in India yearbook: 1987-88.* New Delhi: Ministry of Health and Family Welfare, Government of India.

De Silva, W. I. 1992. Achievement of reproductive intentions in Sri Lanka, 1982–1985: A longitudinal study. *Social Biology* 39(1–2):123–137.

Desai, S. 1991. Why fertility preferences fail to predict fertility? Evidence from longitudinal data in the Philippines. Paper presented at the annual meeting of the Population Association of America, March, in Washington, D.C.

Dixon-Mueller, R. 1993. *Population policy and women's rights.* Westport, Conn.: Praeger.

Freedman, R., et al. 1971. Fertility after insertion of an IUD in Taiwan's family-planning program. *Social Biology* 18(1):46-54.

Freedman, R., A. I. Hermalin, and M. C. Chang. 1975. Do statements about desired family size predict fertility? The case of Taiwan, 1967–70. *Demography* 12(3):407–416.

Freedman, R., A. K. Jain, and T. H. Sun. 1970. Correlates of family limitation in Taiwan after IUD insertion. In G. P. Cernada (ed.), *Taiwan family planning reader: How a program works.* Taichung: Chinese Center for International Training in Family Planning.

Freedman, R., and J. Y. Takeshita. 1969. *Family planning in Taiwan: An experiment in social change.* Princeton, N.J.: Princeton University Press.

Hermalin, A. I., et al. 1979. Do intentions predict fertility? The experience in Taiwan, 1967–74. *Studies in Family Planning* 10(3):75–95.

Huber, S. C., and P. D. Harvey. 1989. Family planning programs in ten developing countries: Cost effectiveness by mode of service delivery. *Journal of Biosocial Science* 21(3):267–277.

Jain, A. K. 1985. The impact of development and population policies on fertility in India. *Studies in Family Planning* 16(4):181–198.

———. 1989. Fertility reduction and the quality of family planning services. *Studies in Family Planning* 20(1):1–16.

———. (ed.). 1992. Conclusion. In *Managing quality of care in population programs*. West Hartford, Conn.: Kumarian Press.

Jain, A. K., J. Bruce, and S. Kumar. 1992. Quality of services, programme efforts and fertility reduction. In J. F. Phillips and J. A. Ross (eds.), *Family Planning Programmes and Fertility*. Oxford: Clarendon Press.

Lapham, R. J., and W. P. Mauldin. 1984. Family planning program effort and birthrate decline in developing countries. *International Family Planning Perspectives* 10(4):109–118.

Mauldin, W. P., and J. A. Ross. 1991. Family planning programs: Efforts and results, 1982–89. *Studies in Family Planning* 22(6):350–367.

Phillips, J. F., et al. 1988. Determinants of reproductive changes in a traditional society: Evidence from Matlab, Bangladesh. *Studies in Family Planning* 19(6):313–334.

Phillips, J. F., and J. A. Ross, (eds.). 1992. *Family planning programmes and fertility*. Oxford: Clarendon Press.

Ross, J. A., and C. B. Lloyd. 1992. Methods for measuring the fertility impact of family planning programmes: The experience of the last decade. In J. F. Phillips and J. A. Ross (eds.), *Family Planning Programmes and Fertility*. Oxford: Clarendon Press.

Shelton, J. D. 1991. What's wrong with CYP? *Studies in Family Planning* 22(5):332–334.

Tietze, C., and S. Lewit. 1968. Statistical evaluation of contraceptive methods: Use-effectiveness and extended use-effectiveness. *Demography* 5(2):931–940.

United Nations. 1987–90. *World population policies*. 3 vols. New York.

———. 1992. *World population monitoring, 1991*. New York.

Visaria, P., L. Visaria, and A. Jain. 1992. *Contraceptive use and fertility in Gujarat*. Ahmedabad: Gujarat Institute of Development Research.

Westoff, C. F., and N. B. Ryder. 1977. The predictive validity of reproductive intentions. *Demography* 14(4):431–453.

Wishik, S. M., and K. Chen. 1973. *Couple-year of protection: A measure of family planning program output*. Manual for Evaluation of Family Planning Programs No. 7. New York: Columbia University, Center for Population and Family Health.

15

Reaching Young People: Ingredients of Effective Programs

Kirstan Hawkins and Bayeligne Meshesha

The foundations for sexual and reproductive health and gender relations are laid early in life through an interplay of familial, social, economic, and cultural forces. Although data are fragmentary, the number of sexually active young people is clearly substantial and probably growing rapidly. Many girls and young women still marry or enter consensual unions very young (United Nations 1989:34) and are exposed to sexual relations before they are physically and emotionally mature. In many other cases, survey data and qualitative evidence suggest that young people around the world are more and more likely to be sexually active outside of marriage, as a result of economic conditions, peer pressure and mass media influences, migration, and other forces of social change.

Demographic and Health Survey (DHS) data show, for example, that in seven of 11 countries in Sub-Saharan Africa, more than half of teenage women (both married and unmarried) aged 15–19 have had sexual relations at least once; in five of these countries, more than half the young women with sexual experience are unmarried (Population Reference Bureau 1992: 31). In 10 of 11 countries of Sub-Saharan Africa, contain-

ing 40 percent of the region's population, the majority of teenage women give birth by age 20 (Barker 1990). World Fertility Survey (WFS) data suggest that unmarried adolescents in Sub-Saharan Africa are about as sexually active as youth in Europe and North America (Ajayi 1991; Population Reference Bureau 1992: n. 32; WHO 1989b). By age 19, more than 90 percent of all Latin American males have reportedly had intercourse, as have 45–60 percent of females (Singh and Wulf 1990). Few data exist on young people's sexual activity in Asia, and variation across countries may be great. About 25 percent of single adolescents may be sexually active, and many, especially girls in South Asia, marry very young (United Nations 1989).

Regardless of age, marital status, or income level, young people are exposed to mass media images of sexuality, violence, and gender roles that influence their values, material aspirations, and interactions with one another, their families, and their communities. Generally ignorant about their own bodies, and unwilling or unable to use most family planning and health services (Ford et al. 1992), sexually active young people are at significant risk of experiencing serious consequences, such as health complications or death from pregnancy and childbirth (United Nations 1989);[1] unwanted pregnancy and unsafe abortion;[2] sexually transmitted diseases (STDs), including AIDS (United Nations 1989);[3] social rejection, including expulsion from home or school; and destructive sexual relations (Hawkins, Ojakaa and Meshesha 1992; Singh and Wulf 1990).

Deteriorating economic conditions in many countries place young people at increased risk of abusive, exploitative, and unsafe sexual encounters. Poverty is often a direct cause of prostitution among the young, some of whom are sold by their families (Pyne 1992). Reports also abound, particularly in countries of Sub-Saharan Africa undergoing economic structural adjustment programs (such as Zimbabwe and Ghana), of young women conceding to pressure from older men and trading sexual favors for school fees, transportation, food, and clothing in order to continue their education, support their families, or simply survive (Hawkins, Ojakaa, and Meshesha 1992; Standing 1989). Violence against and sexual abuse of young people are also widely reported (Heise, Germain, and Pitanguy 1994; Nowrojee 1993). Many, including very young children, who end up living on the street (in Brazil, for example) are victims of violence in the streets and abuse in the family (Filgueras 1992). Meanwhile, the rape and seduction of very young girls is also being reported in many communities; some young women and researchers interpret this as a strategy by men to avoid Human Immunodeficiency Virus (HIV) infection (Hawkins et al. 1991). Young women who seek to enter domestic service find themselves entering commercial sex work, often as a result of initial abuse by their employers (Dixon-Mueller 1993; Heise, Germain, and Pitanguy 1994; IPPF 1991). Many of these women have already been rejected by their own families. Paradoxically, as young people stay in school longer and delay marriage, factors that contribute to lower fertility overall, they are increasingly likely to engage in premarital sexual relations and are thus exposed to the associated risks (United Nations 1989; WHO 1989a).

Without appropriate and effective programs for sexuality and gender education, and without access to family planning and other reproductive health services, young people will remain at risk and, further, will be unprepared as parents to assist their children in coping with this most intimate and complex aspect of human life. Nonetheless, the design and implementation of programs for youth in many countries have been severely constrained by the norms of parents, educators, religious leaders, family planning professionals, policy makers, and politicians. To the extent that conventional population and family planning programs address adolescent sexuality, they have for the most part limited their focus to the consequences of unprotected adolescent sex, especially teenage pregnancy (Dixon-Mueller 1993). "Population education" and "family life education" projects have generally ignored sexuality and gender relations, promoting instead norms of "responsible parenthood" within marriage and abstinence outside it. Conventional education projects rarely, if ever, provide information on sexual feelings, attitudes, and behavior, or on gender roles and expectations; nor do they generally refer young people to contraceptive and other reproductive health services. It is doubtful that such programs do much to prevent either early sexual debut or the consequences of sexual relations for young people. A 16-year-old single mother in Nairobi clearly states the dilemma young people face: "They are always telling us we should plan our families, but no one will tell us how."

The failure of parents and social institutions to provide information on sexuality and services that enable young people to protect themselves from harm and to develop the foundations for healthy, satisfying, and responsible sexuality and reproduction not only leaves them at high risk, but also contravenes basic principles of human rights (see Correa and Petchesky in this volume). Similarly, conventional programs that do not challenge existing sex roles and attitudes toward male and female sexuality reinforce prevailing imbalances of power in gender relations.

In this chapter, we briefly address the societal contexts within which many young people become sexually active; assess current strategies to meet young people's needs; and suggest improved approaches to reaching them. Our primary conclusions are that we must listen to young people themselves to understand their concerns; ensure their participation in formulating solutions; encourage them to establish more egalitarian gender relations, including healthy and responsible sexual relationships; provide them with the information as well as the opportunity to discuss sexuality and gender; and guarantee their access to reproductive health services.

Our focus is on special projects for youth in Southern countries, the area of our experience. Such programs both directly assist the youth involved and serve as examples for broader replication or expansion. They will, perhaps, produce a generation of parents who can help their children. They will not redress the underlying structural conditions that foster early and unsafe sexual activity; nor are they likely to reach young people in the most dire circumstances — those who have been abandoned, exploited as domestic or industrial labor, sexually abused, or sold into prostitution. To prevent such exploitation, and to help youngsters out of these circumstances, substantially more resources must be allocated to health, education, and poverty alleviation programs. Complementary policies and programs are also needed to change a multitude of other predisposing conditions, including sex discrimination and mass media messages, to name only two of the most important.

Reaching Young People

Definitions of childhood and adulthood vary across cultures, as well as within socioeconomic groups and historical periods. In many societies, a period of "adolescence" does not exist. Rather, children are recognized as sexual adults after they have gone through a rite of passage, such as marriage, special lessons, or a particular ceremony — genital mutilation being an extreme example (Population Reference Bureau 1992; Toubia

1993). Demographic studies, social science research, and literature published by family planning and population programs use imprecise definitions of "youth" and various age ranges. These sources rarely provide data on sexual activity for children under 15. Many use the age range 15–24, which covers dramatically different stages of life; others aggregate data for 5- to 14-year-olds and 15- to 24-year-olds, making the calculation of teenage rates impossible. Some large surveys, such as the DHS, a few specialized "young adult reproductive health" surveys, and smaller community-based studies collect data on ages 10–19. (Data from such inquiries are usefully summarized in Barker 1990; Singh and Wulf 1990; and United Nations 1989.)

Marital status is another critical distinguishing characteristic that often is not clearly specified in the literature. All young people should have access to sexuality and gender education, as well as to services to protect their sexual and reproductive health; however, by law or practice, the unmarried are often excluded from these services (United Nations 1989). For a variety of reasons, available data do not permit estimation of "unmet need" for contraception and other reproductive health services among unmarried people, with the consequence that unmarried youth are omitted from basic calculations used to design and implement many family planning programs (Dixon-Mueller and Germain 1993: 332). Young unmarried people who are sexually active are also likely to face special social problems and sanctions that inhibit them from seeking advice and care from parents, teachers, or health professionals.

There are two main reasons that we have little systematic information about young people's sexual experience, feelings, and attitudes. First, asking young people about their sexual experience, especially outside marriage, is regarded as extremely sensitive in most settings. Second, existing research on adolescents in Southern countries has been motivated more by concerns about fertility than by interest in sexuality. These studies provide some information on contraceptive use, abortion, and maternal outcomes, but often do not include data on boys and young men. An important exception is a 1992 study of young people's sexual experience in 11 African countries (WHO 1992).

In most countries, including the United States and the United Kingdom, most children do not receive adequate sex education either in school or at home. A United Nations inquiry (1989) found that among governments acknowledging concern about adolescent fertility, only 22 percent in Africa and 33 percent in Latin America included contraceptive education as part of their public school curricula. Young people's main sources of information — peers and mass media — can be seriously inaccurate and even encourage risky behavior, such as use of ineffective means of contraception or STD prevention (Ajayi 1991; Elangot 1987; IPPF 1985; Makinwa-Adebusoye 1992; Shepherd 1987; United Nations 1989; WHO 1989b).

Almost everywhere, young people are exposed to contradictory social expectations with regard to their sexuality. The virtually universal double standard that values premarital virginity for girls and early sexual experience for boys (Gage-Brandon and Meekers 1992; Singh and Wulf 1990; WHO 1989a; WHO 1989b), along with mass media images that portray women as sexual objects, places severe burdens on both young women and young men. Young women are often pressured into early sexual relations by boys or men who see this as their right; the young woman may perceive the sexual encounter, or the yielding of her virginity, as the means to a relationship or marriage, but in reality the encounter often leads to rejection by the man, or by peers and parents.

Other pressures and contradictions arise in pronatalist cultures. In parts of Sub-Saharan Africa, both virginity and proof of a woman's fertility are seen as prerequisites to marriage (Ford et al. 1992). Boys also face pressure to have premarital sex. In Latin America, cases have been reported of fathers who have taken their sons to prostitutes against their will in order to initiate them into sexual experience and reinforce heterosexual gender roles (Hawkins 1991). In most countries,

boys are teased by their peers if they have not had sex, and frequently fabricate lies to hide their lack of experience (Antrobus, Germain, and Nowrojee 1994; ECOS 1992). Although the burden of responsibility for unwanted pregnancy falls on young women (Obura 1991), they are often powerless either to resist pressure to have sex or to negotiate use of condoms.

Many young people thus find themselves pressured into their first sexual experiences with little accurate information and filled with anxiety, shame, and guilt. Unwanted pregnancy, infection, and other physical and emotional harm are often the results, for young women and young men alike.

Despite the centrality of sexuality and reproduction to human life, few societies prepare either their children or their adults to cope well with these issues. In many cultures, traditional mechanisms to socialize and educate young people about sexuality and sexual behavior are breaking down. In parts of Sub-Saharan Africa, for example, the role of grandparents, aunts, and uncles has been eroded as young people have been separated from their kin by either geographic or cultural distance (Dixon-Mueller and Germain 1993: 332; Kilbride and Kilbride 1990).

In many Asian cultures, where sexuality has always been a taboo subject between parents and children, there exist no prescribed ways for young people to learn about their sexuality. In parts of Asia, early marriage is used to control girls' sexuality and limit it to purposes of reproduction (Ramasubban 1994). So great are the sanctions in some societies that young, unmarried women who have engaged in premarital or extramarital sexual activity, or who have even been raped, may be murdered with impunity by a father or brother, executed, or driven to suicide (Koenig et al. 1988).

In Latin America and the Caribbean, sexuality is typically not openly discussed between parents and daughters. Romantic love and marriage are idealized in popular youth culture, and are in direct conflict with gender norms of male sexual prowess (machismo) and female passivity. Lacking educational and employment opportunities, many young women in these countries perceive pregnancy, even outside marriage, as a way of achieving adult social status and a clearly valued role in the community.

It is evident from work across many cultures that sexuality profoundly affects young people's sense of identity and self-esteem, as well as their physical well-being and social development. A recent International Planned Parenthood Federation (IPPF) meeting with representatives from youth programs in six countries (Ireland, Grenada, Lebanon, India, Thailand, and Ethiopia) confirmed this view. The young people concluded that programs must recognize their right to choose whether or not to be sexually active; to use contraception; to obtain safe abortion; to receive information; and to exercise these choices regardless of economic or political conditions. Moreover, they emphasized the importance of using the language of young people themselves in these programs. How close do current programs come to this standard?

Current Programs and Gaps to Be Filled

The objectives of "population education" and "family life education" as promoted in Southern countries have been primarily to prevent adolescent childbearing by stressing premarital abstinence, encouraging youth to delay marriage, and promoting family planning within marriage. Most population education and family life education are given only at the secondary school level, however, by which time attitudes about sex roles and gender relations have been formed, the majority of young people have left school, and many are married or otherwise sexually active.

The United Nations Educational, Scientific, and Cultural Organization (UNESCO) defines "population education" as "an educational program which provides for the study of the population situation in the family, community, nation, and world, with the purpose of developing the student's rational and responsible attitudes toward that situation" (Sherris 1982). In several countries, including Indonesia, South Korea, the Philippines, and Singapore, population educa-

tion programs date back to the late 1960s and early 1970s, and were designed as one of several elements of policies to reduce population growth. In-school population education programs, funded by the United Nations Population Fund (UNFPA), UNESCO, and the World Bank, as well as by bilateral donors, have usually sought to explain the relationship between population growth and development and to promote small family norms (Sherris 1982). Often population topics are incorporated into social studies, geography, home economics, science, or mathematics courses. Although population education is sometimes viewed as a precursor to sex education, in reality most of these programs omit information on contraception, sexuality, and gender relations, on grounds that such information is too sensitive to impart to the young and the unmarried (Ford et al. 1992; Dixon-Mueller 1993).

"Family life education" has been defined as "an educational process designed to assist young people in their physical, social, emotional, and moral development as they prepare for adulthood, marriage, parenthood, and aging, as well as their social relationships in the socio-cultural context of family and society" (IPPF 1985). Family life education is usually integrated into geography, biology, home economics, and religious or moral studies curricula. Though family life education programs vary greatly in content, for the most part they emphasize conservative values and conventional family forms, and ignore sexuality in order to avoid political or religious opposition (Ford et al. 1992). Family life education programs that do include sexuality generally provide basic information on the biology of reproduction but exclude discussions of sexual feelings, identity, attitudes, behavior, or gender roles. Most teachers are not trained in counseling and interpersonal skills, and are therefore ill equipped to deal with young people's concerns and questions relating to sexuality and gender relations.

Although population and family life education programs have existed in some countries for nearly three decades, little research has been done to assess whether they improve young people's knowledge or change their attitudes on the topics covered. We also know almost nothing about the impact, if any, on their sexual and reproductive health (Ford et al. 1992), or about growth in young people's knowledge or changes in their attitudes. Professionals and policy makers are questioning both the content and the efficacy of such programs. For example, in Kenya, where various family life education programs have been in place for more than 20 years, a study of youth aged 12–19 found that 66 percent had received information on reproduction; of these, only 8 percent could correctly identify a woman's fertile period (Barker 1990: n.50). Given the widespread reliance of young people on the rhythm method or withdrawal to prevent pregnancy, such lack of knowledge carries serious consequences.

Family planning services in Southern countries, even those that have initiated pilot programs in "sex education," often refuse, or are forbidden by law or policy, to provide or make referrals for contraceptive and abortion services for unmarried young people (see, for example, Brandrup-Lukanow et al. 1992; United Nations 1989). In fact, the only "protection" offered to most young people is abstinence, despite the strong forces that may impel them toward sexual relations. Even in programs open to innovation, the attitudes of service providers can be a major barrier to young people's access to services. In some countries, clinic staff are known to deny contraceptives to young, unmarried women unless their fertility has already been proved through a previous pregnancy, and many deny post-abortion contraception to unmarried women. Lack of confidentiality and long waiting times discourage unmarried young people from attending clinics, where they may be spotted by family, friends, or teachers. As a result, many of these young people attempt ineffective or harmful remedies to prevent conception, or obtain contraceptives from pharmacies, if they can afford them, without information or counseling (IPPF 1991). Some conventional family planning services that are open to young people are now experimenting with ways to provide information or counseling on sexuality and gender relations that will assist young people to avoid or end dangerous or irresponsible sexual relationships.

The International Planned Parenthood Federation has strongly advocated greater access for young people, regardless of marital status, to information and services that address their reproductive and sexual health needs, sexuality, and gender relations (IPPF 1993). While much remains to be done to achieve this goal throughout the IPPF network, backed by family planning associations that are willing to experiment, this policy initiative may help to identify means to remove pervasive taboos. To meet the aspirations of young people, these programs will need to surmount opposition from many quarters, including the reluctance of policy makers to deal with sex and challenge gender roles; the taboos against sexual discussions between children and their parents; the moral position that abstinence before marriage is the only appropriate behavior; and the pervasive belief that sex education — and, even more so, provision of contraceptive information and services — leads to promiscuity among the young.

There is no evidence that sexual activity increases among young people who are provided sex education (Ford et al. 1992). Rather, it appears from our experience that sexual activity is delayed with increased awareness, peer support, and greater freedom to discuss sexuality with parents and other adults. For example, some of the youth promoters in the Family Guidance Association of Ethiopia explained that they were not currently sexually active and wished to delay any sexual relations until they had finished their education and were able to commit themselves to marriage. Evidence from the United States also suggests that no strong links exist between sexual education and either the start of sexual intercourse or increased sexual activity (Kirby et al. 1991). Sex education alone can at least provide accurate information about contraception and protection against STDs, without which sexually active youngsters subject themselves to tremendous risk (for example, the use of lime and potassium salt as a vaginal contraceptive in Nigeria). Healthy sexuality, however, requires access to services, not just information. An honest and positive view of sexuality is necessary for young people to manage their sexual and reproductive health: "Half an education is dangerous," reported one mother participating in a sexuality seminar for mothers and daughters in Cameroun (Antrobus, Germain, and Nowrojee 1994). A Canadian study found that teenagers who had negative feelings about sexuality were less likely to practice safe sexual behaviors than were their peers who had positive feelings about sexuality (Fisher 1990).

Proposed Program Approaches

The needs of young people vary according to age; gender; class; religion and culture; urban or rural residence; and whether they are in school or out of school, married or unmarried, sexually active or not sexually active (Ford et al. 1992). Likewise, the programs designed to meet diverse needs are clearly shaped by broader social and economic factors. While no one program model could possibly suit all contexts, some basic principles can be derived from our experience to date.

The starting point for any program is to listen to young people's concerns and understand how they perceive their own needs. Programs such as Gente Joven in Mexico have done this by conducting community surveys and identifying interested and responsible young people to be trained as "peer promoters" according to a clear set of guidelines (Aguilar 1992). All educational materials are geared to needs identified by young people and are pretested to elicit input from youth themselves. The counseling center in Ethiopia, the Kenya Youth Program, and the PROFAMILIA youth clinic in Colombia also utilize groups of peer promoters to provide continual feedback to program managers on the relevance, strengths, and weaknesses of the programs (see Brandrup-Lukanow et al. 1992). Programs must include not just information, but also counseling and services. They must be participatory rather than didactic, and should be continu-

ally evaluated and modified to assure their effectiveness. They must attempt to mobilize parental and community support.

Provision of Sexuality Education, Counseling, and Services

Sexuality education is likely to be most effective when it is interactive and participatory. Mexfam, for example, provides sexual guidance courses to youngsters as well as to parents and teachers, using a participatory technique based on five principles — dialogue, responsibility, life planning, equality between women and men, and mutual respect — adapted from the Center for Population Options Life Planning Education Curriculum (1985). The family planning association of Guatemala, APROFAM, has also adopted this educational methodology and has organized discussion groups between young people and their parents. While separate sessions for boys and girls to discuss gender roles and sexuality are beneficial, there are also advantages to exploring male and female attitudes in mixed sessions. It appears that the best strategy may involve a combination of mixed and separate sessions, depending upon cultural appropriateness. Mexfam uses such a combined approach, whereas the youth program of the Family Guidance Association of Ethiopia has found that separate sessions for boys and girls are needed in order to address their different concerns.

In addition to accurate information and contraceptive services, one-on-one counseling and broader health services are essential. The concerns raised by young people in counseling sessions provide clear indications of the need for supportive interaction as well as services. The Ethiopian Youth Project, for example, has provided services and support to young people on the full range of sexuality-related issues: to young women who are pregnant and seeking abortion; young women with severe gynecologic problems following illegal abortion; young men concerned about girlfriends who have tried to abort their own pregnancies; couples and single women seeking contraceptive advice and services; young men with painful discharge, afraid of AIDS after unprotected sex with prostitutes; teenagers anxious about masturbation, wet dreams, premature ejaculation, penis size, impotence, or talking to girls; youths who have low self-esteem, have difficulty talking about sex, or have questions about virginity; young victims of rape and abduction; young women in domestic service who have been subjected to sexual abuse; and young people worried about attracting a boyfriend or girlfriend, and about unreciprocated love (see Box 1).

Counseling, not simply teaching, empowers young people to resolve conflicts, understand their sexual feelings, and make their own decisions. Thus it requires a nonjudgmental approach based on trust between the counselor and the young person. Although such a relationship is difficult in societies that condemn talk of sexuality and premarital sex, staff must be trained and motivated to build a positive environment in which they and young clients can discuss the meaning of sexuality in the young people's own terms, acknowledging the pleasure as well as the

risks. To be most effective, as it is in the Ethiopia project, counseling must be a dynamic, continuous process of communication that goes beyond the initial question or concern to address the broader tensions and dilemmas young people face. This process is also reflected in plays written and performed by a youth drama troupe attached to the counseling program. For example, in one play, which is also being used to develop educational videos in local languages, a conflict between a girl and her parents is resolved with the help of an uncle, who acts as a bridge between the traditional values of his brother and the new values and peer pressures acting on his niece. In the Mexfam program, coordinators and promoters refer young people to community doctors or psychologists for counseling and other services.

In addition to counseling, young people need health services, including contraceptives; emergency postcoital contraception; diagnosis and treatment of STDs; pregnancy testing; provision of, or referral for, prenatal care if the pregnancy is wanted; and safe abortion if it is not. Provision of

---

BOX 1

Reaching Young People in Ethiopia

Youth in Ethiopia are caught not only in a time of personal transition in the development and understanding of their sexuality and personal relationships, but also in an environment of great social and economic upheaval. In response to high levels of unwanted pregnancy, unsafe abortion, and STD infection among young people, the Family Guidance Association of Ethiopia initiated a youth counseling program in Addis Ababa in 1990.

The project seeks to reach young people of both sexes, in school and out of school, through existing youth recreation centers that are easily accessible to the many young people who have been displaced by war from their families and communities. Staff and peer promoters provide information, education, counseling and contraceptives services. Youth ask for advice and information on a wide array of concerns, including sexual development, relationships and sexual identity, the consequences of botched abortion, pregnancy testing, fear of AIDS or STDs after

unprotected sex with prostitutes, and sexual violence.

Condom distribution from the recreation centers, school counseling programs, and peer promoters have been particularly successful components of the program. Over 20,000 condoms were distributed to young people in 1991. As a result of media campaigns initiated by the project and the government, there also now appears to be a high level of HIV awareness among young people in Addis Ababa.

The first three years of the project have demonstrated that it is possible to talk to young people about sexuality and provide contraceptives where appropriate, in a manner that increases young people's own sense of personal responsibility and without engendering opposition. The program is still in a pilot stage. The major challenge is to replicate its small-scale successes on a wider scale.

Source: Hawkins, Ojakaa, and Meshesha 1992.

services to young people is a highly contentious issue in most communities and requires not only strong program leadership and well-trained providers, but also careful work with parents and community leaders to help them understand the very real dangers that young people face and the consequences of failure to provide services. For example, the first time many young women seek help is when they are pregnant. If abortion services (or referrals) are not available at an affordable cost, these young women are likely to risk a backstreet abortion even after being counseled on the hazards (IPPF 1991). A study in Benin City, Nigeria, found that complications from induced abortion accounted for 72 percent of the deaths among young women under age 19 (United Nations 1989: 94). Youngsters with undiagnosed or untreated STDs face the risk of infertility, which can ruin their lives.

Although parental and community support are essential for program survival, the young person seeking help must be assured of confidentiality. Experience of nongovernmental organizations, such as the Family Guidance Association of Ethiopia and the Colombian family planning association, PROFAMILIA, demonstrates that separate sites for delivery of youth services are necessary to maintain young people's privacy and to develop their trust in service providers. Services must also be physically accessible, free or affordable, and provided at times that do not conflict with jobs or school. Current examples show a wide range of strategies that can be used to make services and information available to young people. These include informal youth networks linked to existing community-based health services, as in Mexico; counseling, education, and reproductive health services based in youth recreation centers, as in Ethiopia and Guatemala; and counseling and information rooms in schools, as has been done in Ethiopia.

Youth Participation and Peer Promotion

In contrast to the lecture technique employed by family life education, participatory education facilitated by young people themselves enables them to explore their own attitudes, values, and feelings regarding sexuality and gender relations. Youth engagement helps to build self-esteem and to develop decision-making skills. Projects operating in widely disparate circumstances demonstrate that young people view peers as their preferred source of information, and that training youth for this role is feasible and effective. In the Mexfam project, for example, trained volunteer youth promoters, directed by a staff coordinator, conduct workshop sessions with young people on topics relating to self-esteem, communication, values and attitudes, sexuality, human reproduction and contraception, and prevention of STDs; distribute nonmedical contraceptives (condoms and foaming tablets); and make referrals to Mexfam community doctors (Aguilar 1992). Similarly, peer promoters in seven Ethiopian schools provide information, condoms, and referrals. In Kenya, youth promoters have provided information to schools and other youth groups about STDs, the risks of unprotected sex, coercion by older men, and contraception.

Participatory work with peers helps young people to understand the contradictory attitudes that they may hold, such as the double standards for male and female sexual behavior described above. It can also assist them in clarifying their own values, developing a sense of responsibility toward themselves and others, overcoming gender stereotypes and negative attitudes about abstinence or condom use, and resolving misunderstandings or miscommunication about sex. Particularly important are attitudes about who may initiate sexual activity, and respect for those who decline to have sex or insist on using a condom. Confusion and misunderstanding on such topics abound among young people. For example, in one discussion group, young men said that women do not want their partners to use condoms because they believe that men use condoms only with prostitutes; in the same group, young women said that men do not like to use condoms because "it is like eating a sweet with the wrapper on." In fact, both the young men and the young women said that they understood the importance of using condoms for protection against HIV infection and pregnancy, and expressed a desire to receive accurate information, as well as to be able to voice their anxieties to their friends so that such myths could be dispelled (Hawkins, Ojakaa, and Meshesha 1991).

Little real evaluation has been done of the effectiveness of peer promotion strategies (Ford et al. 1992). However, anecdotal evidence suggests that peer promoters can have an important catalytic effect among young people, but that contraceptive and health services are imperative, either at the program site or through referral.

Process Evaluation and Documentation

One of the greatest shortcomings of youth programs developed to date is the lack of documentation and evaluation. Quantitative and qualitative monitoring and assessment, both of program development and of program success, are essential to ensure relevance and efficacy and to provide a basis for expansion or replication. A critical factor should be whether and how well the program is meeting the needs identified by young people themselves. For this reason, youth involvement in the evaluation process is essential. Techniques remain to be developed, but they must employ criteria based on principles of gender equity and the rights of young people, not simply on quantitative measures such as those used to evaluate family planning outcomes (see Jain and Bruce in this volume). The Mexfam program is evaluated through monthly reports by program coordinators and through use of an "indicator of the well-informed user," which measures the level of young people's knowledge after they complete an education program. However, it is desirable to incorporate into program design an ongoing process of evaluation that assesses feedback from young people on the relevance, strengths, and weaknesses of current measures.

Building Community Support

Initial work on explaining a program's objectives to parents, teachers, religious groups, the media, and other opinion leaders is essential to overcome opposition based on fear and mistrust, and to enlist support. In Zimbabwe, for example, youth counseling programs have found that teachers and parents will refer young people for help once they have developed an understanding of a program's aims and philosophy. The Mexfam Gente Joven program uses films, plays, and discussion groups to awaken the adults in a community — parents, political leaders, school directors, and other decisionmakers — to the need for youth education. The Ethiopia project supports a youth drama troupe that reaches neighborhood audiences throughout Addis Ababa. Other strategies include discussion groups led by the Guatemalan family planning association to foster mutual understanding between young people and parents; training of teachers in sexuality education by PROFAMILIA, Colombia; and the enlistment of professional medical and media support for contraceptive services to sexually active youth in Ethiopia.

Program Implementation

These four program elements — counseling and services, rather than just information; youth participation; monitoring and evaluation; and community involvement — though increasingly understood by professionals in the field and by international agencies such as UNFPA and the World Health Organization to be essential to program success (Barker 1990; WHO 1990), have yet to be widely implemented. Projects such as those mentioned here, and others like them, are demonstrating on a small scale how to reach young people effectively with information, counseling, and health services directly connected to sexuality. Many unanswered questions remain regarding program design and implementation, however. Who is in need of what kinds of assistance, and in what order of priority? Should we be doing more to reach youngsters 10–14 years old, or concentrate on youth aged 15–19? How do the needs of young people vary by age and gender, and by other social and economic conditions? To what extent should programs serve males and females separately or together? Should priority go to the unmarried? How should we advance the sexual health, rather than just the reproductive health, of young people who are married and therefore eligible for conventional family planning and health services? How can the healthy development of young people's sexuality be supported at the same time that the risks of disease and unwanted pregnancy are clearly identified?

Projects must also address severe imbalances in power between young women and men both in intimate relations and in society. In particular, it is necessary to confront pervasive ideologies of male sexual entitlement, and to develop in boys and men a sense of responsibility for preventing disease, controlling their *own* fertility, and caring for children they father. It is not enough to enable girls and young women to say no; boys and young men must learn to respect the wishes of girls and young women.

Participants in the 1993 youth consultation convened by IPPF, mentioned above, concluded that telling the truth about sexuality is one of the most effective strategies for bringing about change: "Young people, when directly approached and consulted, will express their needs…equal rights in everything for all — young and old."

In the final analysis, meeting young people's needs requires more than projects that involve young people and the influential adults in their lives. We need to change the sexual and gender messages purveyed by the mass media and educational systems to promote caring, responsible, respectful, and egalitarian relations between males and females (Obura 1991). Even further, we must provide education, employment, and other basic opportunities that will give young people hope for their own futures, and strong alternative sources of satisfaction and identity.

Notes

1   Although childbearing can be safe in the late teenage years, pregnancy without access to necessary services and social support becomes a potentially life-threatening condition (Kirby et al. 1991).

2   In Sub-Saharan Africa, 38–68 percent of women treated in hospitals for complications from abortion are less than 20 years old; in Malaysia, about 25 percent are under 20; in many countries of Latin America, more than 10 percent are 19 or younger (WHO 1989b).

3   According to the World Health Organization, one in 20 teenagers contracts a sexually transmitted disease each year (WHO 1989a), and young people are increasingly vulnerable to Human Immunodeficiency Virus (Barker 1990; Hirsch 1990; Singh and Wulf 1990). Girls as young as 12 or 14 in some countries are at high risk — higher than boys of the same age, since men seek virgin sexual partners so as to avoid infection (Barker 1990; Population Reference Bureau 1992).

References

Aguilar, J. A. 1992. MEXFAM'S Gente Joven program. In A. Brandrup-Lukanow, et al. (eds.), *Adolescent sexual and reproductive health: Report of the workshop.* Paris: International Children's Center.

Ajayi, A. 1991. Adolescent sexuality and fertility in Kenya. *Studies in Family Planning* 22(4):205–216.

Antrobus, P., A. Germain, and S. Nowrojee. 1994 (forthcoming). *Challenging the culture of silence: Building alliances to end reproductive tract infections.* New York: International Women's Health Coalition.

Barker, G. 1990. *Adolescent fertility in Sub-Saharan Africa: Strategies for a new generation.* Washington, D.C.: Center for Population Options.

Brandrup-Lukanow, A., et al. (eds.) 1992. *Adolescent sexual and reproductive health: Report of the workshop.* Paris: International Children's Center.

Dixon-Mueller, R. 1993. The sexuality connection in reproductive health. *Studies in Family Planning* 24(5):269–282.

Dixon-Mueller, R., and A. Germain. 1993. Stalking the elusive "unmet need" for family planning. *Studies in Family Planning* 23(5):330–335.

ECOS (Estudos e Comunicaçao em Sexualidade e Reproduçao Humana). 1992. *A hug: Transcript of a videotape on boys' sexuality.* Sao Paulo.

Elangot, F. 1987. Uganda: An AIDS control program. *AIDS Action* 1:6–7.

Filgueras, A. 1992. Sexuality of street youth. In A. Brandrup-Lukanow, et al. (eds.), *Adolescent sexual and reproductive health: Report of the workshop.* Paris: International Children's Center.

Fisher, W. A. 1990. All together now: An integrated approach to preventing adolescent pregnancy and STD/HIV infection. *SIECUS Report* 18(4):1-11.

Ford, N., et al. 1992. Review of literature on health and behavioral outcomes of population and family planning education programs in school settings in developing countries. Occasional Working Paper No. 19. Exeter, England: Institute of Population Studies, University of Exeter.

Gage-Brandon, A., and D. Meekers. 1992. Sexual activity before marriage in Sub-Saharan Africa. Working Paper No. 1992–06. State College: Population Issues Research Center, Pennsylvania State University.

Hawkins, K, et al. 1991. *Review of youth programme strategies: Latin America*. London: International Planned Parenthood Federation.

Hawkins, K., and D. Ojakaa. 1991. *Review of the youth programme: Family Planning Association of Kenya*. London: International Planned Parenthood Federation.

Hawkins, K., D. Ojakaa, and B. Meshesha. 1992. *Review of the youth programme: Family Guidance Association of Ethiopia*. London: International Planned Parenthood Federation.

Heise, L., A. Germain, and J. Pitanguy. 1994 (forthcoming). *Violence against women: The hidden health burden*. Washington, D.C.: World Bank.

Hirsch, J. 1990. *Teenage pregnancy and sexually transmitted diseases in Latin America*. Washington, D.C.: Center for Population Options.

International Planned Parenthood Federation. 1985. *Family life education: A guide for youth organizations*. London: International Planned Parenthood Federation.

———. 1991. *Sexual and reproductive health for young people*. London: International Planned Parenthood Federation.

———. 1993. *Mission statement: Vision 2000*. London: International Planned Parenthood Federation.

Kilbride, J. C., and P. L. Kilbride. 1990. *Changing family life in East Africa: Women and children at risk*. University Park: Pennsylvania State Park Press.

Kirby, D., et al. 1991. Reducing the risk: Impact of a new curriculum on sexual risk-taking. *Family Planning Perspectives* 23(6):253–263.

Koenig, M. A., et al. 1988. Maternal mortality in Matlab, Bangladesh: 1976–85. *Studies in Family Planning* 19(2):69-80.

Makinwa-Adebusoye, P. 1992. Sexual behavior, reproductive knowledge and contraceptive use among young urban Nigerians. *International Family Planning Perspectives* 18:66–70.

Nowrojee, S. 1993. Sexuality and gender: Impact on women's health. Paper presented at the Medical Women's International Association, Near East and Africa, First Regional Congress on the Health of Women and Safe Motherhood, November 29–December 3, in Nairobi.

Obura, A. P. 1991. *Changing images: Portrayal of girls and women in Kenyan textbooks*. Nairobi: Acts Press.

Population Reference Bureau. 1992. *Adolescent women in Sub-Saharan Africa: A chartbook on marriage and childbearing*. Washington, D.C.

Pyne, H. H. 1992. AIDS and prostitution in Thailand: Case study of Burmese prostitutes in Ranong. Master of City Planning Thesis, MIT.

Ramasubban, R. 1994 (forthcoming). Patriarchy and the risks of HIV transmission to women in India. In M. DasGupta, T. N. Krishnan, and L. Chen (eds.), *Health and development in India*. Bombay: Oxford University Press.

Shepherd, G. 1987. Attitudes to family planning in Kenya: An anthropological approach. *Health and Policy Planning* 2(1):80–89.

Sherris, J. D. 1982. Population education in schools. *Population Reports* Series M, Special Topics 6:203-237.

Singh, S., and D. Wulf. 1990. *Today's adolescents, tomorrow's parents: A portrait of the Americas*. New York: Alan Guttmacher Institute.

Standing, H. 1989. *Sexual behavior in Sub-Saharan Africa: A review and annotated bibliography*. Prepared for the Overseas Development Administration.

Toubia, N. 1993. *Female genital mutilation: A call for global action*. New York: Women, Inc.

United Nations. 1989. *Adolescent reproductive behavior: Evidence from developing countries*, vol. 2. New York.

World Health Organization (WHO). 1989a. *The health of youth: Facts for action, youth and AIDS*. Geneva.

———. 1989b. *The health of youth: Facts for action, youth and reproductive health*. Geneva.

———. 1990. *WHO approaches to health in adolescence*. Geneva.

———. 1992. *A study of the sexuality experience of young people in eleven African countries*. Geneva.

16

Fertility Control Technology: A Women-Centered Approach to Research

Mahmoud F. Fathalla

Throughout human history, women have felt a need to regulate and control their fertility. Until the modern era, they had neither the power nor the safe and effective means to do so. As the historical writings of Hippocrates vividly describe (see Box 1 on next page), the lack of tools did not prevent them from trying to "doctor themselves," often risking their health, their future fertility, and even their lives in the process.

In almost every culture historians have found ancient, traditional methods that women have used. Egyptian papyruses dating from 1850 B.C. refer to plugs of honey, gum acacia, and crocodile dung, used as a contraceptive vaginal paste (Speroff and Darney 1992). Women have had at their disposal only one genuinely effective biological method to postpone pregnancy — prolonged breast-feeding. Whatever the effectiveness of these and other methods, their use throughout history demonstrates the serious intent with which women have pursued control of procreation. Similarly, they have desired means to control male sexuality. In the early 20th century, for example, Marie Stopes, a British leader in the family planning movement, noted that a popular demand of women was for a simple pill or drug to make their husbands less, rather than more, passionate (Stopes 1928), and women often said they liked every-

thing about marriage, except "the going to the bed side of it" (Eyles 1922).

Men, on the other hand, had the power and the means to control sexual relations and fertility from the beginning. The biblical story of Onan is a case in point. After the death of Onan's brother, his father tells him to marry Tamar, his brother's widow, "and raise up seed" to his brother. But "Onan knew that the seed should not be his; and it came to pass, when he went in unto his brother's wife, that he spilled it on the ground, lest that he should give seed to his brother. And the thing which he did displeased the Lord: wherefore he slew him also" (Genesis 38:8–10). The actions in the story are those of Judah, Onan, and the Lord. Tamar had no active role to play. The ancient method of withdrawal, or coitus interruptus, has long enabled men to exercise control over reproduction.

The condom, another effective contraceptive method, has also been available to men for a long time. The history of the development of the condom is lost in antiquity, but most versions indicate that the method was developed by men for use by men. A popular version attributes its discovery to a "Dr. Condom," a physician in England in the 1600s (Speroff and Darney 1992). The story goes that Dr. Condom invented the

Reproductive Suffering in History

When the woman is afflicted with a large wound as a consequence of an abortion, or the womb is damaged by strong suppositories, as many women are always doing, doctoring themselves, or when the foetus is aborted and the woman is not purged of the afterbirth, and the womb inflames, closes and is not purged, if she is treated promptly she will be cured but will remain sterile.
— Hippocrates, 400 B.C., cited in McLaren 1990.

The Contraceptive Revolution

Widespread contraceptive use is a recent phenomenon in human history. The first demographic transition was accomplished in the Northern, industrialized countries in the 18th and 19th centuries, largely by men using coitus interruptus. The development of modern contraceptive methods for women began only in the late 19th century. Published reports about the diaphragm first appeared in Germany in the 1880s, written by a gynecologist, Dr. C. Haase, who prescribed the device for unhealthy women to protect them from undesired and risky pregnancies. He had to publish under a pseudonym, Wilhelm P. J. Mensinga (Speroff and Darney 1992). Fertility in Europe and North America declined gradually, and has reached very low levels, in some places below replacement fertility.

A second demographic transition is taking place now, largely in Southern, developing countries. This transition has begun only in the past few decades and has depended substantially on a revolution in contraceptive technology. Among other things, women for the first time have methods that they can use, even independent of the cooperation of their male partners, to regulate their fertility and to enjoy sexual life without fear of unwanted, ill-timed pregnancy. The consequent decline of fertility has been steeper in the Southern countries than in the North. In the United States, it took 58 years for fertility to decline from 6.5 to 3.5 births per woman; the same level of decline took 27 years in Indonesia, 15 years in Colombia, 8 years in Thailand, and a mere 7 years in China (UNFPA 1991). Contraceptive users in the developing world have increased more than tenfold from an estimated 31 million couples in 1960–1965 to 381 million couples in 1985–1990 (UNFPA 1991). Table 1 shows the percentage of married women of reproductive age using contraception in 1960-1965 and 1985-1990.

Before 1960, men and women had very limited choices in contraception: coitally related methods (condom and withdrawal for the male;

sheath in response to Charles II's annoyance at the number of his illegitimate children. Another version attributes the invention to a medieval slaughterhouse worker, who conceived the idea that covering the penis with the thin membrane from an animal would protect promiscuous men from sexually transmitted diseases (Himes 1970).

In many societies, the predominant objection to contraceptive use has been to reproductive control by women, rather than to contraception itself. Male-dominated societies have resented giving control of the process of reproduction to women. Men in patriarchical societies have reasoned that if women had control over their reproduction, they would also have the unthinkable: control over their own sexuality.

Fertility by choice, not by chance, is a basic requirement of women's health, well-being, and quality of life (Fathalla 1993a). A woman who does not have the means or the power to regulate and control her fertility cannot be considered in a "state of complete physical, mental and social well-being," the definition of health in the constitution of the World Health Organization. She cannot have the joy of a pregnancy that is wanted, avoid the distress of a pregnancy that is unwanted, plan her life, pursue her education, undertake a productive career, or plan her births to take place at optimal times for childbearing, ensuring greater safety for herself and better chances for her child's healthy development.

TABLE 1

Contraceptive Prevalence in the Developing World by Region

Region	Percentage Using	
	1960 – 1965	1985 – 1990
East Asia	13	70
South Asia	7	40
Africa	5	17
Latin America	14	60
All developing countries	9	51

Source: UNFPA 1991.

diaphragm, cervical cap, and vaginal spermicides for the female; periodic abstinence for the couple), and permanent methods (male and female sterilization). The contraceptive revolution of the 1960s and 1970s led to significant improvements in existing methods, including the simplification of methods of female sterilization to the extent that they no longer require general anesthesia or hospitalization. Moreover, for the first time in human history, contraception could be taken out of the bedroom and out of the genital area, with the development of systemic hormonal methods. In addition to oral hormonal contraceptives, which are short-acting and administered daily, the development of long-acting hormonal methods and the introduction of the IUD have freed women from taking precaution at every sexual act and provided an alternative to permanent contraception. Women now have methods that offer protection for up to three months (injectables), five years (Norplant®), or eight years (IUDs).

Another major improvement has been in the effectiveness of contraception. While in the past couples had to choose between coitally related methods, which have fairly low levels of effectiveness, and sterilization, which is effective but permanent, women now have a choice of methods that are highly effective and reversible. The fruits of the contraceptive technology revolution have reached hundreds of millions of people all over the world: people from the skyscrapers of Manhattan, to the peri-urban slums of Latin America, to the rural communities of the Indian subcontinent; people of all socioeconomic strata; people of different cultures, religious beliefs, and value systems; and people at different stages in their reproductive lives.

Clinic and supply methods of contraception, defined as those requiring supplies or clinical services — including male and female sterilization, IUDs, the pill, injectables, condoms, and female barrier methods — account for approximately 83 percent of contraceptive practice worldwide (United Nations 1989). These methods, the ones most frequently offered by family planning programs, account for a larger fraction of contraceptive use in developing than in developed countries — about 90 percent and 65 percent, respectively (Table 2 on next page). The share of all contraceptive use accounted for by nonsupply, or traditional, methods — including rhythm, withdrawal, abstinence, douching, and various folk practices — is higher in developed than developing countries (35 percent and 11 percent, respectively). This difference reflects the differing history of contraceptive practice and family planning programs in the two types of countries. In most developed countries, marital fertility reached low levels before modern contraceptives were invented and in the absence of family planning programs. By comparison, beginning in the 1960s, men and women in developing countries had access to contraceptives through family planning programs that promote modern clinic and supply methods (United Nations 1989).

Contraceptives should not be perceived as a temporary measure to ease the world population problem. Contraception will be a permanent feature of life on this planet. Our reproductive function is being voluntarily adapted to dramatic new realities. We are witnessing nothing less than a major evolutionary jump — one that is science-mediated, rather than imposed by nature.

In the early days of the contraceptive technology revolution, the scientific community dreamed

Percentage Distribution of Contraceptive Users by Method in Developed and Developing Countries

Method	Developed Countries	Developing Countries	World
Female sterilization	10	33	26
Male sterilization	5	12	10
IUD	8	24	19
Hormonal pills	20	12	15
Condom	19	6	10
Hormonal injectables	—	2	1
Vaginal barrier methods	3	1	2
Rhythm	13	5	7
Withdrawal	20	3	8
Other methods	2	3	2

Source: United Nations, 1989.

of an ideal contraceptive that would fit the needs of everyone, everywhere, every time. Scientists soon realized that a "magic bullet" was a dream that would never come true. No single method can meet the diverse needs of individuals. Men and women require a wide range of contraceptives, tailored to different human circumstances and desires (Fathalla 1990). Thus, broadening contraceptive choice is a key to improving the quality of family planning services. Moreover, for all its benefits to the quality of life of women, currently available contraceptive technologies have left women with some genuine concerns, as well as unmet needs. Modern methods' qualities of convenience, effectiveness, and usability by women are not without trade-offs. Furthermore, the modern contraceptive revolution, driven largely by demographics, has left women, for the most part, outside the policy-making process; indeed, women have often served as the means to an end, as objects rather than subjects. This has aroused the suspicions of women's groups and resulted in feminist critiques of medicalized contraceptive technology (Dixon-Mueller 1993). Whether justified or not, these concerns must be voiced and be heard.

Who Is in Control?

Women have more at stake in fertility control than men. Contraception empowers women by maximizing their choices and enabling them to control their fertility, their sexuality, their health, and thus their lives. Many women welcome the convenience of long-acting and permanent methods. However, these methods can be and have been used by governments and others to control women rather than to empower them. Such governments fail to recognize that when women are given a real choice, and the information and means to implement their choice, they will make the most rational decision for themselves, for their communities, and ultimately for the world at large.

Safety Concerns

Without safe abortion as a backup, the use of less-effective contraceptive methods will not meet women's needs for fertility regulation (Germain and Dixon-Mueller 1992). As with any drug, an increase in the effectiveness of contraceptives is often accompanied by a decrease in the margin of safety. From a public health point of view, contraceptive drugs and devices have an excellent record of safety. They have been used by hundreds of millions of women over extended periods of time and under varied circumstances. Few drugs have been, and continue to be, subjected to such rigorous scientific scrutiny with respect to safety. This scrutiny is particularly important because, unlike individuals who use drugs to cure illness, women (and men) who use contraception are taking preventive action (Fathalla 1991).

Safety concerns loom particularly large if a service system is more concerned about demographic targets than about the health and welfare of clients. A contraceptive can be safe or unsafe, depending on who is using it and the quality of the service system delivering it. Moreover, the concept of safety must reflect client concerns. Safety cannot be defined simply as the absence of life-threatening complications, but must be assessed from a woman's perspective. So-called minor inconveniences or side effects such as menstrual bleeding disturbances, headache, or weight gain may not threaten life, but may be of extreme concern and often significantly affect a woman's quality of life (WHO/HRP and IWHC 1991).

The Abortion Dilemma

The contraceptive technology revolution has emphasized development of methods that are so effective, they can prevent the need for abortion. The rationale behind this emphasis derives more from political concerns than from health or scientific ones. In fact, the focus on preventing abortion, to the exclusion (until recently) of work to develop postovulatory methods, has had serious consequences for both health and fertility. The politicization of the abortion issue has important implications for the use of barrier methods that take on particular significance in view of the sexually transmitted diseases (STDs) and AIDS pandemics. Where safe pregnancy termination services are available and acceptable, the need for highly effective contraception lessens, and women can more comfortably choose to use barrier methods, which will also protect against infection. Where abortion is illegal or unsafe, women may

more often choose nonbarrier methods, leaving themselves at higher risk of sexually transmitted infections.

A review of current abortion laws shows that 52 countries, with about 25 percent of the world's population, fall into the most restrictive category, prohibiting abortions on any grounds or allowing them only when the woman's life would be endangered were the pregnancy carried to term. Some 42 countries, comprising 12 percent of the world's population, have statutes authorizing abortion on broader medical grounds — to avert a threat to the woman's general health, for example, and sometimes for genetic or juridical reasons, such as incest or rape — but not for social reasons alone or on request. Another 13 countries, home to 23 percent of the world's population, allow abortion on social or sociomedical grounds. Finally, in 25 countries, containing 40 percent of the world's population, abortion is permitted up to a certain point in gestation without requiring specific grounds (Henshaw 1990).

Even where abortion is legal, however, safe pregnancy termination services are not always available or affordable. Unsafe abortion is one of the most neglected health and human rights problems in the world today. Any other crisis claiming 500 lives daily would draw world attention and probably evoke an international uproar. Yet no uproar is heard in defense of the 500 women who lose their lives every day as a result of unsafe abortions, in rightful pursuit of their reproductive freedom (Fathalla 1992a and 1992b). The current technology for pregnancy termination, even for medical pregnancy termination using mifepristone (RU 486), is still clinic-based. Even in countries that permit abortion, its availability is limited by the availability of clinical services. Clinics are an easy target for political opposition, funding cuts, picketing, or far worse. An effective, simple, affordable, and safe technology that a woman can use to terminate pregnancy in the privacy of her home, outside the health care system, has yet to be developed.

An Unfair Burden

Women now have more reliable methods of birth control than ever before, but they have paid a price. They have had to assume full responsibility for the inconveniences and risks involved. As the data in Table 2 suggest, women assume responsibility for about 72 percent of contraceptive use, in comparison with men's 28 percent. Not only do women bear an unfair burden of responsibility in fertility regulation, but many of the methods that women have available for use are associated with potential health hazards. The importance of male participation and responsibility has grown with the emergence of the AIDS pandemic and the increase in other STDs — against which, apart from abstinence, the use of the condom is the only effective strategy.

Reproductive Tract Infections: A Silent Tragedy

Fertility regulation, though essential, is not the only component of reproductive health. Women have other reproductive and sexual health problems, which are often neglected. Of these, the prevention and control of STDs is the one most clearly linked with family planning. Both unwanted pregnancy and infection are transmitted through sexual intercourse, and women often need effective protection against both. Methods are needed that protect against infection while allowing conception to occur, as well as methods that protect against both simultaneously.

Reproductive tract infections, mostly resulting from STDs, are a major cause of morbidity, and seriously undermine the quality of life of many women, especially in developing countries (Germain et al. 1992). The worldwide spread of STDs has been one of the principal challenges to public health in the past few decades (Fathalla 1992a and 1992b). While the burden of a number of traditional first-generation venereal diseases — like gonorrhea, syphilis, and chancroid — has declined, particularly in the industrialized countries, they have been amply replaced by new syndromes associated with *Chlamydia trachomatis*, human herpes virus, human papilloma virus, and the Human Immunodeficiency Virus (HIV).

These agents, regarded as the second generation of sexually transmitted organisms, are more difficult to identify, treat, and control. Moreover, they can cause serious complications, including chronic ill health, disability, and death. Both generations of STDs remain significant health problems in most developing countries. Reliable data on the worldwide incidence of STDs are not available. Minimal estimates by the World Health Organization (WHO) of the annual number of new cases are shown in Figure 1, including 500,000 new cases of AIDS. STDs are now hyperendemic in many developing countries, including the rural areas, where facilities for diagnosis and treatment are usually inadequate.

By definition, STDs affect both men and women. However, STDs have more serious sequelae in women than in men. Early detection and hence early treatment of STDs are easier in men. In women, lesions often occur in the inner genitalia and are thus hidden and quite often remain asymptomatic. Moreover, ascending infection in women can have much graver consequences: it can cause pelvic inflammatory disease, increase the risk of ectopic pregnancy, and result in permanent infertility. Cancer of the cervix is also a potential late sequela. Another ramification is the possible transmission to the fetus of several STD pathogens. Although the risk of transmission is much greater from man to woman than the other way around, the most effective means available for protection against STDs, the use of a condom, is entirely controlled by the man. An effective method of protection that a woman can use without the need for her partner's cooperation simply does not exist. (The female condom, under development, requires male cooperation and is likely to remain prohibitively expensive.)

Contraception-21: The Agenda for Research

To meet women's closely interrelated needs for birth control and disease prevention, a second contraceptive technology revolution must occur. A woman-centered approach to contraceptive research and development will require a clear

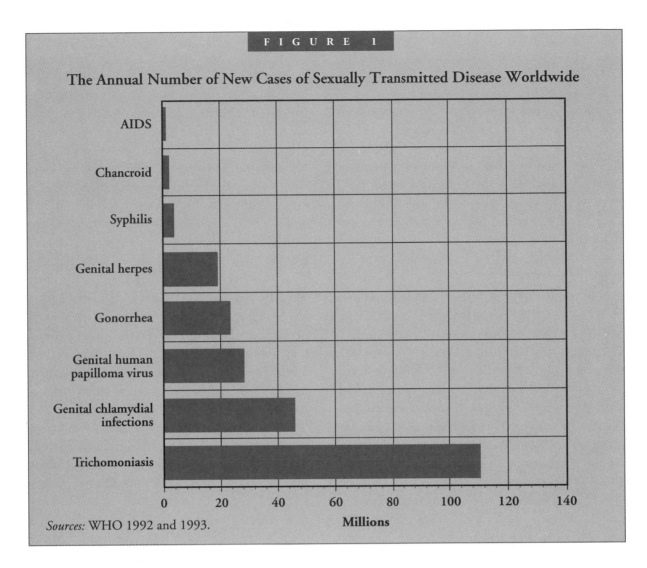

FIGURE 1

The Annual Number of New Cases of Sexually Transmitted Disease Worldwide

Sources: WHO 1992 and 1993.

Millions

mission, a collaborative effort between contraceptive users and researchers, a definition of priorities, a reinvigorated and gender-sensitized science, and sustained resources (Fathalla 1993b).

The Mission

If the first contraceptive technology revolution was demographically driven, with emphasis on the development of methods that were effective, long-acting, and widely available, then contraceptive research and development today is best described as opportunity-driven. Because of poor funding, scientists follow whatever leads present themselves, and industry seeks only to make marginal improvements or modifications in existing products. For the second contraceptive technology revolution, the field must again be

goal-driven, and the goal should be set right, focusing sharply on a sustained effort to develop contraceptives that address the still unmet needs of women. The demographic impact will not be diminished, but enhanced. The message for all concerned about population growth should be clear: *Women know best.* It is their bodies, their lives, and their children's lives that are at stake (Taylor 1993). Respecting women and responding to their needs is one of the best strategies for saving the planet.

A survey of contraceptive research and development has come up with a list of 94 product leads that are currently being pursued (PATH 1993). Many of these are variants of existing methods or alternatives within existing contraceptive approaches. They include four

IUDs, seven hormonal implants, five hormonal injectables, five hormonal pills, six vaccines, and six techniques for female sterilization. Given financial constraints, among other factors, the field should refocus its efforts on those urgent requirements that are met poorly, if at all, by existing technologies — namely, protection against infection, postcoital and postovulatory methods, and male methods. The field must have the courage to drop leads, even if they are scientifically feasible, and to break new scientific ground.

Creating Common Ground

Honest dialogue between the users and creators of the technology is essential. For example, the WHO Special Programme of Research, Development and Research Training in Human Reproduction collaborated with the International Women's Health Coalition to initiate such a dialogue in 1991. The two organizations convened a meeting of women's health advocacy groups from developed and developing countries and scientists engaged in contraceptive research and development. The meeting proved that scientists and women's health advocates can listen to each other and respect each other's views, even when they differ, and established a basis for continuing interaction (WHO/HRP and IWHC 1991).

It is time for this dialogue to move forward, and for institutionalization of mechanisms to ensure that the voices of women are not only heard but also heeded. Women's health advocates should be represented in all decision-making and advisory bodies that are established to guide the research process at all stages, including definition of criteria for safety, determination of research priorities, design and implementation of research protocols, setting and monitoring of ethical standards, and deliberations on whether to advance a fertility regulation method from one stage to the next — especially decisions to move from clinical trial to introduction of a method into family planning programs (WHO 1993).

Priority Needs

An international symposium entitled Contraceptive Research and Development for the Year 2000 and Beyond was convened in Mexico City in March, 1993. (Excerpts of the symposium's declaration appear in Box 2.) The symposium brought together senior managers of all the international, and some national, public-sector agencies that undertake contraceptive research; program directors and senior staff of international and national agencies that support or are otherwise involved in fertility regulation research; and women's health advocates. A clear recommendation was that particular emphasis and priority should be given to methods that coincide with women's perceived needs and priorities, including methods that are under the user's control and that also protect against STDs, postovulatory methods, and safe male methods that enable men to share responsibility for fertility regulation and disease prevention (WHO 1993).

Carl Djerassi, a father of the oral contraceptive, has remarked that if he were to choose one new contraceptive to develop, it would be a once-a-month pill effective as a menses inducer (Djerassi 1991). Whereas currently used oral contraceptives are taken daily for most of the month, a menses inducer would be taken only during months when a woman has had unprotected coitus. Instead of waiting to see whether she misses her period, a woman would take a single pill (containing a short-lived and rapidly metabolized drug) to induce menstrual flow at the expected time. Although not suitable for every woman, such a regimen would be an enormous improvement for many (Rimmer et al. 1992). At most, a woman would take 12 pills annually, rather than the present 250 or more, and the decision to use contraception would be made postcoitally. For some women, including adolescents, a menses inducer would be an attractive backup to barrier contraceptive methods, thus encouraging their wider use. A menses inducer could also provide a technological answer to the abortion controversy, since the user would not know whether she carried a fertilized ovum. It could transfer the issue from

BOX 2

Excerpts from the Declaration of the International Symposium, "Contraceptive Research and Development for the Year 2000 and Beyond"[1]

Among other conditions, the status of women, in society and in sexual relationships, continues to require urgent improvement. Since women bear the brunt of the responsibility for fertility regulation, it is vital to include their perspectives in research on fertility regulations. This would allow scientists to appreciate better women's expectations with regard to methods of fertility regulation. Over the past ten years, the views of women on reproductive rights, reproductive and sexual health, the suitability and safety of fertility regulating methods in different settings, and on the types and quality of family planning information and service delivery programmes have been more effectively articulated. Along with other initiatives, this has led to a wider recognition of fertility regulation as part of broader, interrelated sexual and reproductive health challenges that persist or are increasing. For example, every year there occur 36–53 million induced abortions...[and] an estimated 250 million new cases of STDs, contributing to severe morbidities, infertility, and cervical cancer. WHO projects a three- to fourfold increase in HIV infections from 10–12 million to 30–40 million by the year 2000.... Research is required not only to develop methods suitable for use by different people at different stages of their lives, but also to understand the social and behavioral issues related, for example, to sexuality and gender relations and acceptance and use of fertility regulation. Research is also needed to identify and solve problems associated with the delivery of fertility regulation technologies through family planning programmes, as indeed it is required to monitor the long-term safety of methods.

Recommendations

1. Governments should establish programmes for the conduct of reproductive and sexual health research as a priority component of their national health research agendas, and allocate the funds and develop the human and institutional resources required for carrying out such research....

2. The international donor community should provide greater financial resources as a priority in order to strengthen further the human and institutional capabilities of developing countries to conduct research to address problems of reproductive and sexual health.

3. Women's health advocates and potential users should be represented in all decision-making mechanisms and

advisory bodies that are established to guide the research process....

4. In developing (or introducing) new methods of fertility regulation account should be taken of the adequacy of the health infrastructure and family planning services likely to be available, the potential of the method to be used, and the safeguards needed to ensure that methods will be used safely, effectively, and voluntarily.

5. ...Particular emphasis and priority should be given to methods that coincide with the women's perceived needs and priorities, including among others, methods that are under the user's control and that also protect against STDs, post-ovulatory methods, and safe male methods that enable men to share responsibility for fertility regulation and disease prevention....

6. Governments and donor agencies should increase their support for...research...essential to ensure that all existing new and improved methods, as well as underutilized methods (such as emergency and post-coital contraception, male condoms, and other barrier methods), reach users in ways that assure free and informed choice and safe and effective use.

7. Research on sexuality and gender roles and relationships in different cultural settings is urgently needed....

8. ...A new type of partnership between the public and private sectors is needed that would mobilize the experience and resources of industry while protecting the public interest. National drug and device regulatory agencies should be actively involved as collaborators in all stages of the development process.

9. It should be recognized that unsafe abortion is a major threat to women's lives and health, and research should be undertaken to assure the safety, quality, affordability, and accessibility of abortion services.

10. ...In conducting reproductive and sexual health research special attention should be given to the problems of adolescents in order to develop suitable policies and programmes to meet their reproductive and sexual health needs.

11. Increased attention should be given to the wide and systematic dissemination of research findings to policymakers, opinion leaders, all providers, and users of fertility regulation methods, as well as to the general public, and to the application of research findings to problem solving.

Source: Van Look and Perez-Palacios 1994 (forthcoming).

the public domain to the privacy of the individual's moral code. To have real impact, a menses inducer must be safe enough to be used at home, outside the health care system.

Women have to carry all the burden and risks of pregnancy and childbirth. This, however, is no reason that they should also bear most of the burden of fertility regulation. A sustained research effort is needed to develop contraceptive choices that will enable men to share effectively in the responsibility for fertility regulation. For biological reasons, regulation and control of the reproductive process is more difficult in the male than in the female. Hormonal suppression of spermatogenesis may be feasible, but unless it is accompanied by replacement hormone therapy, sexual potency is suppressed. A better understanding of mechanisms involved in the posttesticular maturation of sperm, without affecting spermatogenesis and testicular hormonal production, utilizing the new tools of molecular and cell biology and biotechnology, could provide promising leads for systemic male contraceptives of the future (see Waites 1993).

Reinvigorating and Reorienting the Science

The Contraception-21 agenda requires that advances in cell and molecular biology and biotechnology be applied to fertility regulation. While such advances have opened new frontiers in the medical and biological sciences, contraceptive research and development have yet to exploit them. Investment in reproductive endocrinology provided most of the leads for the first contraceptive technology revolution; the field is now ripe for another major initiative. At the same time, both new and conventional approaches to research must be gender-sensitive, taking into account especially women's experiences and perspectives.

Resources

Although estimates of global expenditures for contraceptive research and development are difficult to obtain, it is clear, contrary to what some people believe, that contraceptive research and development are poorly funded. The most complete study of the levels and sources of worldwide funding for contraceptive research and development, reporting on trends only up to 1983, estimates that $63 million was spent for contraceptive research in that year (Atkinson, Lincoln, and Forrest 1985). This figure includes funding for the evaluation of long-term safety of existing methods. Of the total, private industry contributed an estimated $22 million, or about 35 percent, and specialized public-sector agencies contributed, out of funds given by international donors, an estimated $26 million, or 41 percent of worldwide expenditure. The remaining $15 million, or 24 percent of expenditures, was provided mainly by national governments that funded mission-oriented research. Developing countries—especially China, India, Chile, and Mexico—contributed about 1 percent of the total. There is no evidence that the overall picture has changed much since then. An assessment in 1993 estimated the worldwide annual funding for contraceptive research and development at $57 million (PATH 1993).

Global expenditure on contraceptive research and development, from all sources, equals less than 3 percent of global contraceptive sales, estimated to be between $2.6 billion and $2.9 billion (PATH 1993). The funding of public-sector programs of contraceptive research and development represents about 3 percent of the international assistance for population and family planning, estimated in 1990 to be $929 million (Michaud and Murray 1994). Another figure to note in these budgetary considerations is that about $230 million is required to bring a new drug for human use from research to the market. Figure 2 shows the complex steps of the process of contraceptive research and development.

Because public resources available for family planning and reproductive health are limited, any major infusion of resources in the contraceptive research and development field will have to come from private industry, which possesses finance and expertise in far greater measure than other sources. The pharmaceutical industry in the de-

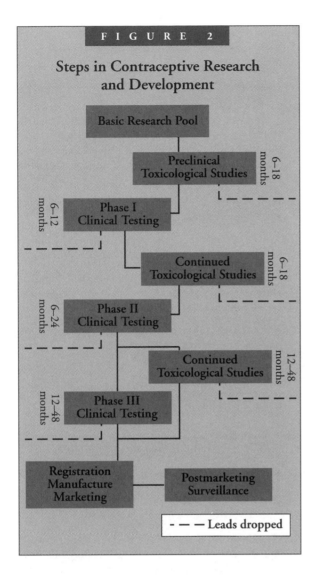

FIGURE 2

Steps in Contraceptive Research and Development

Basic Research Pool

Preclinical Toxicological Studies — 6–18 months

Phase I Clinical Testing — 6–12 months

Continued Toxicological Studies — 6–18 months

Phase II Clinical Testing — 6–24 months

Continued Toxicological Studies — 12–48 months

Phase III Clinical Testing — 12–48 months

Registration Manufacture Marketing

Postmarketing Surveillance

- - - Leads dropped

veloped world invests about 16–19 percent of revenues in research and development of new products (Prices 1992). U.S. and European drug companies report total revenues of over $90 billion per year and a projected annual growth of 9–10 percent by 1999, implying that significant resources might be made available for research activities.

The constraints that earlier led to the retrenchment of industry from the contraceptive field must be addressed. Foremost among these is a perception of the market as being "mature" — that is, saturated in developed countries and not profitable in developing ones — as well as a perceived dearth of new product ideas. Product liability, drug regulatory requirements, and a hostile political climate played a secondary role as disincentives to industry.

The market is changing. High rates of unwanted pregnancy, as well as a heavy reliance on sterilization among the younger population, suggest a latent demand for new contraceptives. Public-sector provision of contraceptives in many developing countries is giving way to a more significant role for the private sector, and as market economies in developing countries evolve, there will be a progressive increase in the share of the private commercial sector, brightening profit prospects. Moreover, drug regulatory requirements have become streamlined, and the political climate, particularly in the United States, seems to be easing.

Conclusion

Will women get the contraceptives they still need to pursue their reproductive rights and reproductive health? The answer is yes, when contraceptive research and development become mission-oriented, when women participate actively in the process, when science is reinvigorated, and when the required resources are mobilized—industrial resources, in particular. Women in the 21st century deserve a better deal. Political will can make it happen, and the time to start is now.

Notes

1 To review the progress made in this field since 1984 and to identify the challenges ahead in preparation for the United Nations International Conference on Population and Development, this international symposium was organized jointly by the Government of Mexico and the Special Programme of Research, Development and Research Training in Human Reproduction, a worldwide research programme co-sponsored by the United Nations Development Programme, the United States Populations Fund, the World Health Organization, and the World Bank. This declaration was adopted by the participants in the symposium and does not necessarily reflect the views and policies of the organizers nor of the organizations, agencies and governments represented at the symposium.

References

Atkinson, L. E., R. Lincoln, and J. D. Forrest. 1985. World-wide trends in funding for contraceptive research and evaluation. *Family Planning Perspectives* 17:196–207.

Bygdeman, M. 1991. The future of antiprogestin. In E. S. Teoh and S. S. Ratnam (eds.), *The Future of Gynaecology and Obstetrics*. Lancaster, U.K.: Parthenon.

Dixon-Mueller, R. 1993. *Population policy and women's rights: Transforming reproductive choice.* Westport, Conn.: Praeger.

Djerassi, C. 1991. New contraceptives: Utopian or Victorian. *Scientific Public Affairs* 6:5–15.

Eyles, M. L. 1922. *The woman in the little house.* London: Grant Richards. Quoted in A. McLaren. 1990. *A history of contraception: From antiquity to the present day.* Oxford: Basil Blackwell.

Fathalla, M. F. 1990. Tailoring contraceptives to human needs. *People* 17:3–5.

———. 1991. Contraceptive technology and safety. *Population Sciences* 10:7–26.

———. 1992a. Family planning: Future needs. *Ambio (A Journal of the Human Environment)* 21:84–87.

———. 1992b. Reproductive health in the world: Two decades of progress and the challenge ahead. In J. Khanna, P. F. A. Van Look, and P. D. Griffin (eds.), *Reproductive health: A key to a brighter future. Special programme of research, development and research training in human reproduction.* Geneva: World Health Organization.

———. 1993a. Contraception and women's health. *British Medical Bulletin* 49:245–51.

———. 1993b. Mobilization of resources for the second contraceptive technology revolution. Paper presented at a symposium, Contraceptive Research and Development for the Year 2000 and Beyond, March 8–10, in Mexico City.

Germain, A., and R. Dixon-Mueller. 1992. Stalking the elusive "unmet need" for family planning. *Studies in Family Planning* 23:330–35.

Germain, A., et al., (eds.). 1992. *Reproductive tract infections: Global impact and priorities for women's reproductive health.* New York: Plenum Press.

Henshaw, S. K. 1990. Induced abortion: A world view, 1990. *Family Planning Perspectives* 22:76–89.

Himes, N. E. 1970. *Medical history of contraception.* New York: Shocken Books.

McLaren, A. 1990. *A history of contraception: From antiquity to the present day.* Oxford: Basil Blackwell.

Michaud, C., and C. Murray. 1994 (forthcoming). Aid flows to the health sector in developing countries. *Bulletin of the World Health Organization* 72(4).

Prices pressure dents profit in US pharmaceutical market. 1992. *Pharmaceutical Business News*, May 15.

Program for Appropriate Technology in Health (PATH). 1993. Enhancing the private sector's role in contraceptive research and development. Paper presented at a symposium, Contraceptive Research and Development for the Year 2000 and Beyond, March 8–10, in Mexico City.

Rimmer, C., et al. 1992. Do women want a once-a-month pill? *Human Reproduction* 7:608–11.

Speroff, L., and P. D. Darney 1992. *A clinical guide for contraception.* Baltimore, Md.: Williams & Wilkins.

Stopes, M. 1928. *Enduring passion.* London: Hogarth. Quoted in A. McLaren. 1990. *A history of contraception: From antiquity to the present day.* Oxford: Basil Blackwell.

Taylor, D. 1993. Mothers know best. *Moving Pictures Bulletin.* Special Issue on Population. London: Central Television Enterprises.

Teoh, E. S., and S. S. Ratnam (eds.). 1991. *The Future of Gynaecology and Obstetrics.* Lancaster, U.K.: Parthenon Publishing Company.

United Nations Fund for Population Activities (UNFPA). 1991. *The state of world population.* New York.

United Nations. Department of International Economic and Social Affairs. 1989. *Levels and trends of contraceptive use as assessed in 1988.* Population Studies No. 110. New York: UNFPA.

Van Look, P. F. A., and G. Perez-Palacios. 1994 (forthcoming). Declaration of the International Symposium, "Contraceptive Research and Development for the Year 2000 and Beyond." In *Contraceptive research and development 1984–1994: The road from Mexico to Cairo and beyond.* New Delhi: Oxford University Press (in press).

Waites, G. M. H. 1993. Male fertility regulation: The challenges for the year 2000. *British Medical Bulletin* 49:210–221.

World Health Organization and International Women's Health Coalition (WHO/HRP and IWHC). 1991. Creating common ground. Report of a meeting between women's health advocates and scientists, February 20–22. Geneva: WHO.

———. 1992. Global health situation and projection. Division of Epidemiological Surveillance and Health Situation and Trial Assessment. WHO/HST/92.1. Geneva.

———. 1993. The HIV/AIDS pandemic: 1993 overview. WHO/GPA/CNP/EVA 93.1. Geneva.

17

Financing Reproductive and Sexual Health Services

Jennifer Zeitlin, Ramesh Govindaraj, and Lincoln C. Chen

An ambitious agenda for reproductive and sexual health has been advanced in the preceding chapters of this section. Meeting this agenda will require substantial resources, irrespective of the strategy adopted. How much would be needed to ensure accessible and affordable reproductive and sexual health services for everyone? From where will the financing come? How should current resources be spent? The answers to these questions are complex and potentially contentious.

Governments and donors classify services that constitute reproductive and sexual health under various budgetary categories; the two most relevant are health and population. In the health sector, reproductive health services include maternal-child health services (MCH); child survival activities such as immunization and oral rehydration; safe motherhood; control of Human Immunodeficiency Virus (HIV) and other sexually transmitted diseases (STDs); contraception; and abortion.[1] Movements to mobilize health resources often underscore the importance of specific diseases — for example, AIDS, tropical diseases, and malnutrition — that deserve high research priority or particularly aggressive interventions.

As described by Jain and Bruce (in this volume), population resources have been concentrated on the provision of contraceptive services. Depending upon the government and donor, population resources may also be invested in related abortion services; MCH services; information, education, and communications programs; training and institutional development; research and evaluation; and demographic data collection and research. Budget breakdowns of population investments vary between countries and agencies, but family planning activities undoubtedly command the bulk of these resources.

Advocates for an enhanced flow of resources to the population field usually stress the importance of contraception provided through family planning programs, primarily for its instrumental role in slowing population growth, and sometimes as an end in itself to promote individual health and rights. The matter of whether and how population funds should be allocated between traditional family planning activities and allied reproductive health objectives has become an arena of vigorous debate. For example, some advocates who accord priority to fertility control alone argue that rapid population growth represents such a serious threat to human well-being that scarce population resources should be directed only to contraceptive services. In their view, stretching limited family planning funds to cover broader reproductive health services would handicap provision of contraceptive services.

Proponents of reproductive health and rights, in contrast, argue that simply increasing resources for contraception may not lead to better health, social, or demographic outcomes. From this perspective, qualitative changes of program objectives and content are required for achieving health and rights objectives, as well as demographic goals. Some would even argue that continuing to invest solely in population control through family planning programs could exacerbate well-known shortcomings in current programs (see Sen, Germain, and Chen in this volume).

The aim of this chapter is to illuminate some of these issues through an exploration of financial investments in reproductive health services in developing countries. We review existing estimates of population resource requirements, consider these estimates in the light of worldwide expenditure patterns for both family planning and health services, and examine the role of international development assistance in both the population and the health sectors.[2]

Our review of available data indicates that we are at a very early stage of information gathering and understanding about how resources flow in support of reproductive and sexual health services in diverse settings around the world. Methodologies currently employed to estimate resource requirements for the population field are inadequate for an analysis of reproductive health — partly because of poor data quality, a focus on demographic targets, and the narrow range of services considered for support by population funds. When we turn to integrated analyses of both health and population expenditures worldwide, we also find severe data deficiencies. Available information, however, clearly highlights the enormous disparity in health and family planning expenditures between and within countries. This disparity seriously compromises access to high-quality services by many people, especially in the lowest-income countries. Because of these financial needs in developing countries, we examine donor health and population budgets. We gener-

ate for the first time a rough estimate of donor investments in the range of reproductive health services and conclude that donor policies, whether for advancing health and rights or for demographic objectives, should emphasize equity-oriented, gender-sensitive human development aimed at building skills and capacities within developing countries.

Resource Requirements for Population Activities

The resurgence of interest in population has been accompanied by several major international efforts to mobilize financial resources in support of population activities in developing countries. In the 1989 Amsterdam Declaration, world leaders estimated that $9 billion annually would be required from all sources to support population activities by the year 2000 (UNFPA 1990). Therefore, they called upon the international community to "increase significantly the proportion of development assistance going to population activities." In the 1991 Rafael Salas Lecture at the United Nations, Robert McNamara arrived at a similar requirement — $8 billion — and recommended that foreign donors enhance population assistance to developing countries from current levels to $3.5 billion annually by the turn of the century (McNamara 1992).

Estimates of global resources required for population activities by the year 2000 have been generated by many agencies in the population field (see Table 1). These projections, mostly based upon the estimated cost of contraceptive services, vary from $600 million (in constant 1988 dollars), for just the supply of contraceptive commodities, to $11.5 billion, for more comprehensive population activities. Two of the lowest estimates exclude China, while all of the higher estimates include China; some of the higher estimates also incorporate the costs of allied health services.

The estimates are computed by multiplying the anticipated number of contraceptive users in the year 2000 by the unit cost of providing services. The numbers of anticipated users are generally derived from the fertility targets of the

Projected Resource Requirements for Population Programs in the Year 2000

Estimation Source	Target Contraceptive Prevalence Rate (%)	Cost per User Per Modern Method User (1988 $U.S. billions)	Calculation Basis[10]	Annual Cost Year 2000 (1988 $U.S. billions)
United Nations[1]	59	17.95	ABCD	9.0
UNFPA[2]	59	1.10	A	0.6
World Bank[3]	58	19.55	ABCD	8.3
U.S. Agency for International Development[4,9]	52	19.72 – 20.25	ABCD	5.2 – 5.4
Population Council[5]	59	1.23	A	0.6
Family Health International[6,9]	48.9 – 49.5	14.10	ABCD	3.6
Research Triangle Institute[8]	Africa: 23 Asia: 57 Latin America: 55	15.00 10.00 10.00	ABCD	7.8
Population Action International[7]	75	16.00	ABCD	11.5

Notes
1. Van Arendonk 1990   2. UNFPA 1993   3. Bulatao 1985
4. Gillespie 1988   5. Mauldin and Ross 1991   6. Janowitz et al. 1990
7. Population Crisis Committee 1990   8. Kocher and Buckner 1991   9. Excluding China
10. (A) Commodity Costs   10. (B) Services   10. (C) Research/Info/Training
10. (D) others

Source: Lande and Jeller 1991.

UN's median variant population projections. The corresponding desired contraceptive prevalence rates range from 49 percent to 59 percent and translate to between 320 million and 567 million contraceptive users by the year 2000. Population Action International (PAI)[3] uses a contraceptive prevalence rate of 75 percent, which would achieve more rapid population declines; this yields 720 million users by 2000. The selection of this target has a considerable impact on the resulting cost estimates (Janowitz 1993).

To determine the average cost per user, the most common method has been to divide actual expenditures on family planning programs by the current number of users. A major limitation of this approach is the absence of comprehensive data on family planning expenditures. Estimates are based on incomplete data of poor quality, some of which are 10 or even 15 years old. Data from the private sector are rarely available, so most estimates cover only government programs. Moreover, the composition of activities included under the "population" category differs among countries, compromising comparability among national totals. In particular, government budgets reflect only the family planning services already in place; thus, if family planning services are inadequate or some services, such as abortion, are omitted, the cost estimates are correspondingly biased.

A second method involves extrapolation of the service costs in countries that have detailed data to other countries with scarce or no data. Extrapolation permits a normative assessment of the services that should be available to women, but it oversimplifies by ignoring the fact that the cost of services depends heavily on the context in which they are provided. Differences in price structure, population density, infrastructure development, and health system organization are only some factors that influence the costs of services.

These estimates suffer from several additional shortcomings. First, they are sensitive to assumptions about the evolution of costs associated with the expansion of services, changes in contraceptive method mix, and involvement of the private commercial sector (Janowitz, Bratt, and Fried 1990; UNFPA 1993). Most estimates assume that average costs will remain constant, an unlikely scenario. The marginal cost of providing services to each additional user depends on geographic and population density, private-sector development, and many other factors. In most settings, marginal costs may decline as programs expand, thereby reducing average costs (Knowles and Wagman 1991); in others, however, marginal costs may rise as programs attempt to reach more isolated population subgroups (World Bank 1991).

Second, these projections are based on a "supply" rather than a "demand" approach, as fertility targets are used to estimate future needs for contraceptive service provision. A common justification for using demographic projections to forecast demand is the concept of "unmet need" (Sinding 1992; Westoff and Moreno 1992). In Demographic and Health Surveys (DHS) and World Fertility Surveys (WFS), a substantial number of women who were not using contraception reported that they did not want any more children or that they wished to delay their next pregnancy. These women, plus those who were pregnant but said that their pregnancy was unwanted or ill timed, have an "unmet need" for contraception. The number of women in the developing world, excluding China, who have an unmet need has been estimated at 100 million

(Sinding 1992). Clearly, many women who wish to limit their fertility do not have effective access to services; it is uncertain, however, whether the mere provision of financial resources for the supply of services would meet their needs. Many economic, social, and cultural factors determine whether unmet need, however defined, will translate into real demand for contraceptive services. Moreover, the concept of unmet need ignores the range and quality of services, as well as unmarried women and men, and adolescents (Dixon-Mueller and Germain 1992).

Third, a "supply" approach makes potentially inappropriate assumptions about method mix (Gillespie et al. 1988; Janowitz, Bratt, and Fried 1990; UNFPA 1993). Specifically, the cost projections usually assume little change of contraceptive mix. When changes are assumed, the potential shifts are usually from less-costly, traditional methods to more expensive, modern methods. Another alternative, more consistent with a reproductive health approach, would attempt to identify the preferences of clients if a full range of methods and services were made available. Such a demand approach could also incorporate health and other concerns of clients, such as service quality or the availability of barrier methods to protect against sexually transmitted diseases.

From a reproductive health perspective, however, the chief limitation of current estimates is that most calculations are based exclusively on contraceptive services and demographic targets. In contrast to policies that incorporate human development objectives such as reduction of maternal and infant mortality, all current population program estimates assume that the principal objective of resource mobilization should be the attainment of global fertility targets. They thus omit the prevention and treatment of other reproductive health problems — maternal malnutrition, unsafe motherhood, infertility, unsafe abortion, and HIV and other STDs. Only one study, by Kocher and Buckner (1991), has attempted to evaluate resource needs for broader maternal and child health. Its estimates of only

"MCH" costs in the year 2000 vary between $4.1 billion, for limited-effort programs, and $7.6 billion,[4] for moderate efforts. These figures, however, are based on extremely limited data and address neither the fundamental questions of health needs nor the cost impact of alternative implementation strategies.

A reappraisal of existing estimates of resource requirements for reproductive health and the adoption of more sophisticated analytic tools for projecting resource needs is needed. Current projections of resource requirements for population programs are seriously constrained by data availability, tenuous assumptions, and bias toward a supply approach. Moreover, applying an international average for a full package of service costs — covering personnel, facilities, and other variables — to any country belies the diversity and heterogeneity that characterize the range of national and subnational settings. When projections are stretched to address broader reproductive health needs, these limitations become even more serious.

Health and Population Expenditures

Estimates of reproductive health expenditures must include both population and health budgets. The amount being provided by population budgets for contraception must be supplemented by health budget investment, direct and indirect, in reproductive health services. This type of integrated analysis has, to our knowledge, never been undertaken. Some work has been initiated by researchers at the Harvard Center for Population and Development Studies. An analysis of levels and patterns of health and population financing worldwide was commissioned by the World Bank in support of the *World Development Report 1993* (Michaud and Murray 1994; Murray, Govindaraj, and Chellaraj 1993). This work integrates estimates of health and family planning expenditures in developing countries, as well as the pattern of external development assistance in both the health and the population sectors.

One of these studies (Murray, Govindaraj, and Chellaraj 1993) estimated that global resources for health and family planning in 1990 came to $1.7 trillion, an amount equivalent to 8 percent of world income. Governments, parastatal institutions, and social security agencies financed more than $1 trillion, or nearly 60 percent, of this total; private institutions and consumers contributed the rest. Of these global expenditures, only $170 billion, or 10 percent, was spent by the developing countries of Africa, Asia, and Latin America (half coming from governments and half from private sources). Developing countries' spending for health and family planning averaged approximately 4 percent of gross national product (GNP). This proportion is half the level of the worldwide average and less than one-third the level in advanced industrialized countries like the United States.

Inequity

The distribution of health and family planning expenditures was highly inequitable among countries. The 22 percent of the world's population who live in the established market and former socialist economies spent more than $1.5 trillion in 1990, or 90 percent of the world's total health and family planning resources (see Figure 1 on next page); the United States alone consumed $800 billion of these funds. As noted, developing countries, where 78 percent of the world's people live, spent only $170 billion. The huge expenditure disparities between Northern and Southern countries are well illustrated by their respective per capita expenditure levels. People in Northern countries spent about $1,860 per capita annually, in comparison to only $41 per capita for people in Southern countries, a 40-fold difference. The difference is even more marked if the comparison is stretched from the highest-spending Northern country, the United States, at nearly $3,000 per capita, to so-called "low-income" developing countries, which average only $14 per capita, about a 200-fold difference. In some lowest-income countries, per capita health and family planning expenditures are under $5, or less than 0.025 percent of the U.S. figure.

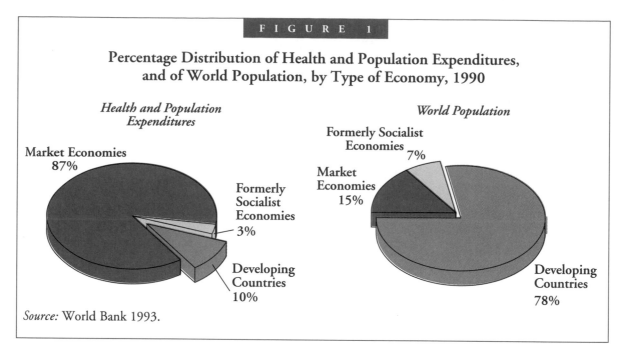

FIGURE 1

Percentage Distribution of Health and Population Expenditures, and of World Population, by Type of Economy, 1990

Health and Population Expenditures

Market Economies
87%

Formerly
Socialist
Economies
3%

Developing
Countries
10%

World Population

Formerly Socialist
Economies 7%

Market
Economies
15%

Developing
Countries
78%

Source: World Bank 1993.

Clearly, for many developing countries, current expenditure levels are insufficient to support universal access and good-quality reproductive health services. For many populations, even the so-called basic package of public health and clinical services advocated by the 1993 *World Development Report* is unaffordable where health budgets are constrained. The combined per capita cost of the public health package ($4.20) and the essential clinical package ($7.80) is $12, unreachable where average per capita health expenditure is only $14 and where governments typically spend only about $5.50 per person on health (World Bank 1993).

Diversity

Table 2 shows the estimated public-sector expenditures for family planning and health activities in the developing world. Family planning expenditures in the table were calculated using a lower and upper range of estimated average per-user costs in each region (Kocher and Buckner 1991). Data on family planning expenditures were not available for the Asian ex-Soviet republics, which the World Bank now includes in the developing country category; regional aggregates were thus used after appropriate adjustment. These data suffer from many of the same weaknesses described earlier on population resource projections.

TABLE 2

Regional Population and Health Public-Sector Expenditures in Developing Countries, 1990 ($U.S. millions)

Region	Population Expenditures	Health Expenditures
Sub-Saharan Africa	250 – 500	9,637
Asia	2,900 – 5,800	40,250
Latin America and Caribbean	375 – 750	26,218
All Developing Countries	3,525 – 7,050	76,105

Sources: For population expenditures, Kocher and Buckner (1991); for health expenditures, World Bank (1993).

The data in Table 2 show that estimates of total current family planning expenditures in the developing world range from $3.5 billion to $7.1 billion, or from about 4 percent to 9 percent of total government health and family planning expenditures. This proportion varies substantially across regions, with Asian countries allocating between 7–14 percent of health expenditures to family planning programs, African countries between 3–5 percent, and Latin American and Caribbean countries between 1–3 percent. These crude figures camouflage additional diversity across developing countries in the per capita funding of family planning programs; budgetary shares between population and health sectors also vary tremendously. Among 29 countries for which data are available, for example, the proportion of government budgets allocated to family planning programs ranges from zero to one-third (Ross et al. 1992).

In addition to government and nongovernmental organizations (NGOs), the commercial sector is an important provider of contraceptive services. Private-sector expenditures are poorly captured in currently available data, and this precludes generation of comprehensive national expenditure data. DHS data, however, provide some preliminary information on sources of contraceptives and certain basic reproductive health services. As shown in Table 3, the extent of private service provision is highly variable across developing countries. Moreover, price structures and levels in the private sector vary dramatically from country to country: IUDs range from $300 in Côte d'Ivoire to $0.17 in Indonesia; female sterilization in the private sector costs $645 in Peru, but only $1.50 in Turkey (Ross and Isaacs 1988).

National-level data on government health investments in the broad range of reproductive health services are even more elusive. Health sector budgets are rarely disaggregated according to the types of health problems addressed. In a few countries, MCH or family planning program expenditures are separated from total health expenditures. In India, for example, family planning expenditures make up 15 percent of total health spending, and MCH expenditures make up 1 percent (Griffin 1992). One thorough analysis of MCH and family planning expenditures in Sri Lanka found that the Ministry of Health devoted about 21 percent of its total resources to MCH, of

---

TABLE 3

Selected Developing Countries Categorized according to Percentage of Contraceptive Users Served by the Commercial Private Sector

≤10%	11–50%	>50%
El Salvador	Belize	Bolivia
Kenya	Cameroon	Brazil
Mali	Colombia	Dominican Republic
Mauritius	Ecuador	Egypt
Niger	Guatemala	Paraguay
Sri Lanka	Haiti	
Swaziland	Indonesia	
Tanzania	Jamaica	
Uganda	Nigeria	
Zimbabwe	Peru	
	Thailand	
	Togo	
	Zambia	

Source: Robey et al. 1992:19

which two-thirds went into maternal health (WHO 1982).

Investment Strategies

Quantitative data on amounts spent by governments and donors can mask great diversity in how funds labeled as "population" or "health" are actually invested. The organization of financing and service delivery systems determine the efficiency, effectiveness, and equity of population and health programs. The importance of going beyond amounts spent is illustrated by the cases of India and Zimbabwe, both of which spend a significant proportion of health budgets on population. In the former, population funds channeled from the central government are almost entirely devoted to "family welfare," the label used for contraceptive services. Very little of India's population budget is expended on allied reproductive health services, such as HIV or STD control, nor even on a full range of contraceptive services, since female sterilization is the principal focus of the program. In Zimbabwe, by contrast, reproductive health and contraceptive services are fully integrated.

External Assistance

Given the worldwide disparities in health and family planning expenditures, and the inability of many countries to afford minimal levels of reproductive health services, foreign aid can play a critical role. It is important to recognize, however, that health and population sector assistance by donor governments and international agencies is only part of an overall development assistance program. Thus, consideration of health and population aid should always occur within the context of overall foreign assistance levels and allocation patterns. Sadly, only a few industrialized countries have attained the internationally agreed upon foreign aid target of 0.7 percent of GNP. Japan is now the largest donor country, having overtaken the United States, which despite its larger economy provides only 0.2 percent of its GNP in development assistance. Moreover, health and population assis-

tance are only two of the social investments required for human development. It is thus important to consider health and population aid as components of the overall donor assistance being provided for social and human development.

As shown in Table 4 and Figure 2, health and population assistance disbursed in 1990 totaled

TABLE 4	
Population Aid Disbursements by Major Donors, 1990 ($U.S. millions)	
Source	Disbursement
Bilateral donors *(direct bilateral disbursements)*	
United States	280
France	143
Norway	26
Germany	16
United Kingdom	15
Sweden	14
Other	64
Subtotal	*558*
Multilateral donors	
UNFPA	180
World Bank (International Development Association and International Bank for Reconstruction and Development)	124
WHO/Special Programme for Research Development and Research Training in Human Reproduction	28
Subtotal	*332*
Large foundations/NGOs	
William and Flora Hewlet Foundation	2
IPPF	4
MacArthur Foundation	5
Ford Foundation	6
Rockefeller Foundation	11
Population Council	18
Subtotal	*46*
Total for Population	*936*

Source: Michaud and Murray 1994.

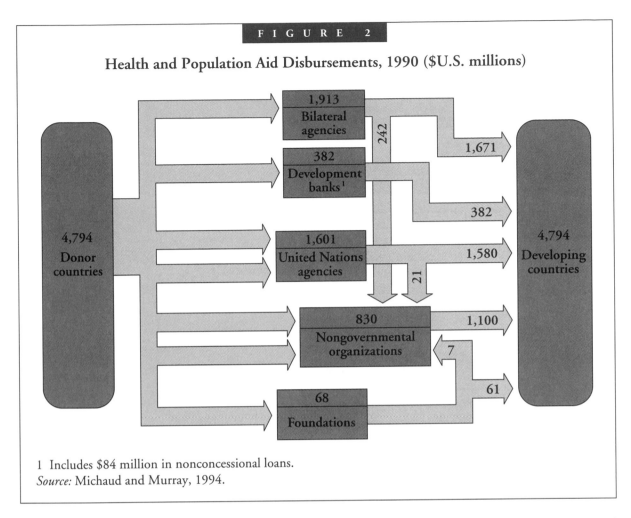

FIGURE 2

Health and Population Aid Disbursements, 1990 ($U.S. millions)

4,794 Donor countries

1,913 Bilateral agencies

382 Development banks[1]

1,601 United Nations agencies

830 Nongovernmental organizations

68 Foundations

242

21

1,671

382

1,580

1,100

7

61

4,794 Developing countries

1 Includes $84 million in nonconcessional loans.
Source: Michaud and Murray, 1994.

$4.8 billion, including $936 million for population programs. The predominant sources of these funds were industrialized country governments, although private sources were also significant. These funds were channeled either directly to developing country governments or NGOs, or through various international agencies and organizations. In the population sector, about 60 percent was provided by bilateral donors, 36 percent by multilateral donors, and 4 percent by private foundations or NGOs. The largest bilateral donors were the United States, France, Norway, Germany, the United Kingdom, and Sweden. UNFPA and World Bank provided nearly all of the multilateral aid (Michaud and Murray 1994).

It is important to underscore that 97 percent of total health and family planning expenditures in the developing world are provided by national governments and local consumers. Foreign aid constitutes only 3 percent of total expenditures. The bulk of the economic burden in paying for services thus is absorbed by developing country governments and consumers. The role of donors is far more financially significant in the population than the health sector. Foreign aid to family planning may account for up to one-quarter of resources spent on such programs in the public sector. This fact may account for the general impression that population programs are "donor-driven."

Of these total health and population sector funds, how much is invested in reproductive health? Although data are crude, a rough picture of the pattern of donor funding for reproductive health may be constructed by making assumptions about what portions of population and health assistance may be labeled as supporting reproductive health activities. These estimates are shown in Figure 3 and Table 5. Of the total health and population aid of $4.8 billion, about $2.2 billion, or 46 percent, could be classified as related in some way to reproductive health; this estimate is based upon the crude assumption that all population assistance may be classified as going to reproductive health and that health funds supporting nutrition, MCH, child survival, AIDS or STD prevention and treatment, and safe motherhood are similarly classified. Population and health aid, therefore, each contribute about half of the external aid for reproductive health. In addition to $936 million for population activities, donors provided support for services relating

to nutrition ($445 million), MCH ($360 million), child survival ($285 million), and AIDS and other STDs ($184 million). Direct donor support for the "safe motherhood" initiative was only $4 million, or less than 0.2 percent of external assistance for reproductive health.

The category of unspecified general health services accounts for 46 percent of total external assistance to health and population. Most of these funds presumably support hospital-based services. Some portion of this amount may be directed toward reproductive health. However, the magnitude of this additional spending cannot be assessed.

Conclusion

We have attempted to gain economic insights into investments in reproductive health services in developing countries and have found a paucity of data. Yet understanding the sources, volume, and patterns of expenditures for reproductive health is absolutely essential for strengthening strategies to attain high-quality and universally accessible services.

We do not know how much would be needed to meet either reproductive health or family planning costs in the year 2000. Current projections of resource requirements for population programs are too imprecise, too supply-oriented, and based upon fragile assumptions. The methodologies oversimplify or neglect many critical dimensions of reproductive health programs, such as quality of service delivery, availability of an appropriate constellation of services, full choice in contraceptive methods, and abortion services. From a reproductive health perspective, enhancing resources for the population sector would be meaningless without a qualitative shift in the investment strategies of population funds toward meeting the reproductive and sexual health needs of clients.

Our analyses underscore also the wide disparities in reproductive health expenditures between countries. Among the low- and lowest-income countries, serious gaps exist with regard to the sufficiency of financing for even rudimentary

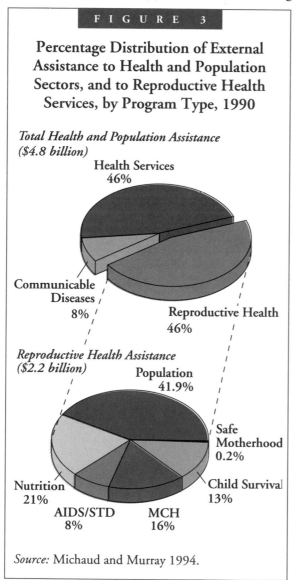

FIGURE 3

Percentage Distribution of External Assistance to Health and Population Sectors, and to Reproductive Health Services, by Program Type, 1990

Total Health and Population Assistance ($4.8 billion)

Health Services 46%

Communicable Diseases 8%

Reproductive Health 46%

Reproductive Health Assistance ($2.2 billion)

Population 41.9%

Safe Motherhood 0.2%

Child Survival 13%

MCH 16%

AIDS/STD 8%

Nutrition 21%

Source: Michaud and Murray 1994.

TABLE 5

External Assistance to Health and Population Sectors, by Program Type, 1990 ($U.S. millions)

Program	Disbursements	Percentage of Total Health and Population Aid
Reproductive health		46
Population programs	936	20
Nutrition	445	9
MCH	360	8
Child survival	285	5
AIDS/STD	184	4
Safe motherhood	4	<1
Communicable diseases		8
Tropical diseases	146	3
Leprosy	87	2
Blindness	33	1
Tuberculosis	20	<1
Others	93	2
Chronic diseases	19	<1
Health services		46
General (unspecified)	1,958	41
Hospitals	223	5
Total	4,794	100

Source: Michaud and Murray 1994.

reproductive and sexual health services. The role of bilateral and multilateral donors assumes particular importance in these settings. More information and stronger research, however, are required to improve the efficiency and effectiveness of both foreign and domestic investments in reproductive health.

Future work should seek to fill four important gaps in current information and knowledge. First, the objectives of reproductive health policies and programs, beyond the reduction of fertility, should be clearly specified and innovative approaches to assessing program outcomes developed. The chapters in this volume by Jain and Bruce, and Aitken and Reichenbach, assert that the objectives must include social and health concerns, not simply the traditional focus on fertility regulation. Further,

clearly defined program outputs are required for cost-effectiveness analyses (Simmons 1987).

Second, an underlying methodological structure for understanding resource flows in reproductive health is necessary for guiding data collection and analysis. Data on government reproductive health expenditures are extremely scarce, and private-sector data are practically nonexistent. Separating the reproductive health component of government expenditures is exceedingly difficult because of definitional ambiguity, accounting procedures, and joint costs (Janowitz and Bratt 1992). There is thus a compelling need for systems of cost estimates, including household surveys of reproductive health expenditures. Such economic studies should be country-specific, as priorities and decisions vary with local circumstances shaped by disease prevalence, levels of fertility and mortality, and institutional capacity.

Third, future work should address the hypothesis that it is socially beneficial and cost-effective to invest both health and population resources in reproductive health. As discussed by Aitken and Reichenbach, the 1993 *World Development Report* clearly concluded that reproductive health interventions are among the "best buys" in generating health returns for each dollar invested. The high ranking of reproductive health activities should be confirmed empirically in field settings and also widely disseminated among policymakers. This analysis will rely heavily on the development of appropriate outcome measures for evaluating programs with multiple health and fertility impacts.

Finally, more field studies are needed to demonstrate that the provision of integrated, comprehensive reproductive health services will generate higher benefits at lower cost than programs that provide each service vertically. Again, Aitken and Reichenbach review the preliminary evidence that an integrated approach to reproductive health can enhance both the efficiency and the effectiveness of interventions. Several small-scale experimental programs are demonstrating that high-quality care can yield high benefit-cost ratios, and that the provision of integrated reproductive health services as a package can be efficient and effective (for example, see Box 1).

Progress in all these areas will depend critically upon work within developing countries. Nearly all of the analytic work undertaken thus far has

---

B O X   1

Are Reproductive Health Services Affordable?

Are reproductive health services affordable? Financial analyses on this question especially for large-scale national programs have not been undertaken, and thus the experiences of private non-governmental organizations (NGOs) may be able to shed light on this question.

One NGO that has had extensive operational experience is the Bangladesh Women's Health Coalition (BWHC). Founded in 1980 to meet a critical gap in reproductive services for Bangladeshi women (menstrual regulation (MR)), the BWHC has dramatically expanded its services in scope and coverage. Services offered through 10 clinics now include contraception and referral for sterilization; gynecological and pre- and postnatal care; general adult and child health; child immunization; counselling, laboratory tests and referrals. In 1992-93, BWHC served over 100,000 clients. BWHC is managed by female staff committed to good quality, effective and caring services and counselling. A newly designed record system follows each client, not just episodic ser-

vices, to track clients' health on a continuing basis. BWHC also provides health education, adult literacy, and information on women's legal rights to women clients and clinical training to approximately 60 government paramedics (FWVs) annually.

Although information and client choice, counselling, follow-up, and referral require staff time, they are neither luxuries nor unaffordable. One study concluded that the average cost was $3.75 per post MR contracepting client and $5.68 per returning client, figures well within the range of costs reported for regular family planning programs in developing countries.

More studies on the experiences of the BWHC, other NGOs, and national programs are needed to determine the affordability of reproductive health services in diverse settings around the world.

Sources: Kay and Kabir 1988;
Kay, Germain, and Bangser 1991.

been based outside of the countries where data must be generated and decisions ought to be made. Since most programs will be implemented at the national and subnational levels, it is important to strengthen data collection and analytic capacity within developing countries. Global estimates, while useful, fail to accommodate diversity and could alienate, rather than promote, local ownership of investment decisions. A sustained long-term program, therefore, is needed to build economic research capability among developing country scientists in their own institutions. It will be through their work that we will come to better understand the health impact of alternative reproductive health financing strategies.

The policies of donors are critical to such capacity strengthening. Global estimates by the donor community may be useful for mobilizing population or reproductive health funding from industrialized country governments, but the problems and work to be done are mostly in developing countries. Donor funds should be invested directly in developing country scientists, policy analyses, and institutions. Such support should promote integrated analyses of population, health, and development budgets, including whenever possible the private sector. Enhancing such economic analyses would strengthen efforts to establish more effective, efficient, and equitable reproductive health services for women, and men, in the developing world.

Notes

1 For the sake of brevity, in much of this chapter we will use the term *reproductive health* as a more economical representation of the concept of reproductive and sexual health.

2 In the remainder of this chapter, the terms *population* and *family planning* may be used interchangeably. This is intended to be a rough equivalency in budgetary terms, as most population resources are devoted to family planning. It is not the intention of the authors to confuse the substantive meaning of these two terms, only to convey their similarity in fiscal matters.

3 Formerly the Population Crisis Committee.

4 The following assumptions, based on UNICEF estimates, were used to derive the totals presented here:

moderate MCH effort (at a cost of $1.50 per mother-child unit), breast-feeding promotion (costing $0.25 per mother-child unit), and immunization (at $4.00 per child).

References

Bulatao, R. A. 1985. Expenditures on population programs in developing regions: Current levels and future requirements. World Bank Staff Working Paper No. 679, Population and Development Series No. 4. Washington, D.C.: World Bank.

Dixon-Mueller, R., and A. Germain. 1992. Stalking the elusive "unmet need" for family planning. *Studies in Family Planning* 23(5):330–35.

Gillespie, D. G., et al. 1988. Financing the delivery of contraceptives: The challenge of the next twenty years. Paper prepared for the conference on the Demographic and Programmatic Consequences of Contraceptive Innovations, sponsored by the Committee on Population of the National Academy of Sciences, October 6–7, in Washington, D.C.

Griffin, C. 1992. *Health care in Asia: A comparative study of cost and financing*. Washington, D.C.: World Bank.

Janowitz, B. 1993. Why do projections of the cost of family planning differ so widely? *Studies in Family Planning* 24(1):62–65.

Janowitz, B., and J. H. Bratt. 1992. Costs of family planning services: A critique of the literature. *International Family Planning Perspectives* 18(4):137–144.

Janowitz, B., J. H. Bratt, and D. B. Fried. 1990. Investing in the future: A report on the cost of family planning in the year 2000. Research Triangle Park, N.C.: Family Health International.

Kay, B.J., and S.M. Kabir. 1988. A study of costs and behavioral outcomes of menstrual regulation services in Bangladesh. *Social Science Medicine* 26(6):597-604.

Kay, B.J., A. Germain, and M. Bangser. 1991. *Quality/Calidad/Qualité*, No.3. New York: Population Council.

Knowles, J. C, and A. E. Wagman. 1991. The relationship between family planning costs and contraceptive prevalence: Will FP costs per user decline over time? Chapel Hill, N.C: Futures Group.

Kocher, J. E., and B. C. Buckner. 1991. Estimates of global resources required to meet population goals by the year 2010. Research Triangle Park, N.C.: Research Triangle Institute, Center for International Development.

Lande, R. E., and J. S. Jeller. 1991. *Paying for family planning*. Population Reports Series J, No. 39. Baltimore, Md.: Johns Hopkins University Population Information Program.

Mauldin, W.P., and J. A. Ross. 1991. Family planning programs: Efforts and results, 1982–1989. *Studies in Family Planning* 22(6): 350–367.

McNamara, R. 1992. Robert McNamara on Global Population Policy. *Population and Development Review* 18(1):200–202.

Michaud, C., and C. Murray. 1994 (forthcoming). Aid flows to the health sector in developing countries. *Bulletin of the World Health Organization* 72(4).

Murray, C., R. Govindaraj, and G. Chellaraj. 1993. Global domestic expenditures on health. Background Paper for *World Development Report 1993*. Washington, D.C.: World Bank.

Population Crisis Committee. 1990. *Population Crisis Committee: A twenty-five year history*. Washington, D.C.: Population Crisis Committee.

Robey, B., S. O. Rutstein, L. Morris, and R. Blackburn. 1992. *The reproductive revolution: New survey findings*. Population Reports Series M, No. 11, Special Topics. Baltimore, Md.: Johns Hopkins University Population Information Program.

Ross, J. A., and S. L. Isaacs. 1988. Costs, payments and incentives in family planning programs. Washington, D.C.: World Bank.

Ross, J., et al. 1992. *Family planning and child survival programs as assessed in 1991*. New York: Population Council.

Simmons, G. 1987. Cost effectiveness and efficiency: The methodological issues. In R. J. Lapham and G. B. Simmons (eds.), *Organizing for effective family planning programs*. Washington, D.C.: National Academy Press.

Sinding, S. W. 1992. Getting to replacement: Bridging the gap between individual rights and demographic goals. Paper presented at the IPPF Family Planning Congress, October 22–24, in New Delhi.

United Nations Population Fund (UNFPA). 1990. The Amsterdam Declaration. *Population and Development Review* 16(1):185–192.

———. 1993. *Contraceptive commodity requirements in developing countries in the 1990s*. New York.

Van Arendank, J. 1990. Cited in Lande, R.E., and J.S. Jelter. 1991. *Paying for family planning*. Population Reports Series J, No. 39. Baltimore, Md.: Johns Hopkins University Population Information Program.

Westoff, C. F., and L. Moreno. 1992. Demand for family planning: Estimates for developing counties. In J. F. Phillips and J. A. Ross (eds.), *Family planning programs and fertility*. Oxford: Clarendon Press.

World Bank. 1991. *Indonesia: Family planning perspectives in the 1990s*. Washington, D.C.

———. 1993. *World development report 1993: Investing in health*. New York: Oxford University Press.

World Health Organization (WHO). 1982. National study on resource allocation for MCH/FP in Sri Lanka. Geneva.

Abbreviations and Acronyms

ACHR	Advisory Committee on Health Research (WHO)
Agenda 21	Global action plan adopted by the United Nations Conference on Environment and Development in Rio de Janeiro in 1992
ANM	Assistant Nurse-Midwife
APROFAM	Family Planning Association of Guatemala
BRAC	Bangladesh Rural Advancement Committee
BWHBC	Boston Women's Health Book Collective
BWHC	Bangladesh Women's Health Coalition
CBR	Crude Birth Rate
CEDAW	Convention on the Elimination of All Forms of Discrimination Against Women (United Nations)
CEDPA	Centre for Development and Population Activities
CEPAL	The UN Economic Commission for Latin America
CPR	Contraceptive Prevalence Rate
CYP	Couple Years of Protection
DALY	Disability-Adjusted Life Years
DAWN	Development Alternatives with Women for a New Era (from Southern countries)
DHS	Demographic and Health Survey
DHYL	Discounted Healthy Years of Life
Economic Covenant	The International Covenant on Economic, Social, and Cultural Rights
ECOS	Estudos e Comunicaçao em Sexualidade e Reproduçao Humana (Studies in Communication in Sexuality and Human Reproduction)
EPI	Expanded Program on Immunization (WHO)
FAO/ASPBAE	Food and Agricultural Organization/Asia South Pacific Bureau of Adult Education
FHI	Family Health International
FINRRAGE	Feminist International Network of Resistance to Reproductive and Genetic Engineering
GDP	Gross Domestic Product
GNP	Gross National Product

GPA	Global Program on AIDS (WHO)
HARI Index	Helping Individuals Achieve their Reproductive Intentions
HDI	Human Development Index (UNDP)
HIV	Human Immunodeficiency Virus
HRP	Special Programme for Research, Development, and Research Training in Human Reproduction (WHO)
ICASC	International Contraception, Abortion, and Sterilization Campaign
ICPD	International Conference on Population and Development, Cairo, 1994
ICRW	International Center for Research on Women
ILO	International Labor Organization
IPPF	International Planned Parenthood Federation
IWHC	International Women's Health Coalition
IWY	International Women's Year
LACWHN	Latin American and Caribbean Women's Health Network
MCH	Maternal and Child Health
MexFam	Mexican Foundation for Family Planning
NAS	National Academy of Sciences
NGO	Non-Governmental Organization
OPEC	Organization of Petroleum Exporting Countries
PAHO	Pan American Health Organization
PAI	Population Action International
PAISM	Integrated Women's Health Program (Brazil)
PATH	Program for Appropriate Technology in Health
PID	Pelvic Inflammatory Disease
Political Covenant	The International Covenant on Civil and Political Rights
PQLI	Physical Quality of Life Index
PrepCom	Preparatory Committee for the ICPD
Profamilia	Colombian Family Planning Association
RRNN	Reproductive Rights National Network (R2N2)
RTI	Reproductive Tract Infection
RU-486	Patent name for mifepristone which, used with a prostaglandin, acts as an abortifacient
SEWA	Self Employed Women's Association (India)
SIDA	Swedish International Development Authority
SIECUS	Sex Information and Education Council of the U.S.
STD	Sexually Transmitted Disease
TFR	Total Fertility Rate
UNCED	UN Conference on Environment and Development
UNDP	United Nations Development Programme
UNESCO	United Nations Education, Scientific, and Cultural Organization
UNFPA	United Nations Population Fund
UNICEF	United Nations Children's Fund

USAID	United States Agency for International Development
WDP	World Development Program
WEDO	Women, Environment, and Development Organization
WFS	World Fertility Survey
WGNRR	Women's Global Network for Reproductive Rights
WHO	World Health Organization
WHO/HRP	WHO's Special Programme on Research, Development, and Research Training in Human Reproduction
WLMLN	Women Living under Muslim Laws Network
WPPA	World Population Plan of Action
WRRC	Women's Resource and Research Center (Philippines)

Index

NOTE: Figure and table page numbers are in italics; bold page numbers refer to information in boxes.

Abortion
  and adolescents, 215, 216, 218, **218**, 219
  in the ancient world, **224**
  and coercion, 41
  and ethics, 17, 19, 21-22
  and family planning, 36, 196, 200-201, 202-203, 204, *204*, 205, 216
  and fertility control, **224**, 227, **231**
  and financial issues, 52-53, 235, 238, 244
  and the Harare Statement by Parliamentarians, **12**
  and health workers, 185
  and human rights, 94, 96, 97, 98, 99, 100
  as a legal issue, 36, 227
  politicization of issue of, 36, 227
  and reconsidering population policies, 3-4, **12**
  and reproductive health and sexual services, 29-30, 36, 37, 51, 109, 112, 178, *179*, 185, *186*
  statistics about, 227
  and the Women's Declaration on Population Policies, **33**
  and the women's health movement, 47, 49, 51, 52-53, 54, 56, 57
Abstinence, 19, 42, 215, 216
Abu, K., 163, 164
Accountability, **34**
Acharya, M., 140
Activists. *See* External change agents
Adamchak, D. M., 197
Adams, A., 8, 111, 131, 155, 161-71
Adekunle, A. O., 41
Adolescents
  and abortion, 215, 216, 218, **218**, 219
  and abstinence, 215, 216

and the community, 219, 220
and contraceptives, 213, 214, 215, 216, 217-218, **218**, 219-220
and counseling, 217-219, 220
current programs concerning, 215-217
definition of, 213
and the double standard, 41, 214, 219, 221
education/information about, 10 212, 213-214, 215-217, 218-220, 221
evaluation of programs concerning, 220
and family planning, 10, 42, 95, 212, 213, 215-217
and gender relations, 10, 212, 214, 215, 221
and the Harare Statement by Parliamentarians, **12**
and human rights, 94, 95, 212, 215, 220
implementation of programs concerning, 220-221
and individual confidentiality, 219
and marriage, 214-215
and men's responsibilities, 39
and parenting, 212
and parents, 219
and peers, 214, 216, 217, **218**, 219-220
and population education, 10, 212, 215-217
and pregnancies, 10, 211, 212, 214-215, **218**, 219-220
and premarital sex, 211, 212, 214
proposed program approaches concerning, 217-220
and prostitution, 212, 214, 218, 219
reaching young people about, 213-215, **218**
and reconsidering population policies, 10, **12**
and reproductive decisions, 215
and reproductive health and sexual services, 10, 30, 37, **38**, 42, *179*, 213-221
and self perception, 215, 218
and sex education, 218-219
and societal contradictions, 214
and status, 214-215
and STDs, 10, 212, 214, 216-218, **218**, 219-220
and violence, 10, 212

youth participation in programs concerned with, 219-220

See also specific country

Advocacy, **33**, **34**. *See also specific organization, conference, or document*

Africa

adolescents in, 211, 212, 214

autonomy in, **156**, 164, 166, 170

children in, 162, 164, 165, *165*, 169, 170, 171

contraceptives in, **155**, 161, 168-69

development in, 64

economic issues in, 67, 79, 164, **164**, 168, 170

education in, 161, 166, 168

empowerment in, 8

equality in, 80

family in, 166, **168**, 169, 214

fertility control in, 162, 167-68, *225*

fertility rates in, 80, 161, 162

and financial issues, 239, *240*, 241

gender relations in, 80, 142, 161-71, 212

household dynamics in, 8, 161-71

life cycle of women in, 166, *167*, 168-70, **169**, 171

male responsibilities in, 142

marriage in, **155**, **156**, 161, 162, 163-64, 165-66, **166**, 170

mortality in, 80, 162

parenting in, 142, 143, *144*, 165

patriarchal societies in, 162, 163-64, 169, 170

reproductive decisions in, 8, **155**, **156**, 161-71

reproductive health and sexual services in, 179-180, *181*, 183, *184*

reproductive and sexual rights in, 114

status in, **156**, 161-71

STDs in, 114, 179-180

structural constraints in, **140**, *141*, 142, 143

well-being in, 79, 80

widows in, 162, 163, *169*, 170

women's health movement in, 51-52, 54

women's relationships with women in, 8, 164-66, 170

women's roles in, 163-68, **168**, 169-71, *169*

See also specific country or people

Agarwal, B., 66, 142, 145

Ageism, 37

"Agency" freedom, 77

Agenda 21, 56

Agounke, A. M., 161

Aguilar, J.A., 219

AID. *See* U.S. Agency for International Development

AIDS

and abortion, 227

and adolescents, 212, 217-218, **218**

effects of epidemics of, 28

and family planning, 37

and fertility control, 227, 228

and financial issues, 235, 244

and gender relations, 42

and reconsidering population policies, 4, 9, 28

and reproductive health and sexual services, 9, 28, 37, 41, 42, *179*, **180**, *182*, 188

and reproductive rights, 111, 119

and research, 42

and the Women's Declaration on Population Policies, **33**

and the women's health movement, 51

Aird, J. S., 98

Aitken, I., 10, 35, 36, 37, 57, 177-189, 245, 246

Ajayi, A., 211, 214

Akan people, 167-68

Akhtar, F., 131, 132

Alternative Communication Network (Santiago, Chile), 55

Amin, S., 154

Amniocentesis, 17, 51

Amsterdam Declaration (1989), 236

Anand, S., 6, 7, 27, 28, 53, 75-83, 97, 151, 183

Antrobus, P., 28, **31**

APROFAM (Guatemala), 217

Aral, S. O., 41

Argentina, 49

Aristotle, 76

Arizpe, L., 69

Asia

adolescents in, 211, 214

development in, 8, 64

economic issues in, 8, 67

empowerment in, 8, 127, 129-137

equality in, 80

feminism in, 108

fertility control in, *225*

fertility rates in, 80

and financial issues, 239, *240*, 241

gender relations in, 80, 154

life expectancy in, 80

marriage in, 214

mortality rates in, 80

parenting in, 143, *144*

reproductive decisions in, 154

reproductive health and sexual services in, 178, *181*, 183, *184*

well-being in, 80

widows in, 143

women's health movement in, 48, 51

See also specific country

Asian and Pacific Women's Resource Collection Network, 48
Atkinson, L. E., 232
Autonomy, 151, 153-154, 155-157, **155**, **156**, 164, 166, 170

Banerji, D., 98, 99
Bang, A., 41
Bang, R., 41, 114
Bangladesh
    contraceptives in, 154
    control of income/resources in, 154
    empowerment in, 132
    family planning in, 52, 184-185, 189, 198
    gender relations in, 79, 80
    health workers in, 184-185, 187
    life expectancy in, 80
    literacy in, 79
    Matlab experiment in, 198
    reproductive decisions in, 154, 157
    reproductive health and sexual services in, 184-185, 187, 189
    structural constraints in, *141*, 145
    support networks in, 157
    well-being in, 79, 80
    women's health movement in, 52
Banister, J., 98
Barker, G., 211, 213, 220
Barnes, J., 76
Barroso, 53-54
Basic needs
    and development, 65, 66, 68, 71
    and empowerment, 8, 9
    and the environment, 71
    and human development, 7-8
    and reconsidering population policies, 4, 7-8, 9
    and structural constraints, 139, 144-147, *146*
    and well-being, 76
Basu, A. M., 119, 140, 154
Basu, K., 140, 154
Batliwala, S., 8, 127-137, 142, 157, 183
Bayles, M. D., 18
Becker, G., 163
Behrman, J. R., 142
Belizan, J. M., 178, *241*
Bender, D., 162
Benmayor, R., 118
Bennett, L., 140
Berelson, B. B., 96, 189

Berer, M., **31**, 37, 114
Berlin, Isaiah, 77
Bhasin, Kamla, 108
Bhatia, S., 187
Bhende, A., 41
Birth control. *See* Contraceptives; Fertility control; *specific method*
Bisharat, L., 166
Blaikie, P., 69
Blake, J., 28
Bledsoe, C., 165, 166, 168
Bodily integrity, 6-7, 30, **32**, 42, 95, 97, 100, 107-108, 109, 113-115, 118
Bok, S., 6, 15-25, 96
Boland, R., 6, 29, 30, 89-103, 111, 118
Bolivia, *241*
Bolton, P., 142
Bongaarts, J., 27, 198, 199, 200
Borkar, A., 130
Bose, A., 99
Boston Women's Health Book Collective, 52
Botswana, 119, *141*, 143, *144*
Boulier, B., 198
Brady, M., 37
Brandrup-Lukanow, A., 216, 217
Bratt, J. H., 245
Brazil
    abortion in, 49, 51
    adolescents in, 212
    contraceptives in, 49-50
    development in, 65
    economic issues in, 65, 79
    feminism in, 49, 111-112
    fertility decline in, 111-112
    and financial issues, *241*
    mortality in, 49
    parenting in, *144*
    reproductive health and sexual services/rights, in, **40**, 54, 111-112
    sterilization in, 111-112
    violence in, 212
    well-being in, 79
    women's health movement in, 48, 49-50, **50**, 51, 54-55
Breast-feeding, 223
Brennan, K., 97
Bridewealth, 164, **164**
Briggs, C., 30

Briscoe, J., 145
Brown, L. R., 96
Browne, Stella, 108
Bruce, J.
    and adolescents, 220
    and empowerment, 153, 154
    and family planning, 193-207
    and financial issues, 235, 245
    and gender relations, 163, 170
    overview of chapter by, 9-10
    and reproductive health and sexual services/rights,
        9-10, 27, 30, 36, 39, 114, 115, 183, 188
    and structural constraints, 140
    and the women's health movement, 54
Brunham, R. C., 179
Brydon, L., 130
Bucharest, Romania: population conference (1974) in,
    4, 67, 91, **92**, 94, 97, 101
Buckner, B. C., 238, 240
Bumpass, L. L., 143
Bunch, C., 94, 110, 111
Burkina Faso, *141*
Burundi, *144*
Buvinic, M., 140, 143

Cairo, Egypt: ICPD (1994) in, 27, 29, **31-34**, 51-52,
    53, 55, 56-57, 58, 102, 119, 120
Caldwell, J., 139, 152, 161, 162
Caldwell, P., 161, 162
Callahan, D., 22
Cameroun, 51, 217, *241*
Canada, 56-57, 217
Capabilities approach, 75-76, 77, 82
Caplan, A., 99
Caribbean, *144*, 214-215, *240*, 241
Castillo, S., 39
Castle, S., 8, 111, 131, 155, 161-71
Catholic church, 21, 51, 52
Catholics for a Free Choice, 52
CBR. *See* Crude birthrate
CEDAW. *See* Convention on the Elimination of All
    Forms of Discrimination against Women
    (CEDAW)
Central African Republic, *141*
CEPIA, 58
Chadney, J. G., 98
Chand, M., 142
Chandrasekaran, C., 198

Change
    and reconsidering population policies, 8-10
    strategies for, 8-10, 55-57
    and the women's health movement, 55-57
    See also Empowerment
Change agents
    external, 131-132, 134, 136-137
    mothers as, 140
Chant, S., 130
Chatterjee, M., 49
Chen, K., 197
Chen, L., 3-12, 79, 145, 146, 236
Chen, M. A., 157
Chesler, E., 108
Child abuse. *See* Violence
Child care
    and autonomy, 164
    and education, 152
    and employment, **143**, 154
    and empowerment, 9, **143**, 152, 154
    and gender relations, 116-117, 164, 169, 170
    and human development, 8
    and men, 9, 142
    by other children, 169
    and reconsidering population policies, 8-9
    and reproductive decisions, 169
    and structural constraints, 142, **143**, 145
    and the Women's Declaration on Population
        Policies, **33**
    and women's roles, 170
    See also specific country or people
Child health
    and education, 139
    and employment, 139, 140
    and the individual vs. society, 145
    model of, *146*
    and overburdened mothers, 139-142, **140**, *141*
    and reproductive health and sexual services, 29-30,
        37, **38**, 178, *179*, 180, *181*, *182*, 183, 188, 189
    and structural constraints, 139-142, **140**, *141*, 145,
        146
Child Survival Movement, 4
Children
    costs of, 170
    as domestic labor, 170
    foster, 165, *165*, 169, 170, 171
    and human rights, 90
    and male responsibilities, 28, 39-40
    morbidity of, 195
    mortality of, **38**, 67, 152, 162, 178, 195
    rights of, 91

value of, 171
See also Child care; Child health; *specific country or people*

Chile, 49, 51, 55, 79-80, 232

China
abortion in, 98, 99
contraceptives in, 98
development in, 65
economic issues in, 65, 77-79
equality in, 79-80
and ethics, 17, 21-22, 23
family planning in, 52, **98**, 199
fertility control in, 224, 232
financial issues in, 236
gender relations in, 79-80
human rights in, 23, 96, 98-99, **98**, 99, 100-101
life expectancy in, 79, 80
literacy in, 79, 80
mortality rates in, 80
reproductive and sexual rights in, 113
socioeconomic rights in, 23
sterilization in, 98, 99
well-being in, 77-80
women's health movement in, 49, 52

Chlamydia trachomatis, 228

Claro, A., 7, 8, **31**, 36, 53, 68-69, 102, 109, 119

Classism, **32**, **34**, 147

Cleland, J., 152

Cobbah, J. A. M., 97

Cochrane, S. H., 152

Coercion
and abortion, 41
definition of, 100
and development, 68
and ethics, 6, 20-22
and gender relations, 41
and human rights, 90-91, 96, 97-98, 100
and reconsidering population policies, 11
and reproductive and sexual rights, 29, 41, 113, 116
and well-being, 82, 83
and the Women's Declaration on Population Policies, **32**, **33**, **34**
and the women's health movement, 47

Coeytaux, F., 37

Cognitive growth model of education, 152

Coitus interruptus, 223

Colombia, **40**, 49, 143, *144*, 217, 219, 220, 224, *241*

Comilla Declaration, 54, 55

Committee on Women, Population and the Environment, 55, 64

Community
and adolescents, 219, 220
and empowerment, 9
and fertility control, 167-68
and gender relations, 167-68
and human development, 8
and reconsidering population policies, 8-9, 10
and reproductive health and sexual services, 10
women's roles in the, 167-68

Comprehensive Program for Women's Health Care (PAISM), 49, **50**

Condoms, **34**, 36, 39-40, **40**, 219-220, 223-224, 228

Conly, S., 68

Consciousness-raising, 8, 135-137, **136**

Consequential welfarism, 81

Conservatism, 4

Consortium for Action to Protect the Earth, 64

Contraception-21, 228-233

Contraceptive prevalence rate (CPR), 196-197, 198, 200, 237

Contraceptive Research and Development for the Year 2000 and Beyond (Mexico City, March 1993), 230, **231**

Contraceptives
and adolescents, 213, 214, 215, 216, 217-218, **218**, 219-220
and autonomy, **155**
barriers to, 157
benefits of, 226
and control of income/resources, 154, 226
in developed countries, *226*
in developing countries, 224, 225, *225*, *226*, 228, 232, 233
and development, 67, 68
and education, 152, 153
effectiveness of, 225, 226
and empowerment, 9, 152, 153, 154, **155**, 157
and equality, 116, 117
and ethics, 19, 21
examples of, **231**
and family planning, 39, 67, 195-197, 203, 204, *204*, 206, 216, 225, 226, 235-236
and fertility rates, 194
and financial issues, 68, 235-237, 238-239, 241, *241*, 242, 244
and gender relations, 39-40, 168-69, 223, 224, 228, 230, **231**, 232
and the Harare Statement by Parliamentarians, **12**
and human rights, 96, 98, 99, 100
as a major aspect of population policies, 3
and men, 39-40, **40**, 117

modern revolution in, 222-228

oral, 99

reasons for using, 168-69

and reconsidering population policies, 3, 4, 9, 10, **12**

and reproductive health and sexual services, 10, 36, 37, 39-40, **40**, 41, 178, *179*, 182-183, 185, *186*, 188, 189

and reproductive and sexual rights, 29, 30, 36, 37, 39-40, **40**, 41, 112, 113, 114, 115, 116, 117

research/testing of, 36, 49, 100, 117, 228-233, *233*

safety concerns about, 226-227

safety of, 36, 47

statistics about, 224, 225, *225*, *226*

and status, **155**

and "unmet need," 183

and the Women's Declaration on Population Policies, **33, 34**

and the women's health movement, 47, 49-50, 51, 53, 54, 57

and women's rights, 95

See also specific method or country

Convention on the Elimination of All Forms of Discrimination Against Women (CEDAW), 94-95, 116

Cook, R. J., 94, 95, 101, 111, 117

Copelon, R., 111

Corea, G., 28, 30, 41, 42

Correa, S.
  and adolescents, 212
  and development, 69
  and empowerment, 127
  and human rights, 91, 93, 102
  overview of chapter by, 6-7
  and reproductive and sexual rights, **31**, 107-20
  and the Women's Declaration on Population Policies, **31**
  and the women's health movement, 53, 57

Costa Rica, 39-41, 65, 79-80

Counseling, **33**, 35, 37, **38**, 39, **40**, 217-219, 220

Couple years of protection (CYP), 196-197, 205

CPR. *See* Contraceptive prevalence rate

Crane, B. B., 93, 94

Crenshaw, K., 110, 111

Crude birthrate (CBR), 196

Cuba, 65

Cutright, P., 198

Cyclofem, 50

CYP. *See* Couple years of protection

Dahlgren, G., 29

Dankelman, I., 70

Darney, P. D., 223, 224

Das Gupta, M., 152

Dasgupta, P., 82

Daughters-in-law, 169-70, *169*, 170

David, H. P., 97

Davidson, J., 70

Davis, K., 28

Dawit, S., 41

DAWN. *See* Development Alternatives with Women for a New Era (DAWN)

De Silva, W. I., 203

Deaton, A. S., 79

Decade of Women: United Nations, 4

Decision making
  and autonomy, 151, 156
  barriers to women's, 111
  and control of income/resources, 154
  and development, 68
  and ethics, 6-7
  feminist's dilemma about, 112
  and gender relationships, 151, 156
  and human development, 11
  and inequalities among women, 117
  and marriage, **155**
  and personhood, 115
  and reconsidering population policies, 6-7, 8, 9, 11, 43
  and reproductive and sexual rights, 6-7, 28-29, 30, 112, 115, 117
  and self perception, 156
  and structural constraints, 146
  and the Women's Declaration on Population Policies, **32, 33, 34**
  and the women's health movement, 47
  See also Empowerment; Reproductive decisions

Declaration on Contraceptive Research and Development for the Year 2000 and Beyond, 55

Declaration of the International Symposium on Contraceptive Research and Development (Mexico City, 1993), 58

Declaration of Mexico on the Equality of Women and Their Contribution to Development and Peace (1975), 95

Demeny, P., 67

Demographics
  and development, 67-69
  and freedom, 81-82
  and gender relations, 161-62
  and the household, 161-62

and reconsidering population policies, 28
and reproductive and sexual rights, 28, 29, 37
and well-being, 81-82
and the Women's Declaration on Population
    Policies, 32
and the women's health movement, 53
"Dependency" school, 65
Desai, S.
    and development, 70
    and empowerment, 154, 157
    and family planning, 203
    and gender relations, 164, 171
    and human development, 8
    overview of chapter by, 8
    and reproductive health and sexual services, 183, 188
    and reproductive and sexual rights, 109
    and structural constraints, 139-147
    and the women's health movement, 53
Developed countries, 20, 80, 143, *184, 226. See also
    specific country*
Developing countries
    external assistance to, 11-12, 242-244, *242, 243,
    244, 245*
    factors influencing reproductive decisions in, 152
    "unmet need" in, 238
    women's health movement in, 48-52
    See also Development; *specific country or topic*
Development
    and basic needs, 65, 66, 68, 71
    and contraceptives, 67, 68
    and decision making, 68
    and demographics, 67-69
    and the "dependency" school, 65
    and economic issues, 64-71
    and education, 67, 68
    and the environment, 63, 64, 66, 69-71
    and equity, 65, 66
    evolution of debate about, 64-67
    and external assistance, 7, 64, 68
    and family planning, 65, 67, 68, 70, 207
    and feminism, 63, 64, 70-71, 118-120
    and fertility decline, 67, 68, 71
    and funding, 68, 70, 71
    and gender relations, 64, 65, 68-69, 70, 71
    government role in, 64, 66
    and human development, 7
    and human rights, 68-69
    and the individual vs. society, 66
    and justice, 66
    means and ends of, 75-76
    and mortality, 67, 68, 71

and NGOs, 63
and political issues, 66, 68, 71
and reconsidering population policies, 4, 7, 28, 63-71
and reproductive and sexual rights, 28, 29, 68, 71,
    109, 118-120
and rights of the poor, 66
and social issues/movements, 65, 66, 67-68, 69-70
and socialism, 65
and structural adjustment programs, 65-66
and structural constraints, 139
and the "trickle-down" approach, 64-65, 66
and women as objects, 32
and the Women's Declaration on Population
    Policies, 32
and the women's health movement, 57
See also Empowerment
Development Alternatives with Women for a New Era
    (DAWN), 52, 109, 113, 114, 115, 120, 129
Discrimination, 32, 90, 91, 94-95, 96
Diversity
    and ethics, 6-7
    and financial issues, 240-242
    and human rights, 117
    and reconsidering population policies, 6-7
    and reproductive and sexual rights, 6-7, 107-108,
    113, 117-118
    in the women's health movement, 48, 53-54, 55
Divorce, 143, 164
Dixon-Mueller, R.
    and adolescents, 212, 213, 214, 215
    and empowerment, 153, 157
    and family planning, 206
    and fertility control technology, 226
    and financial issues, 238
    and reproductive health and sexual services, 183, 187
    and reproductive and sexual rights, 28, 29, 30, 35,
    36, 41, 42, 110, 113
    and the women's health movement, 48, 49, 54, 55
Djerassi, Carl, 230
Dogon communities (Mali), 165
Dominican Republic, 115, *144, 241*
Donnelly, J., 97
Dos Santos, R. B., 189
Double standard, 41, 214, 219, 221
Dreze, J. P., 80, 143
Due, J. M., 28
Dunlop, Joan, 31
Dwyer, D., 140, 153, 154
Dyson, T., 156, 166

Earth Summit. *See* Rio de Janeiro, Brazil: environment and development conference (1992) in

East and Southeast Asia—Pacific Regional Women and Health Network, 51

Economic issues
  and the "dependency" school, 65
  and development, 64-71
  and education, 132, 168
  and empowerment, 8, 128, 129-137, **136**
  and the environment, 64, 71
  and equality, 79-81, 117, 119
  and ethics, 19-22, 23
  and freedom, 75-83
  and gender relations, 164, **164**, 168, 170
  and human development, 7-8
  and human rights, 5, 23, 90-91, 94, 96, 100
  and life expectancy, 77-79, *79*
  and reconsidering population policies, 4, 7-8
  and reproductive health and sexual services, 177, 180-183, *182*
  and reproductive and sexual rights, 27, 28-29, 100, 112, 113, 117, 119
  and status, 164, **164**
  and structural constraints, 139-147
  and the "trickle-down" approach, 64-65, 66
  and well-being, 75-83, *79*
  and the Women's Declaration on Population Policies, **32, 34**
  and the women's health movement, 47
  and women's roles, 168, 170
  See also Employment; Financial issues; Funding; Poverty; Resources

ECOS, 41

Ecuador, *144*

Edemikpong, N. B., 41

Education
  and access to health care, 153
  and adolescents, 212, 214, 215-217, 219-220, 221
  and autonomy/freedom, 82, 83, 166
  barriers to women's, 157
  and child care, 152
  and child health, 139
  and contraceptives, 152, 153
  and development, 67, 68
  and economic issues, 132, 168
  and empowerment, 5, 8-9, 132, 151, 152-153, 157
  and ethics, 19
  and family planning, 67, 153
  and family size, 152
  and fertility decline, 82, 195
  and gender relations, 29, 152, 166, 168
  and human rights, 90, 100

  and marriage age, 152
  models of, impacting attitudes/behavior of women, 152
  and mortality, 67, 152
  need for improvement in women's, 68
  participatory, 219-220
  and reconsidering population policies, 4, 5, 8-9, 10
  and reproductive decisions, 151, 152-153, 157
  and reproductive health and sexual services, 10
  and reproductive and sexual rights, 29, 37, 41, 112
  and sexuality, 29
  sources of women's, 153
  and structural constraints, 139
  and well-being, 82, 83
  and the Women's Declaration on Population Policies, **33**
  and the women's health movement, 54-55
  and women's roles, 168
  See also specific country or people

Egypt, 54, 115, **188**, 199, 223, *241*. *See also* Cairo, Egypt

Ehrlich, A. H., 63, 96

Ehrlich, P. R., 63, 96

Eisenstein, Z., 110, 111

Ekwempu, F., 41

El Salvador, *241*

Elangot, F., 214

Elias, C., 36, 42, 114

Elliott, B., 178

Elmendorf, M., 146

Elshtain, J. B., 110

Elson, D., 28

Embree, J. E., 179

Employment
  advantages/disadvantages of, 153-154
  and autonomy/freedom, 79, 153-154
  and child care, **143**, 154
  and child health, 139, 140
  and empowerment, 8, **143**, 151, 153-154, 157
  and equality, 79
  and family size, 154
  and gender relations, 153, 154
  and reconsidering population policies, 8
  and reproductive decisions, 151, 153-154, 157
  and reproductive and sexual rights, 29, 112
  and resources, 140
  and sexual abuse, 212
  and structural constraints, 139, 140, **143**
  and well-being, 79
  and the Women's Declaration on Population Policies, **32, 33**
  and women's roles, 153-154

Empowerment
   and autonomy, 151, 153-154, 155-157, **155**, **156**
   and basic needs, 8, 9
   benefits of, 11
   and child care, 9, **143**
   and the community, 9
   as a concept, 127-129
   and consciousness-raising, 8, 135-137, **136**
   and contraceptives, 9, 152, 153, 154, **155**, 157
   and decision making, 8, 9, 151, 154, **155**, 156
   definition of, 8, 129
   in developing countries, 127-128, 152, 154, 155-156
   and economic issues, 8, 128, 129-137, **136**
   and education, 5, 8-9, 132, 151, 152-153, 157
   and employment, 8, **143**, 151, 153-154, 157
   and equality, 8, 130, 136
   and external change agents, 131-132, 134, 136-137
   and the family, 8, 129, 139
   and family planning, 153
   and family size, 152, 154, 157
   and feminism, 127-128
   and fertility, 8-9
   and gender relations, 8, 9, 127-137, 151, 152, 153, 154, 155-157, **155**
   as a goal, 127, 130
   and the government, 9
   and households, 8
   and human development, 8
   and the integrated development approach, 8, 136, **136**
   and interests/needs, 128, 134, 137
   and legal traditions, 156, **156**
   and lessons for an empowerment strategy, 136-137
   and marriage, **155**, **156**
   and men, 9, 29, 130-131
   and NGOs, 134-136, 137
   obstacles to, 137
   as a panacea, 127
   and patriarchal societies, 129-130, 131, 134, 136
   and political issues, 131, 134, 137
   as a process, 129, 130, 131-134
   and reconsidering population policies, 3, 5, 8-9, 11, 43
   and relationships among women, 8, 9
   and reproductive decisions, 8, 151-157
   and reproductive health and sexual services, 9
   and reproductive and sexual rights, 28, 29, 30, 42, 112- 113, 116, 119, 127, 129, 137
   and research, 9
   and resources, 8, 9, 129-137, **136**, 154, 155, 157
   and self perception, 132, 151, 156, 157
   and sexuality, 9
   and status, 5, 8, 128, 130, 136, 151-157, **155**, **156**
   as a strategy, 5, 157

   and structural constraints, 139, **143**
   and support networks, 156, 157
   and technology, 9
   and women as objects, 8
   and the Women's Declaration on Population Policies, **32**
   and the women's health movement, 8, 47, 53
   and women's rights, 9
   and women's roles, 153-154, 155-157
Entitlement theory of justice, 77
Environment
   and basic needs, 71
   data about population and the, 7-8, 69
   and development, 63, 64, 66, 69-71
   and economic issues, 64, 71
   and ethics, 17, 19-22
   and feminism, 63, 64, 70-71
   and freedom, 82-83
   and gender relations, 70, 71
   and human rights, 96, 97
   and the individual vs. society, 66
   locale-specific vs. global approaches to, 69
   and political issues, 71
   and reconsidering population policies, 4, 7-8
   and reproductive and sexual rights, 71
   and social issues/movements, 66, 69-70
   and well-being, 82-83
   and the Women's Declaration on Population Policies, **32**
   and the women's health movement, 7-8, 57
Epstein, T. S., 155
Equality
   and contraceptives, 116, 117
   and development, 65, 66
   and economic issues, 79-81, 117, 119
   and employment, 79
   and empowerment, 8, 130, 136
   and ethics, 6-7, 17
   and financial issues, 239-240
   and freedom, 79-81, 82
   and gender relations, 75, 79-81
   and human development, 7-8
   and human rights, 90, 91, 93, 94, 95, 96, 100
   and inequalities among women, 117
   and men's responsibilities, 39
   and personhood, 116-117
   and political issues, 119
   and reconsidering population policies, 6-9
   and reproductive choice, 94
   and reproductive health and sexual services, 9, 183
   and reproductive and sexual rights, 28, 39, 107-108, 109, 112, 113, 116-117, 118, 119

and well-being, 75, 79-81, 82
and the Women's Declaration on Population
    Policies, **32, 33**
and the women's health movement, 48, 53, 56
and women's rights, 94, 95
Eschen, A., 189
Esrey, S. A., 145
Establishment, and the women's health movement,
    55-56, 57
Ethics
    and coercion, 6, 20-22
    and decision making, 6-7
    and diversity, 6-7
    and ends and means issues, 16-22, 25
    and the environment, 17, 19-22
    and equality, 6-7
    and feminism, 7, 107-108, 113-118
    and gender relations, 6
    and the government, 7
    and the Harare Statement by Parliamentarians, **12**
    and human development, 6-7
    and human rights, 6, 17, 19, 20, 21, 22, 23-24, 25
    and incentives, 6, 8
    and the individual vs. society, 6, 7, 17, 25
    and legal issues, 6
    "lifeboat," 20-21
    and moral space, 6
    need for emphasis on, 15-25
    questions concerning, 6
    and reconsidering population policies, 3, 5, 11, **12**
    and reproductive choices, 6
    and reproductive and sexual rights, 6-7, 19, 107-
        108, 113-118
    and research, 6
    and resources, 6-7
    and socioeconomic issues, 19-22, 23
    and women as objects, **32**
    and the Women's Declaration on Population
        Policies, **32-33**
Ethiopia, adolescents in, 215, 216, 217-218, **218**,
    219, 220
Europe, 49, 101, 211. *See also specific country*
Evaluation
    of family planning, 9
    of programs for adolescents, 220
    and quality of care, 35, 36
    of reproductive health and sexual services, 30, 35, 36
    and the Women's Declaration on Population
        Policies, **34**
Expert Group Meeting on Population and Women
    (Botswana, 1992), 119

External assistance
    decreases in, 28
    and development, 7, 64, 68
    and family planning, 68
    and human development, 7
    by program type, *245*
    and reconsidering population policies, 7, 10, 28
    for reproductive health and sexual services, 10, *244*
    to developing countries, 11-12, 242-244, *242, 243,*
        244, 245
External change agents, 55, 131-132, 134, 136-137
Eyles, M. L., 223
Ezeh, A. C., 111

Fabros, M. L., 109
Fainzang, S., 170
Family
    and adolescent roles, 214
    as basic unit of society, 90, 91, 93, 94, 95
    and empowerment, 8, 129, 139
    and human rights, 90, 91, 93, 94, 95
    natal, 166, **168**, 169
    and reconsidering population policies, 8
    and rights, 110
    size of, 171
    and value of children, 171
    and women's rights, 95
    See also Family planning; Patriarchal societies
Family Guidance Association (Ethiopia), 216, 218,
    219
Family Health International, *237*
Family life education, 10, 215-217. *See also* Family
    planning
Family planning
    and abortion, 36, 196, 200-201, 202-203, 204,
        204, 205, 216
    and adolescents, 10, 42, 95, 212, 213, 215-217
    agendas for, 71
    aims/goals of, 19-20, 22
    case study about, 203
    and contraceptives, 39, 67, 195-197, 203, 204, *204,*
        206, 216, 225, 226, **231,** 235-236
    criticisms of, 65, 68, 70
    definition of, 9, 195
    in developing countries, 179, 193-194, 199, 206, 241
    and development, 65, 67, 68, 70, 207
    and education, 67, 153
    and empowerment, 153
    and ethics, 19-20, 21, 22
    evaluation of, 9, 196-207
    and family size norms, 196

and feminism, 120
and fertility control, 225, 226, **231**
and fertility decline, 27, 193-207
and financial issues, 22, 65, 68, 70, 235-236, 237, 241, 243
and freedom, 82
functions of, 195
and gender relations, 42, 68, 93
and the Harare Statement by Parliamentarians, **12**
and human rights, 93, 95, **98**, 99, 100
and the ICPD, 119
and the individual, 195-207, *202*
as a major aspect of population policies, 3
and men, 29, 39, **40**
and morbidity, 195, 200-201, 202-203, 204, 206
and mortality, 195, 200
need for reform of, 5, 65
objectives of, 195-196, 199-200, 206
and political issues, 68
and poverty, 67
proposals concerning, 200-205
and quality of care, 30, 35, *35*, 68, 183, 196
and reconsidering population policies, 4, 5, 9, **12**, 28, 29-30
and reproductive health and sexual services, 5, 9, 10, 27, 28, 29-30, *35*, 36-37, 39, **40**, 42, 177, 179, 183, 184-185, 188, 189, 193-207
and resources, 28
and sex education, 216
and STDs, 36, 37
and technology, 36
and unwanted/unplanned pregnancies, 195-196, 199-201, 202-203, 204, 206
and well-being, 82
and the Women's Declaration on Population Policies, **32**
and the women's health movement, 47, 49, 52, 53, 57, 68, 70
and women's rights, 95
See also specific country or program

Family size, 11, 28-29, 152, 154, 157, 196

Fathalla, M., 10, 36, 183, 223-233

Feinberg, J., 18

Feminism
and developing countries, 127-128
and development, 63, 64, 70-71, 118-120
and empowerment, 127-128
and the environment, 63, 64, 70-71
and the Establishment, 55, 57
and ethics, 7, 107-108, 113-118
and family planning, 120
and fertility decline, 107

and human rights, 102, 107
and NGOs, 120
and political issues, 110-111
and reconsidering population policies, 7
and reproductive and sexual rights, 107-120
and rights, 7
and social rights, 107
and the women's health movement, 48, 49, 51, 52, 53-55, 57, 119-120

Fertility, 4, 8-9, 39, 164. *See also* Fertility control; Fertility decline; Fertility rates; Reproductive decisions

Fertility control
and abortion, 224, 227, **231**
and adolescents, **231**
advantages of, 224
in the ancient world, **224**
and Contraception-21, 228-233
in developing countries, 224, 225, *225*, *226*, 228, 232, 233
drugs for, 227
expenditures for, 232
and family planning, 225, 226, **231**
and gender relations, 162, 223, 224, 228, 230, **231**, 232
history of, 223-224, **224**
and human rights, 93-94
international meetings about, 230, **231**
methods of, 223-225, *226*, **231**
and morbidity, 228
and patriarchical societies, 224
and the pharmaceutical industry, 233
and public-private partnerships, **231**
and reproductive and sexual rights, 29
and reproductive tract infections, 228
research and development concerning, 228-233, *233*
statistics about, 228
and STDs, 227, 228, *229*, 230, **231**
and sterilization, 225
and unwanted/unplanned pregnancies, 228, 233
and the Women's Declaration on Population Policies, **32**
and women's roles, 167-68
See also specific country, people, or method

Fertility decline
and child morbidity, 195
and child mortality, 195
and current population policies, 5
in developing countries, 82, 224
and development, 67, 68, 71
and education, 82, 195

and family planning, 27
and feminism, 107
and freedom, 82-83
and health services, 82
and reproductive and sexual rights, 107, 111-112, 113
and resources, 195
and status, 162-71
and well-being, 82-83
and the women's health movement, 47, 53
See also Family planning
Fertility rates, 162, 194. *See also* Total fertility rate (TFR); *specific country*
Filgueras, A., 212
Financial issues
  and the basic package of health services, 240
  and budget categories, 235-236
  data about, 236, 239, 244, 245
  and developing countries, 236-247, *240, 241, 242, 243, 244, 245*
  and diversity, 240-242
  and equality, 239-240
  and expenditures, 243, 244
  and external assistance, 11-12, 242-244, *242, 243, 244, 245*
  and human development, 29
  and investment strategies, 242, 244-11
  and private vs. public expenditures, 241, *241*
  projected resource requirements for the year 2000, *237*
  and reconsidering population policies, 10
  and reproductive health and sexual services, 10, 30, **40**, 180-183, *182*, 189, 235-247, *244*, **246**
  and reproductive and sexual rights, 29
  and social benefit-cost analysis, 246
  and type of economy, *240*
  and "unmet need," 238
  and the Women's Declaration on Population Policies, **34**
  and the women's health movement, 53
  See also Funding; Health: as a budget category; Population: as a budget category; Resources; *specific topic, e.g.* AIDS
Finkle, J. L., 93, 94
First birth, 166
Fisher, W. A., 217
Ford Foundation, 37, *242*
Ford, N., 211, 215, 216, 217, 220
Foreign aid. *See* External assistance
Forgacs, D., 128
Foster children, 165, *165*, 169, 170, 171

France, 52, *242*, 243
Francis, C., 42
Frank, O., 180
Frankenberg, E., 27, 39
Freedman, L. P., 95, 111, 113, 114, 115, 117
Freedman, R., 187, 203
Freedom
  "agency," 77
  and demographics, 81-82
  and economic issues, 75-79, 82-83
  and education, 82, 83
  and employment, 79
  and environment, 82-83
  and equality, 79-81, 82
  and family planning, 82
  and fertility decline, 82-83
  and gender relations, 79-82, 83
  and health services, 82
  and human development, 7
  and human rights, 93, 97, 100
  and the individual vs. society, 81
  and justice, 81, 83
  and life expectancy, 77-79
  and literacy, 77-79
  and mortality, 77-79
  negative/positive, 77, 81, 82
  and the priority of liberty, 77
  and reconsidering population policies, 7, 11
  and reproductive health and sexual services/rights, 81-82, 83, 183
  and rights, 77, 83
  and well-being, 75-83
Freire, P., 128
Fricke, T. E., 166
Friedman, M., 110
Fulani communities (Mali), 164, **164**, 165, *165*, 166, **168**
Fullilove, M. T., 41
Funding
  for abortion, 52-53
  for contraceptives, 68, 228-233
  and development, 68, 70, 71
  for family planning, 22, 65, 68, 70
  of population education, 215
  for reproductive health and sexual services, 30, **38**, 71
  for research and development, 228-233
  and the Women's Declaration on Population Policies, **34**
  for the women's health movement, 57-58
  See also External assistance; Financial issues

Gabriela (women's coalition), 57

Gage-Brandon, A., 142, 214

Galey, M. E., 95, 101

Gambia, 168-69

Garcia-Morena, C., 7, 8, **31**, 36, 68-69, 102, 109, 119

Gender relations
  and abortion, 41
  and adolescents, 10, 212, 214, 215, 221
  and autonomy, 155-157, **155**, 164, 166
  and child care, 116-117, 164, 169, 170
  and decision making, 151, 156
  and demographics, 161-62
  in developing countries, 79
  and development, 64, 65, 68-69, 70, 71
  and economic issues, 64, 164, **164**, 168, 170
  and education, 29, 152, 166, 168
  and employment, 153, 154
  and the environment, 64, 70, 71
  and family planning, 42, 68, 93
  and fertility control, 162
  and freedom, 79-82, 83
  and the Harare Statement by Parliamentarians, **12**
  and household dynamics, **33**, 161-71
  and human development, 7-8
  and human rights, 91, 92-94, 110-111
  and justice, 81
  and the media, 42
  and population education, 215
  and reconsidering population policies, 6, 7-9, 10, **12**
  and reproductive decisions, 152, 154, 162-71
  and reproductive health and sexual services, 9, 10, *179*, 183
  and reproductive and sexual rights, 28-29, 37, 39, 41-42, 92-93, 112, 114, 116-117
  and research, 42
  and resources, 155, 162-71
  and responsibilities, 39-41, 139, 183
  and rights, 110
  and self perception, 156
  and sexuality, 39-41
  and spousal communication, 152
  and status, 155-157, **155**, 162-71, **164**
  and structural constraints, 139, 142-143, **143**, *144*, 146, 147
  and well-being, 75, 79-82, 83
  and the Women's Declaration on Population Policies, **32**, **33**
  and the women's health movement, 47, 53, 54, 56
  See also Contraceptives; Fertility control; Empower-ment; Equality; Sexually-transmitted diseases (STDs); Women's roles; *specific country or people*

Genital mutilation, **33**, 41, 51, 53, 112, 113

Gente Joven (Mexico), 217, 220

Germain, A.
  and adolescents, 213, 214
  and development, 68-69
  and fertility control technology, 226, 228
  and financial issues, 236, 238
  and human rights, 102
  and male responsibilities, 10
  overview of chapter by, 9, 10
  reconsidering population policies by, 3-12
  and reproductive health and sexual services, 9, 10, 177- 178, 183
  and reproductive and sexual rights, 27-43
  and the women's health movement, 48, 49, 54, 55, 57

Germany, *242*, 243

Ghadially, R., 41

Ghana, *144*, 161, **165**, 167-68, 170, 212

Gillespie, D. G.., 238

Gilligan, C., 111

Global Campaign for Women's Human Rights, 102

Goetz, A. M., 140

Goldscheider, F. K., 143

Gollub, E. L., 39

Goody, J., 162, 163, 165

Gordon, J. E., 189

Gordon, L., 108

Government
  development role of, 64, 66
  and empowerment, 9
  and ethics, 7
  and quality of life, 11
  and reconsidering population policies, 4, 7, 9, 11, 82
  and reproductive and sexual rights, 113
  subsidies by the, 82
  and the Women's Declaration on Population Policies, **32**
  women's health movement's criticisms of, 47

Greece, 223, **224**

Grenada, 215

Griffin, C., 241

Gross, J., 41

Grown, C., 53, 65, 129, 130

Guatemala, 217, 219, 220, *241*

Guha, A., 98

Guha, R., 145

Gupte, M., 130

Gwatkin, D. R., 98

Haiti, *241*

Hamblin, J., 42

Handwerker, W. P., 41

Harare Statement by Parliamentarians, 11, **12**

Hardin, G., 20, 63

Hardy, E. E., 35

HARI index (Helping Individuals Achieve their Reproductive Intentions), 200-205, *204*, *205*

Hartman, B., 55, 57, 65

Harvard Center for Population and Development Studies, 239

Harvey, P. D., 197

Hawkesworth, M. E., 130

Hawkins, K., 10, 37, 39, 42, 184, 211-221

Haws, J. M., 95

HDI. *See* Human development index, 77

Health
    as a budget category, 235-247, *240*, *244*
    definition of, 224

Health workers, 10, **34**, 35, **38**, 49, 184-185, *184*, 187, **187**, 189

Heise, L., 41, 42, 111, 212

Helie-Lucas, M., **31**

Heller, A., 110

Helzner, J., 56

Henshaw, S. K., 227

Hermalin, A., 198, 203

Heyzer, N., **31**, 140

Heyzer, Noeleen, **31**

Himes, N. E., 224

HIV. *See* Human Immunodeficiency Virus (HIV)

Holmes, H., 91

Holmes, K., 36, 179

Homosexuality, 113, 114

Honduras, 142

Hoskins, M., 145

Households
    and demographics, 161-62
    and empowerment, 8
    and gender relations, **33**, 161-71
    and human development, 8
    and reconsidering population policies, 8-9
    refining the concept of, 162-63
    and structural constraints, 140-147
    and the Women's Declaration on Population Policies, **33**
    women's roles beyond, 166-68
    women's roles in, 163-66, 169-71

Huber, S. C., 197

Huezo, C. M., 30

Human development
    and basic needs, 7-8
    and decision making, 11
    definition of, 29
    and reconsidering population policies, 3, 5, 6-8, 11, 28-29, 42
    tradition focus of, 11
    See also Empowerment; Freedom; Well-being

Human development index (HDI), 76, 77

Human Immunodeficiency Virus (HIV)
    and adolescents, 212, **218**, 219-220
    effects of epidemics of, 28
    and family planning, 36
    and fertility control, 228
    and financial issues, 235, 238, 242
    and the ICPD, 119
    and reconsidering population policies, 4, 9, 28
    and reproductive health and sexual services, 9, 28, 36, 41, 178, 179, *179*, 180, **180**, *181*, *182*, 183, 188, 189
    and reproductive and sexual rights, 114
    and the "unmet need," 183
    and the women's health movement, 51, 53

Human rights
    and abortion, 94, 96, 97, 98, 99, 100
    and adolescents, 94, 95, 212, 215, 220
    basic documents concerning, 89-91, 101
    and children, 90
    conferences/documents about, 5, 90, 91, 102-3. *See also specific conference or document*
    and contraceptives, 96, 98, 99, 100
    criticisms of, 109
    and culture, 96-97
    and developing countries, 93-94
    and development, 68-69
    and discrimination, 90, 91, 96
    dissemination of information about, 102
    and diversity, 117
    and economic issues, 5, 23, 90-91, 94, 96, 100
    and education, 90, 100
    enforcement of provisions about, 101
    and environment, 96, 97
    and equality, 90, 91, 93, 96, 100
    and ethics, 6, 17, 19, 20, 21, 22, 23-24, 25
    and the family, 90, 91, 93, 94, 95
    and family planning, 93, **98**, 99, 100
    and feminism, 102, 107
    and fertility control, 93-94
    and freedom, 93, 97, 100
    and gender relations, 91, 92-94, 110-111

and the individual vs. society, 89, 90-91, 96-99, 109-113
and the law, 101, 102, 108
and marriage, 90
monitoring of, 101
and mortality, 97
and national sovereignty, 90-91, 93
and NGOs, 101, 102
and patriarchy, 91
and political issues, 23, 89, 90-91, 100, 108, 109-110
population documents about, 91-94, **92**
and quality of care, 100
and reconsidering population policies, 3, 4, 5, 6, 11, 28, 99-103
and religious groups, 101
and reproductive and sexual rights, 28, 29, 42, 89, 91, 92-94, 99-100, 109-113, 117, 118, 178
and responsibility, 92-93
and sex education, 100
and sexuality, 110-111
and social rights, 5, 23, 89, 91
and status, 93, 100
and STDs, 100
and sterilization, 97-98, 99, 100
and structural adjustment programs, 101
and technology, 99
universal, 102, 118
and unwanted/unplanned pregnancies, 97, 100
violations of, 89
and violence, 100, 102
as a Western invention, 23, 96
and women's conferences/rights, 91, 94-96
and the Women's Declaration on Population Policies, **32, 33**
See also specific document, or country
Human Rights Conference (Vienna, 1993). *See* Vienna, Austria: human rights conference (1993) in
Huston, P., 108

Ibo people, **156**, 167-68
ICASC. *See* International contraception, Abortion and Sterilization Campaign
ICPD. *See* Cairo, Egypt: ICPD (1994) in
ICRW. *See* International Center for Research on Women (ICRW)
Identification model of education, 152
ILO. *See* International Labour Office (ILO)
IMF. *See* International Monetary Fund (IMF)
Incentives, 6, 22, **33**, 115-116
Income. *See* Resources

India
abortion in, 51
adolescents in, 215
change in, 132
children in, **143**, 152, 154
contraceptives in, 51, 189, 197
economic issues in, 81
education in, 81, 152
employment in, 81, **143**, 154
empowerment in, 129, 132, **133**, 134, **143**, 152, 153, 154, 157
equality in, 80, 81
family planning in, 52, 114, 184-185, 197, 199, 241
fertility control in, 232
financial issues in, 241, 242
gender relations in, 41, 80, 81, 129, **143**
government role in, 81
health services in, 81, 153
health workers in, 184-185, **187**
human rights in, 97-98
life expectancy in, 80, 81
literacy in, 81
mortality in, 80, 153
reproductive decisions in, 152, 153, 154, 157
reproductive health and sexual services in, 184-185, **187**, 189
reproductive and sexual rights in, 114
SEWA in, **143**
STDs in, 41, 114
sterilization in, 97-98
structural constraints in, 142, **143**, 145
support networks in, 157
well-being in, 80, 81
women's health movement in, 48, 49, 51, 52
Individual vs. society
and child health, 145
and development, 66
and the environment, 66
and ethics, 6, 7, 17, 25
and freedom, 81
and human development, 7
and human rights, 89, 90-91, 96-99, 109-113
and reconsidering population policies, 4, 6, 7, 11
and reproductive and sexual rights, 107, 109-113, 118
and structural constraints, 145
and well-being, 81
and the women's health movement, 47
Indonesia
adolescents in, 215
contraceptives in, 99
family planning in, 52, 99, 199

fertility control in, 224
financial issues in, 241, *241*
human rights in, 23, 99
Norplant in, 99, 115
parenting in, *144*
socioeconomic rights in, 23
structural constraints in, *141*
women's health movement in, 52
Industrialized countries, 13, 228, 239, 243. *See also
specific country*
Infants
and infanticide, 99
mortality of, 67, 76, 97
Infertility, 36, 54, 178, 179-180, *179*
Infrastructure, 8-9, 29, **33**, **34**, 144-145. *See also*
Structural constraints
Integrated development approach, 8, 136, **136**
Integration of health services, 8, 10, 187-189
Inter-American Commission of Human Rights, 101
Intergenerational justice, 18
International Bill of Rights, 90-91
International Center for Research on Women
(ICRW), 42
International Conference on Human Rights (Teheran,
1968). *See* Teheran, Iran: human rights conference
(1968) in
International Conference on Population and
Development (ICPD) (Cairo, 1994). *See* Cairo,
Egypt: ICPD (1994) in
International Conference on Population (Mexico City,
1984). *See* Mexico City, Mexico: population
conference (1984) in
International Conference on Women and
Development (United Nations, 1995), 29
International Contraception, Abortion and
Sterilization Campaign (ICASC), 52
International Covenant on Civil and Political Rights
(United Nations, 1966), 90-91, 101
International Covenant on Economic, Social and
Cultural Rights (United Nations, 1966), 90-91
International Day of Action for Women's Health, 54-55
International Declaration of Human Rights (United
Nations, 1948), 90, 91
International Drinking Water and Sanitation Decade
(1980s), 145
International Labour Office (ILO), 65, 66, 76
International Monetary Fund (IMF), 66
International Planned Parenthood Federation (IPPF),
30, 37, 214, 215, 216, 219, 221, *242*

International Population Conference (Mexico City,
1984). *See* Mexico City, Mexico: population
conference (1984) in
International Reproductive and Sexual Rights Action
Group, 54
International Women and Health Meetings, 52, 54
International Women's Health Coalition (IWHC),
36-37, 48, 52, 54, 55, 56, 58, 230
International Women's Year (IWY, 1975), 95, 113
IPPF. *See* International Planned Parenthood
Federation (IPPF)
Ireland, 215
Isaacs, S. L., 95, 100, 111, 113, 114, 115, 117, 241
Isis International, 48, 51, 52, 55
Isiugo-Abanihe, U. C., 165
Islam, 53
IUD (intrauterine device), 35, 98, 99, 100, 203, 204,
204, 225, 229, 241
Ivory Coast, *141*, 241
IWHC. *See* International Women's Health Coalition
(IWHC)

Jain, A., 9-10, 36, 100, 115, 188, 193-207, 220, 235,
245
Jain, D., 142, 154
Jamaica, 65, 79-80, *241*
Jamison, D. T., 181, 182
Janowitz, B., 12, 237, 238
Japan, 76, 242
Jaquette, J. S., 49
Jayawardena, K., 49, 108
Jeffery, P., 111, 166
Johnston, A., 8-9, 93, 139, 151-157
Jolly, R., 67
Jones, D. V., 24
Joseph, A., 132
Journet, O., 170
Justice, 17, 18, **32**, 66, 77, 81, 83

Kabeer, N., 140
Kabir, S., **31**, 35, 189
Kabra, S. S., 98
Kadirgamar-Rajasingham, S., 130
Kannabiran, K., 131
Kasolo, J., **31**
Kay, B. J., 35, 189
Kelly, J., 110

Kendell, C., 142

Kennedy, P., 63

Kent, G., 145

Kenya, 41, 129, *144*, 146, 198, 199, 216, 217, 219, *241*

Keysers, L., **31**, 56

Khan, Nighat, 108

Khattab, H., 35, 111

Kilbride, J. C., 214

Kilbride, P. L., 214

King, M., 21

Kirby, D., 216

Kisekka, M., 54

Kissling, F., **31**

Knowles, J. C., 238

Koblinsky, M. A., 178

Kocher, J. E., 238, 240

Koenig, M. A., 214

Kramer, M. S., 178

Krishnan, T. N., 67

Kristof, N. D., 98, 99

Kritz, M. M., 154

Kutzin, J., 182, 183

Kyte, R., 56

LACWHN. *See* Latin American and Caribbean Women's Health Network (LACWHN)

Ladipo, O. A., 41

Laguna, *141*

Lapham, R. J., 198

Larsen, T., 98

Latin America
  abortion in, 54
  adolescents in, 211, 214-215
  development in, 64, 67
  economic issues in, 67
  feminism in, 49, 51
  fertility control in, *225*
  financial issues in, 239, *240*, 241
  gender relations in, 142, 214
  male reproductive needs in, **40**
  male responsibilities in, 142
  parenting in, 142, 143, *144*
  reproductive health and sexual services in, **40**, *181*, 183, *184*
  structural constraints in, *141*, 142, 143, *144*
  women's health movement in, 48, 49-51, **50**, 54, 55

Latin American and Caribbean Women's Health Network (LACWHN), 48, 49, 55

Law, S. A., 91

League of Nations, 89-90

Lebanon, 215

Ledbetter, R., 98

Lee, L. T., 96

Legal issues, 6, 36, 101, 102, 108, 156, **156**

Lele, U., 28

Leslie, J. M., 140

Lesthaeghe, R. J., 162, 170

LeVine, R. A., 152

Levirate (widow inheritance), 163

Liberia, *144*

Liberty, 17, 77. *See also* Freedom

Lieberson, J., 96

Life cycle, 166, *167*, 168-70, **169**, 171

Life expectancy, 76, 77-79, *79*, 80

Life Planning Education Curriculum (Center for Population Options), 217

"Lifeboat" ethics, 20-21

Lineage, 162, 170

Liskin, L., 36, 39

Literacy, 76, 77-80

Little, P., 69

Lloyd, C., 39

Lloyd, C. B., 142, 143, 161, 198

Lopez, I., 112

Low-birth-weight babies, 178

Lynan, P. J., 39

MacArthur (John D. and Catherine T.) Foundation, 37, *242*

McCarthy, J., 112

McNamara, Robert, 236

Madunagu, B., **31**

Maggwa, A. B. N., 41

Mahmud, S., 8-9, 93, 139, 151-57

Maine, D., 112, 186

Mair, L., 168

Makabenta, L., 99

Makinwa-Adebusoye, P., 154, 214

Malaysia, 23, 52, 54

Mali, *144*, **165**, 166, 169, *241*. *See also* Fulani communities

Management information systems, **33**

Manguyo, F. W., **31**

Marcelo, A., **31**

Marie Stopes Society of Sierra Leone (MSSL), **38**

Marriage
and adolescents, 214-215
age at, 95, 152, 162
and autonomy, **155**, **156**
and decision making, **155**
delay of, 42, 215
and empowerment, **155**, **156**
forced, **155**
and human rights, 90
idealization of, 214
and lineage, 170
and natal families, 166, **168**
and reproductive decisions, **155**, **156**
and reproductive and sexual rights, 28
societal contradictions about, 214
and status, **155**, **156**
women's health movement's concerns about, 53
and women's rights, 95
See also Polygyny; Widows; *specific country or people*

Martin, I., 94, 102

Mason, K., 153, 155, 161

Matamala, M., 49

Mathews, J., 57

Matlab experiment (Bangladesh), 198

Mauldin, W. P., 27, 39, 197, 198

Mauldon, J., 143

Mauritius, *241*

Mbizvo, M. T., 197

Media, **33**, 41, 42, 102, 214, 221

Medical Women's International Association First Regional Congress (Nairobi, 1993), 52

Meekers, D., 214

Men
and contraceptives, 39-40, **40**
and empowerment, 9, 29, 130-131
and family planning, 29, 39, **40**
and parenting, 9, **33**, **38**, 142-143, **143**, *144*
and reproductive health and sexual services, 9, *182*, 183
and reproductive and sexual rights, 28, 29, 30, **38**, 39- 41, **40**, 42
responsibilities of, 9, 10, 28, 29, 30, **33**, 39-41, **40**, 42, 47-48, 53, 142-143, **143**, *144*, 183
sexuality of, **33**, 39-41, **40**, 183
and sterilization, 39
and structural constraints, *141*, 142-143, **143**, *144*
and time-use studies, *141*
and unwanted/unplanned pregnancies, **40**
and the Women's Declaration on Population Policies, **33**
and the women's health movement, 47-48, 53

Menarche, 166, 168

Mencher, J., 140, 143

Menopause, 37, 166, 168

Menses inducers, 10, 230

Menstruation, 41-42, **188**

Mernissi, F., **31**

Meron, T., 101

Merrick, T., 29

Merrills, J. G., 94

Meshesha, B., 10, 37, 42, 184, 211-221

Mexfam program (Mexico), 217, 219, 220

Mexico, 49, 51, 54, 189, 217, 219, 220, 232

Mexico City, Mexico
contraceptive conference (1993) in, 58, 230, **231**
population conference (1984) in, 4, 68, 91-94
women's conference in (1975), 95, 113

Michaud, C., 232, 239, 243

Middle East, 49

Miedzian, M., 41

Mifepristone, 227

Miles Doan, R. M., 166

Miller, V., 71

Mintzes, B., 115

Misra, A., 129

Mitchell, J., 54

Molyneux, M., 128

Moore, M., 156, 166

Moral space, 6, 18-19

Morbidity
of children, 195
and family planning, 195, 200-201, 202-203, 204, 206
and fertility control, 228
and fertility decline, 195
and reproductive health and sexual services, 37, 178, *179*, 180, **180**
and STDs, 228

Moreno, L., 238

Morocco, *144*

Morsy, S., 112

Mortality
of children, **38**, 67, 152, 162, 178, 195
and development, 67, 68, 71
and education, 67, 152
and family planning, 195, 200
and fertility decline, 195
and freedom, 77-79
and human rights, 97

of infants, 67, 76, 97
and reproductive decisions, 162
and reproductive health and sexual services, 37, **38**,
178, *179*, 180, **180**, 183
and reproductive and sexual rights, 111, 112
and well-being, 76, 77-79
and the women's health movement, 49, 51
Moseley, R., 102
Moser, C., 128
Mosley, W. H., 145, 181, 182
Mothers: overburdening of, 139-142
Mothers-in-law, *169*
Mozambique, 65, 79
Mtsogolo, B., 39
Mujer/Fempress (publication), 55
Murphy, C. F., 94
Murray, C., 232, 239, 243

Nag, M., 100, 153
Nairobi, 52, 212
Narayanan, R., 98
Natal family, 166, **168**, 169
National Feminist Network for Reproductive Health
and Rights (Brazil), 49
National Research Council, 117
National sovereignty, 90-91, 93
Ndiaye, S., 161
Nedelsky, J., 110
Nekyon, F., **31**
Nelson, C., 129
Nelson, N., 154
Nepal, *141*
New International Economic Order, 65
New York City, 118
NGOs. *See* Nongovernmental organizations (NGOs)
Ngugi, E. N., 41
Nicaragua, 65
Niger, *241*
Nigeria, 48, 51, 54-55, 117-118, 154, 170, 216-217,
219, *241*.
See also Ibo people; Yoruba people
Njenga, E., **31**
Nondiscrimination. *See* Discrimination
Nongovernmental organizations (NGOs)
and adolescents, 219
and development, 63
and empowerment, 134-136, 137

and the environment, 63
and feminism, 120
and financial issues, 241, *242*, 243
and human rights, 101, 102
and reproductive health and sexual services, 177
and reproductive and sexual rights, 120
and rights, 111
and the Women's Declaration on Population
Policies, **34**
and the women's health movement, 48, 49, 51, 57
See also specific organization
Norplant, 49, 50, 99, 115, 118
North America, 49, 211
Norway, 56-57, *242*
Nowrojee, S., 9, 10, 27-43, 183, 212
Nowrojee, V., 41
Nozick, R., 77, 81

Oakley, A., 54
Obligations, 23-24, 25
Obura, A., 41, 220
Okin, S. M., 110
Okongwu, A., 143
Okun, D., 146
Olsen, F., 109
O'Neill, C., 42
O'Neill, Onora, 23
Open Forum for Reproductive and sexual rights and
Reproductive Health (Chile), 49
Oppong, C., 163, 170
Oral contraceptives, 99, 225
Oral rehydration therapy, 142, 145, 146-147
Ordway, J., 36, 54, 55, 68-69, 177-178
Osborn, R. W., 185
Otsea, K., 37
Over, M., 182

Page, H., 165
PAISM. *See* Comprehensive Program for Women's
Health Care (PAISM)
Pakistan, 79, 80
Palam, V. T., 153
Papanek, H., 157
Paraguay, *241*
Parenting
and adolescents, 212
and men, **33**, **38**, 142-143, **143**, *144*
responsibilities of, 28-29

and structural constraints, 139-143, **140**, *141*, **143**, *144*, 145

and the Women's Declaration on Population Policies, **33**

Parliamentarians, Harare Statement by, 11, **12**

PATH. *See* Program for Appropriate Technology in Health (PATH)

Patriarchal societies

    and empowerment, 129-130, 131, 134, 136

    and fertility control, 224

    and human rights, 91, 101

    and reproductive decisions, 162, 169, 224

    and reproductive and sexual rights, 114, 118

    women's roles in, 163-64, 170

Pearce, Tola Olu, 112, 117-118

Pebley, A. R., 154

Peer support. *See* Support networks

Peers, and adolescents, 214, 216, 217, **218**, 219-220

Perlez, J., 41

Personhood, 6-7, 107-108, 109, 113, 115-117, 118

Peru, 50-51, *141*, *144*, 147, 241, *241*

Petchesky, R. P.

    and adolescent sexuality, 212

    and development, 69

    and empowerment, 127

    and human rights, 91, 93, 102

    overview of chapter by, 6-7

    and reproductive and sexual rights, 28, 30, **31**, 41,

    and reproductive and sexual rights, 107-20

    and the Women's Declaration on Population Policies, **31**

    and the women's health movement, 53

Pharmaceutical industry, 233

Philippines, 48, 49, 51, 54, 109, *141*, 203, 204-205, *205*, 215

Phillips, J. F., 189, 198

Physical Quality of Life Index (PQLI), 76

Pies, C., 116

Piot, P., 182

Pitanguy, J., **31**, 41, 48, 49

Political issues

    and abortion, 36, 227

    and development, 66, 68, 71

    and empowerment, 131, 134, 137

    and the environment, 71

    and equality, 119

    and family planning, 68

    and feminism, 110-111

    and human rights, 23, 89, 90-91, 100, 108, 109-110

and reconsidering population policies, 43

and reproductive and sexual rights, 28, 30, 36, 42, 43, 113, 119

and rights, 110-111

and the Women's Declaration on Population Policies, **34**

and the women's health movement, 49, 57

Polygamy, 143

Polygyny, 161, 162, 163, 164, 165-66, 170

Population

    as a budget category, 235-247, *237*, *240*, *244*

    definitions of, **16**

Population Action International, 237, *237*

Population Council, 37, 56, *242*

Population education, 10, 212, 215-217

Population policies

    abstract nature of, 15

    agendas for, 71

    aims/goals of, 19-22, **32**, 68-69, 194, 238

    and the capabilities approach, 75-76, 77, 82

    contemporary, 3-5

    data about, 18

    definition of, 194

    and the "dirty hands" argument, 22

    documents about, 91-94

    and ends and means issues, 16-22, 25

    evolution of, 4

    fundamental premises of, 3, 4

    and the future, 15, 18

    global nature of debate about, 17, 20

    implementation of new, 100-103

    and the individual vs. society, 4, 17, 25, 66, 81, 89, 90-91, 96-99, 107

    and the instrumental vs. intrinsic views of people, 6, 75, 76, 77, 82

    interest groups concerned with, 4-5, 15-16, 27, 107

    language of, 15

    as a long-term vision, 194-196

    new approach to, 3-12, 24-25, 27-28, **31-34**, 42-43, 99-100

    and obligations, 23-24, 25

    opposition to reform of current, 100-101

    and type of government, 65

    and women as objects, 8, **32**, 53, 99, 157

    and the Women's Declaration on Population Policies, **31-34**

Potter, J. E., 189

Poverty, 27, 28, **32**, 64, 67-69, 212

Power, 107, 168, 170, 171, 212. *See also* Empowerment; Gender relations

Pregnancies
    need for sfe means of terminating, 227
    and reconsidering population policies, 3-4
    and reproductive health and sexual services, 29-30,
        37, 178, *186*, 188
    and status, 215
    See also Abortion; Teenage pregnancies; Unwanted/
        unplanned pregnancies
Premarital sex, 211, 212, 214
Preventive health care, 37
Price, M., 129
PRO-PATER (Brazil), **40**
PROFAMILIA (Colombia), **40**, 217, 219, 220
Program for Appropriate Technology in Health
    (PATH), 229, 232
Prostitution, 212, 214, 218, 219
Protacio, N., 111
Provider-client relations, 10, 35, 184-185, 189
Public assistance, 118, 142
Public health programs, **34**
Puerto Rico, 52
Pyne, H. H., 9, 10, 27-43, 183, 212

Quality of care
    and evaluation, 35, 36
    and family planning, 30, 35, *35*, 183, 196
    and human rights, 100
    and reconsidering population policies, **12**
    and reproductive health and sexual services, **12**, 30,
        35, *35*, 36, **38**, **40**, 183-189, *184*, *186*, **187**, **188**
    and reproductive and sexual rights, 119
    and the Women's Declaration on Population
        Policies, **34**
    and the women's health movement, 47, 53, 54, 57
Quality of life, 11, **32**, 75-83, *79*, 115

Racism, **32**, **34**
Rackner, L. F., 91
Rafael Salas Lecture (UN, 1991), 236
Ramasubban, R., 41, 42, 111, 214
Ramusack, B. N., 108
Rape, 41, 113, 212
Ravallion, M., 77, 79
Ravindran, T. K., 112, 115
Rawls, J., 18, 77, 81
Ray, S., 37
Reanda, L., 91

Recommendations for the Further Implementation of
    the Plan of Action (1984), 91-94, 96
Reichenbach, L., 10, 35, 36, 37, 57, 177-189, 245,
    246
Reid, E., 42
Reifenberg, A., 102
Reinke, W. A., 185
Religious groups, 30, 68, 101, 107, 110, 111, 118
Renteln, A. D., 97
Reproductive choice, 6, **32**, 83, 94, 95
Reproductive decisions
    and access to health services/information, 153, 156
    and adolescents, 215
    and autonomy, 155-157, **155**, **156**, 166
    and child care, 169
    and development, 68, 71
    and education, 151, 152-153, 157
    and employment, 151, 153-154, 157
    and empowerment, 8, 151-157
    and family size, 152
    and gender relations, 152, 154, 162-71
    and the life cycle, 168-70
    and lineage, 162, 170
    and marriage, 152, **155**, **156**
    and mortality, 162
    and natal families, 169
    and patriarchal societies, 162, 169, 224
    and reconsidering population policies, 8
    and resources, 154, 157, 162-71
    and self perception, 151, 156
    and status, 151-157, **155**, **156**, 162-71
    and support networks, 156
    See also Fertility control; *specific country or people*
Reproductive Health Matters (publication), 55
Reproductive health and sexual services
    and abortion, 29-30, 36, 37, 51, 178, *179*, 185,
        186
    access to, 183-189, *184*, *186*, **187**, **188**
    and adolescents, 10, 30, 37, **38**, 42, *179*, 213-221
    affordability of, **246**
    barriers to broadening scope of, 30
    and bodily integrity, 30
    and child health, 29-30, 37, **38**, 178, *179*, 180,
        181, *182*, 183, 188, 189
    and the community, 10
    and contraceptives, 10, 36, 37, 39-40, **40**, 41, 178,
        179, 182-183, 185, *186*, 188, 189
    and cost-effectiveness, 10, 180-183, *182*, 189
    definition of, 177-178
    and demographics, 37

and developing countries, 10, 39, 178, 179, 180, *181*, 183
and development, 68, 71
and economic issues, 177, 180-183, *182*
and education, 10, 37, 41
and equality, 9, 183
evaluation of, 30, 35, 36
and family planning, 5, 27, 28, 29-30, *35*, 36-37, 39, **40**, 42, 177, 179, 183, 184-185, 188, 189, 193-207
and fertility, 39
and financial issues, 10, 30, **38**, **40**, 71, 180-183, *182*, 189, 235-247, *244*, **246**
and freedom, 183
functioning systems for, 185-187, *186*
and gender relations, 9, 10, 37, 39, 41-42, *179*, 183
and the Harare Statement by Parliamentarians, **12**
and health workers, 10, 35, **38**, 184-185, *184*, 187, **187**, 189
and human rights, 178
impacts of, *179*, 183
and infertility, 178, 179-180, *179*
and integration of health services, 10, 187-189
justification for, 193
and morbidity, 37, 178, *179*, 180, **180**
and mortality, 37, **38**, 178, *179*, 180, **180**, 183
and NGOs, 177
objectives of, 30, 35-37, 245
and parenting, **38**
and pregnancies, 29-30, 37, **40**, 41, 177-178, *179*, 182, *186*, 188
and provider-client relations, 10, 35, 184-185, 189
and quality of care, **12**, 30, 35, *35*, 36, **38**, **40**, 183-189, *184*, *186*, **187**, **188**
and reconsidering population policies, 3, 5, 9-10, **12**, 28, 29-30, 43, 194
and religious groups, 30
and research, 9, 10, 42
and resources, 30, 35, 183
and responsibilities, 9, 183
and sexuality, 9, 29-30, 37, **40**, 41-42
and STDs, 10, 28, 29-30, 36, 37, 39, **40**, 41-42, 178, 179- 180, *179*, 180, **180**, *181*, 182, *182*, 183, *186*, 188, **188**, 189
and sterilization, 29, 30, 35, 39
and technology, 36-37
and types of services, 9-10, 53, 185-187, *186*, 235
and the "unmet need," 183
and violence, *179*
and well-being, 9
and the Women's Declaration on Population Policies, **32**
and the women's health movement, 51, 53, 54, 57
See also Reproductive and sexual rights

Reproductive and sexual rights
and abortion, 109, 112
and bodily integrity, 6-7, 30, 42, 107-108, 109, 113-115, 118
and coercion, 29, 113, 116
and contraceptives, 29, 30, 36, 37, 39-40, **40**, 41, 112, 113, 114, 115, 116, 117
and culture, 118
and decision making, 6-7, 28-29, 30, 112, 115, 117
and demographics, 28, 29, 37
and development, 28, 29, 68-69, 71, 109
and diversity, 6-7, 107-108, 113, 117-118
and economic issues, 27, 28-29, 100, 112, 113, 117, 119
and education, 29, 37, 41, 112
and employment, 29, 112
and empowerment, 28, 29, 30, 42, 112-113, 116, 119, 127, 129, 137
and the environment, 71
epistemological and historical premises for, 108-109
and equality, 6-7, 28, 39, 107-108, 109, 112, 113, 116- 117, 118, 119
and ethics, 6-7, 19, 107-108, 113-118
and family planning, 114, 120
and family size, 28-29
and feminism, 107-120
and fertility control, 29
and fertility decline, 107, 111-112, 113
and financial issues, 29
and "free and responsible" choice, 28
and freedom, 81-82
and gender relations, 28-29, 37, 39, 41-42, 92-93, 112, 114, 116-117
and government, 113
and homosexuality, 114
and human development, 28-29, 42
and human rights, 28, 29, 42, 89, 91, 92-94, 99-100, 109- 113, 117, 118
and the ICPD, 119
and incentives, 115-116
and the individual vs. society, 107, 109-113, 118
language about, 119-120
and marriage, 28
and men, 28, 29, 30, **38**, 39-41, **40**, 42
and mortality, 111, 112
and NGOs, 120
origin of term, 108
and patriarchal societies, 114, 118
and personhood, 6-7, 107-108, 109, 113, 115-117, 118
and political issues, 28, 30, 36, 42, 43, 113, 119
and power, 107
and public assistance, 118
and quality of care, 119

and quality of life, 115
and reconsidering population policies, 6-7
and relationships among women, 116
and religious groups, 107, 111, 118
and research, 36
and resources, 28, 30, 107, 118
and responsibilities, 28-29, 30, **33**, 39-41, **40**, 42
and self determination, 108, 109, 112, 118
and service provision, 29-30
and sexuality, 28, 29-30, 37, **40**, 41-42
and social issues, 28-29
and social issues/rights, 107, 114-15, 119
and status, 112
and STDs, 111, 114
and sterilization, 111-112, 113
and structural adjustment programs, 109, 119
and structural constraints, 29
and a support network, 111
and technology, 36-37
universal, 117, 118
and unwanted/unplanned pregnancies, 111, 113, 116
and violence, 29, 41
and well-being, 28, 81-82
and the Women's Declaration on Population Policies, **32**, **33**, **34**
and women's health groups, 119-120
and the women's health movement, 49, 52, 53, 56, 58
and women's rights, 108, 119-120
See also Reproductive health and sexual services
Reproductive tract infections, 54, 100, 114, *186*, 228. See also Sexually-transmitted diseases (STDs)
Research
about contraceptives, 36, 49, 228-233, *233*
and empowerment, 9
and ethics, 6
about fertility control, 228-233, *233*
and financial issues, 13, 228-233
and gender relations, 42
and reconsidering population policies, 4, 6, 9, 10
and reproductive health and sexual services, 9, 10
and reproductive and sexual rights, 36, 42
and STDs, 36, 42
and the Women's Declaration on Population Policies, **34**
and the women's health movement, 49, 54
See also Technology
Research Triangle Institute, *237*
Resources
allocation of, 28, 43
and contraceptives, 154

and decision making, 154
and employment, 140
and empowerment, 8, 9, 129-137, **136**, 154, 155, 157
and ethical issues, 6-7, 18
and family planning, 28
and fertility decline, 195
and gender relations, 155, 162-71
and reconsidering population policies, 6-7, 8, 9, 10-11, 28, 43
and reproductive decisions, 154, 157, 162-71
and reproductive health and sexual services, 28, 30, 35, 183
and reproductive and sexual rights, 107, 118
and rights, 110, 111
and status, 162-71
and structural constraints, 140, 145-147, *146*
and well-being, 76
and the Women's Declaration on Population Policies, **32**, **34**
See also Financial issues; Funding
Responsibilities
and ethics, 6, 23-24, 25
and gender relations, 39-41, 139, 183
and human rights, 92-93
and infrastructure, 144-145
of men, 9, 10, 28, 29, 30, **33**, 39-41, **40**, 42, 142-143, **143**, *144*, 183
parental, 28-29, 145
and reconsidering population policies, 6, 9, 10
and reproductive and sexual rights, 9, 28-29, 30, **33**, 39- 41, **40**, 42, 183
and structural constraints, 139, 142-143, **143**, 144-145, *144*
and the Women's Declaration on Population Policies, **32**
Riding, A., 102
Rights
abstract nature of, 110
of children, 91
classical liberal, 110
and development, 66
as an entitlement, 112, 118
and ethics, 6
and the family, 110
and feminism, 7
and freedom, 77, 83
and gender relations, 110
language about, 109-110, 118
local context for, 111
and NGOs, 111
and political issues, 110-111
of the poor, 66

and reconsidering population policies, 5, 6, 11

and religious groups, 110

and resources, 110, 111

and support networks, 111

and well-being, 77, 83

See also type of rights

"Rights of the Client" (IPPF), 30

Rimmer, C., 230

Rio de Janeiro, Brazil
environment and development conference (1992) in, 17, 54, 55, 56, 63
women's health movement in, 58

Robertson, A. H., 94

Rockefeller Foundation, *242*

Rockefeller, John D. 3rd, 91, **92**

Rodda, A., 129

Rodriguez, G., 152

Rogow, D., 39

Romania, 21-22, 52, 96, 97. *See also* Bucharest, Romania

Rosenberg, M. J., 39

Rosenfeld, M., 110

Ross, J. A., 27, 39, 197, 198, 241

Rowbotham, S., 49

Ruminjo, J., 39

Ryder, N. B., 203

Sabatier, R., 42

Safe Motherhood Initiative, 4

Safilios-Rothschild, C., 153, 156

Saith, A., 98

Sanger, Margaret, 108

Saudi Arabia, 79

Savara, M., 40, 41

Schmetzer, U., 98, 99

Schneider, E. M., 110

Schools. *See* Education: and adolescents

Schuler, M., 130

Schultz, T. P., 79, 82

Scott, D., 90

Scott, J., **31**

Segal, S., 39

Self determination, 108, 109, 112, 118

Self Employed Women's Association (SEWA), **143**

Self-development model of education, 152

Self-perception, 41, 132, 151, 156, 157, 164, 215, 218

Sen, A., 75-76, 77, 80, 81, 82, 157, 163

Sen, G., 3-12, 27, 28, 53, 63-71, 117, 120, 129, 130, 236

Senanayake, P., 37

Senegal, 79, *144*, **165**

Service provision, 2-30, **33**

Sex education, 42, 49, 100, 114-15, 216, 218-219. *See also* Family planning; Population education

Sexual abuse, 212. *See also* Violence

Sexual pleasure, 30, 42, 114-115

Sexual rights. *See* Reproductive and sexual rights

Sexuality
and development, 109
and education, 29
and empowerment, 9
and gender relations, 39-41
and human rights, 110-111
and the ICPD, 119
and the media, 42
of men, **33**, 39-41, **40**, 183
and reconsidering population policies, 9, 43
and reproductive and sexual rights, 9, 29-30, 37, **40**, 41-42
as a taboo subject, 214
and the Women's Declaration on Population Policies, **32**, **33**
and the women's health movement, 47, 49, 51, 53, 56
See also Adolescents; Homosexuality; Reproductive health and sexual services; Reproductive and sexual rights

Sexually-transmitted diseases (STDs)
and abortion, 227
and adolescents, 10, 212, 214, 216-217, **218**, 219
and condoms, 228
in developing countries, 228
effects of, 228
and family planning, 37
and fertility control, 227, 228, *229*, 230, **231**
and financial issues, 235, 238, 242, 244
and gender relations, 41-42, 228
and human rights, 100
and the ICPD, 119
in industrialized countries, 228
and men, 28, **40**
and morbidity, 228
and reconsidering population policies, 4, 9, 10, 28
and reproductive health and sexual services, 9, 10, 29-30, 36, 37, 39, **40**, 41-42, 178, 179-180, *179*, **180**, *181*, 182, *182*, 183, 188, **188**, 189
and reproductive and sexual rights, 111, 114
and reproductive tract infections, 228

and research, 36
statistics about, 228, *229*
and the "unmet need," 183
and the Women's Declaration on Population Policies, **33, 34**
and the women's health movement, 47, 53, 54, 57
Sharma, K., 130
Shaw, R. P., 69
Shelton, D., 35, 96, 197
Shephard, B., 56
Shepherd, G., 214
Sherris, J. D., 215
Shue, H., 18, 23
Si Mujer, 37
Sierra Leone, **38**, 79, 165, 166
Simmons, G., 245
Simmons, R., 36, 184, 185, 188, 189
Sinding, S. W., 19, 238
Singapore, 52, 215
Singh, H., 98
Singh, S., 211, 212, 213, 214
Social Development Summit, 57
Social issues/rights
and development, 67-68, 69-70
and the environment, 69-70
and ethics, 7, 19-22, 23
and feminism, 107
and financial issues, 246
and human rights, 5, 23
and reconsidering population policies, 5, 7
and reproductive and sexual rights, 28-29, 107, 114-15
and the women's health movement, 56
Social movements, 65, 66. *See also* Women's health movement
Socialism, 65
Society. *See* Individual vs. society
Society for Women and AIDS in Africa, 51
Soin, K., **31**
Sontheimer, S., 70
South Korea, 215
Southern countries. *See* Developing countries
Speroff, L., 223, 224
Spicehandler, J., 36
Sri Lanka
development in, 65
economic issues in, 65, 77-79
education in, 79

equality in, 79-80
family planning in, 203, 204, *205*, 241-242
financial issues in, 241-242, *241*
gender relations in, 79-80
government role in, 79
health care in, 79
life expectancy in, 79
literacy in, 79, 80
parenting in, *144*
well-being in, 77-80
Sridhar, C. R., 40, 41
Stacey, M., 129
Standard of living, 11, 90
Standing, H., 212
"Statement on women, Population and Environment: Call for a New Approach" (Committee on Women, Population and the Environment, 1993), 55
Status
and adolescents, 214-215
and autonomy, 155-157, 166
and contraceptives, **155**
definition of, 155-156
and economic issues, 164, **164**
and empowerment, 5, 8, 128, 130, 136, 151-157, **155, 156**
and ethics, 22
and fertility decline, 162-71
and gender relations, 155-157, **155**, 162-71, **164**
and human rights, 93, 100
and legal traditions, 156, **156**
and marriage, **155, 156**
and reconsidering population policies, 4, 5, 8
and reproductive decisions, 151-157, **155, 156**, 162-71
and reproductive and sexual rights, 112
and teenage pregnancies, 214-215
and women's rights, 95
and women's roles, 155-157
See also Gender relations; *specific country*
STDs. *See* Sexually transmitted diseases (STDs)
Stein, Z. A., 39
Stereotypes, 29, **33**, 41, 95
Sterilization
and ethics, 19, 21-22
and fertility control, 225, 230, 233
and financial issues, 242
and human rights, 97-98, 99, 100
and men, 39
and reproductive health and sexual services, 29, 30, 35, 39
and reproductive and sexual rights, 111-112, 113

and the women's health movement, 47, 49, 52
and women's rights, 95
Stopes, Marie, 223
Structural adjustment programs, 27-28, **32**, 53, 65-66,
101, 109, 119
Structural constraints
and basic needs, 139, 144-147, *146*
and children, 139-142, **140**, *141*, 145, *146*
and class issues, 147
and decision making, 146
in developed countries, 143
in developing countries, 143
and development, 139
and economic issues, 139-147
and education, 139
and employment, 139, 140
and empowerment, 139, **143**
and gender relations, 139, 142-143, **143**, *144*, 146,
147
and the household, 140-147
and human development, 8
and the individual vs. society, 145
and infrastructure, 144-145
and men, *141*, 142-143, **143**, *144*
and parenting, 139-143, **140**, *141*, **143**, *144*
and public policies, 142, 145-147, *146*
and reconsidering population policies, 8-9
and reproductive and sexual rights, 29
and resources, 140, 145-147, *146*
and responsibilities, 139, 142-143, **143**, 144-145,
144
and time-use studies, *141*
and the Women's Declaration on Population
Policies, **33**, **34**
Summit on Social Development, 29
Sundari Ravindran, T. K., **31**
Support networks, 111, 156, 157
Swaziland, *241*
Sweden, 42, 56-57, *242*, 243
Sweet, J., 143

Taiwan, 203, 204-205, *204*, *205*
Takeshita, J. Y., 203
Tanzania, *141*, *241*
Taylor, C. E., 189
Taylor, D., 229
Technology, 4, 9, 10, 16-17, **33**, **34**, 36-37, 53-54,
99. *See also* Research
Teenage pregnancies, 39, *179*, 211, 212, 214-215,
219-220

Teheran, Iran: human rights conference (1968) in, 91,
92, 94
TFR. *See* Total fertility rate
Thaddeus, S., 186
Thailand, 115, *144*, 215, 224, *241*
Third World. *See* Developing countries
Thomas, D., 140
Thompson, J., 23
Time-use studies, *141*
Tobago, *144*
Todd, D., 99
Togo, *241*
Total fertility rate (TFR), 196, 198, 199, 200
Toubia, N., 41, 213
Traore, B., 161
"Trickle-down" approach, 64-65, 66
Trinidad, *144*
Trubek, D. M., 90
Trusteeship, 18
Tunisia, *144*
Turkey, 241
Tushnet, M., 109
Tweedie, J., 99

Uganda, 52, *241*
UNCED. *See* United Nations Conference on
Environment and Development (1992)
UNESCO, 80, 215
UNFPA. *See* United Nations Fund for Population
Activities (UNFPA)
Unger, R., 109
UNICEF, 66
Union of Concerned Scientists, 20
United Kingdom, 55, 56-57, 214, *242*, 243
United Nations
Charter of the, 90, 91
Conference on Environment and Development (Rio
de Janeiro, 1992). *See* Rio de Janeiro, Brazil:
environment and development conference (1992)
in and the Convention on the Elimination of All
Forms of Discrimination Against Women
(CEDAW), 116
Decade for Women: Equality, Development and
Peace, 4, 95
and financial issues, *237*
and human rights, 21, 90-91, 101, 102
and the International Bill of Rights, 90-91

International Conference on Women and
 Development (1995), 29
International Covenant on Civil and Political
 Rights (1966), 90-91, 101
International Covenant on Economic, Social and
 Cultural Rights (1966), 90-91
International Declaration of Human Rights (1948),
 21, 90, 91
and the International Women's Year (IWY), 95
Rafael Salas Lecture (1991) at the, 236
and reproductive and sexual rights, 116, 119
and the Social Development Summit, 57
and women's conferences, 57, 95
and the Women's Convention (1981), 94-95, 101
and the women's health movement, 51-52, 56-57
World Conference on Human Rights (Vienna,
 1993). *See* Vienna, Austria: human rights
 conference (1993) in
United Nations Development Programme (UNDP),
 66, 76, 80
United Nations Fund for Population Activities
 (UNFPA), 215, 220, 224, 236, *237*, 238, *242*, 243
United States
 abortion in the, 52-53
 adolescents in the, 214, 216
 current population policies in the, 4
 divorce in the, 143
 family planning in the, 68, 203, 204, *205*
 fertility control in, 224, 233
 and financial issues, 239, 242, *242*, 243
 gender relations in, 41
 and human rights, 94
 parenting in the, 143
 political issues in the, 68
 religious issues in the, 68
 reproductive choices in the, 68
 reproductive and sexual rights in the, 54
 research and development in, 233
 structural constraints in, 143
 women's health movement in the, 52-53, 54, 57
Universal rights, 102
"Unmet need," 183, 238
Unwanted/unplanned pregnancies
 and adolescents, 10, 212, 214, **218**
 and family planning, 195-196, 199-201, 202-203,
  204, 206
 and fertility control, 228, 233
 and financial issues, 238
 and human rights, 97, 100
 and men, **40**
 and reconsidering population policies, 10
 and reproductive health and sexual services, 10, 29,
  30, **40**, 41, 177-178, *179*, 182

and reproductive and sexual rights, 111, 113, 116
and reproductive tract infections, 228
See also Abortion
Uruguay, 49
U.S. Agency for International Development (AID), *237*

Vasectomies, 39-40, **40**, 98
Vienna, Austria: human rights conference (1993) in,
 22, 23, 90, 96, 101, 102, 110
Vietnam, 65
Villar, J., 178
Violence
 and adolescents, 10, 212
 and gender relations, 29, 41
 and the Harare Statement by Parliamentarians, **12**
 and human rights, 100, 102
 and reconsidering population policies, 9, 10, **12**
 and reproductive health and sexual services, 9, 10, *179*
 and reproductive and sexual rights, 29, 41
 and sexual abuse, 212
 and the Women's Declaration on Population
  Policies, **33**
 and the women's health movement, 49, 51
Visaria, P., 197

Wagman, A. E., 238
Wainerman, C. H., 154
Waite, L. J., 143
Waites, G. M. H., 232
Waldron, I., 80
Walker, M. U., 18
Walters, S., 128
Walzer, M., 22
Wambua, L., 42
Ware, H., 142
Wasserheit, J., 36, 41, 42, 54, 114, 179
Wasserstrom, J., 99
WEDO. *See* Women's Environment & Development
 Organization (WEDO)
Weeks, J., 108
Weil, D. E. C., 28
Weiner, J., 69, 109
Weiss, E. B., 18
Weitzman, L., 143
Welfarism: consequential, 81
Well-being
 and demographics, 81-82
 and freedom, 75-83, *79*
 and human development, 7

and male responsibilities, 28
and reconsidering population policies, 7, 9, 11
and reproductive health and sexual services, 9
and reproductive and sexual rights, 28
and the Women's Declaration on Population Policies, **32**, **33**
and the women's health movement, 47, 48
See also Quality of life

Wertheimer, A., 21

Westoff, C., 203, 238

Westrom, L., 179

WGNRR. *See* Women's Global Network for Reproductive and sexual rights (WGNRR)

White, T., 98

Whittaker, M., 189

WHO. *See* World Health Organization (WHO)

Widows, 143, **156**, 162, 163, *169*, 170

William and Flora Hewlet Foundation, *242*

Williams, P. J., 110, 111, 116

Winikoff, B., 37

Winn, M., 41

Wishik, S. M., 197

WomanHealth (Philippines), 51

Women
commonalities among, 16
fertility control as an unfair burden to, 228
impact of population policies on, 16, 17
inequalities among, 117
isolation of, 111
as mothers, 139-142
as objects, 8, **32**, 53, 99, 157
overburdening of, 139-142
relationships among, 8, 9, 116, 164-66, 170
as sexual objects, 214
social construction of "proper," 41-42
value of, 164, **164**

Women in Action (publication), 55

Women Living under Muslim Laws Network, 52

Women's Action Agenda, 55, 56

Women's Caucus (ICPD Preparatory Committee), 53, 56-57

Women's Convention (United Nations, 1981), 94-95, 101

Women's Declaration on Population Policies, 30, **31-34**, 53, 55, 56-57, 58, 102

Women's Environment & Development Organization (WEDO), 55, 56

Women's Global Network for Reproductive and Sexual Rights (WGNRR), 48, 52, 53, 54, 55, 57, 109

Women's health groups, 5, **33**, 64, 65, 68, 69-70, 71, 119-20

The Women's Health Journal/La Revista, 55

Women's health movement
and abortion, 47, 49, 51, 52-53, 54, 56, 57
activities of the, 48, 54-55
agendas for the, 7, 52-50
central tenet of the, 47
challenges facing the, 57-58
and coercion, 47
and contraceptives, 49-50, 51, 53, 54, 57
criticisms of the, 48-49
and decision making, 47
and demographics, 53
in developing countries, 48-52
and development, 57
diversity in the, 48, 53-54, 55
and economic issues, 47
and education, 54-55
emergence/growth of the, 47, 48
and empowerment, 8, 47, 53
and the environment, 7-8, 57
and equality, 48, 53, 56
and the Establishment, 55-56, 57
and external change agents, 55
and family planning, 49, 52, 53, 57
and feminism, 48, 49, 51, 52, 53-55, 57
and fertility decline, 53
and financial issues, 53, 57-58
and gender relations, 47, 53, 54, 56
as a global movement, 52
and the ICPD, 51-52, 53, 55, 56-57
and male responsibilities, 47-48, 53
members of the, 48
and mortality, 49, 51
and NGOs, 48, 49, 51, 57
and political issues, 49, 57
publications of the, 55
and quality of care, 47, 53, 54, 57
and reconsidering population policies, 4, 7-8, 9
and reproductive health and sexual services, 9, 51, 53, 54, 57
and reproductive and sexual rights, 49, 52, 53, 56, 58
and research, 49, 54
and sex education, 49
and sexuality, 47, 49, 51, 53, 56
and socioeconomic issues, 56
statements and declarations by the, 55
and STDs, 47, 51, 53, 54, 57
and sterilization, 49, 52
and strategies for change, 55-57
and structural adjustment programs, 53
and technology, 53-54

and the United Nations, 51-52, 56-57
and violence, 49, 51
and well-being, 48
Western influence on the, 48
and the Women's Declaration on Population
   Policies, **34**
and women's rights, 49, 50-51, 55
Women's Health Project in South Africa, 54
Women's Health Research Network (Nigeria), 54
Women's movements, **33**, 65, 66. *See also specific
   movement*
Women's Network for Sexual and Reproductive
   Rights (Colombia), 49
Women's rights
   basic documents/conferences about, 94-96
   and contraceptives, 95
   and discrimination, 94-95
   and empowerment, 9
   and equality, 94, 95
   and the family, 95
   and family planning, 95
   and the Harare Statement by Parliamentarians, **12**
   and human rights, 91, 94-96
   and the ICPD, 119
   and marriage, 95
   and reconsidering population policies, 9, **12**
   and reproductive choice, 94, 95
   and reproductive and sexual rights, 108, 119-120
   and status, 95
   and sterilization, 95
   and the Women's Convention (1981), 94-95
   and the Women's Declaration on Population
      Policies, **32**, **34**
   and the women's health movement, 49, 50-51, 55
Women's roles
   and autonomy, 155-157, 170
   and child care, 170
   in the community, 167-68
   and economic issues, 168, 170
   and education, 168
   and employment, 153-154
   and empowerment, 153-154, 155-157
   and gender relations, 163-66, 170
   in households, 163-66, 169-71
   and the life cycle, 168, 169, *169*, 170, 171
   and natal families, 166, **168**, 169
   in other households, 166
   in patriarchal societies, 163-64, 170
   and power, 168, 170, 171
   and status, 155-157
   See also Status
Wong, S., 98, 99

World Bank
   and adolescent sexuality, 215
   and development, 65, 66, 67-68
   and financial issues, *237*, 238, 239, 240, *242*, 243, 246
   and human rights, 96
   and reproductive health and sexual services, 37, 41,
      177, 180, 181, 182
   and structural constraints, 139, 145, 146, 147
   and well-being, 80
World Development Report 1992 (World Bank), 147
World Development Report 1993 (World Bank), 41,
   139, 147, 180-181, 239, 240, 246
World Health Organization (WHO)
   and adolescents, 220
   and fertility control, 224, 227, 228, 230
   and financial issues, 242, *242*
   Human Reproduction Programme, 55
   Human Resource Programme, 36, 55, 56
   and reproductive health and sexual services, 178,
      185, 187
   and reproductive and sexual rights, 37, 42
   Special Programme of Research, Development and
   Research Training in Human Reproduction, 55
   and structural constraints, 145
   and the women's health movement, 55, 56
World Population Conference (Bucharest, 1974). *See*
   Bucharest, Romania: population conference (1974) in
World Population Plan of Action (WPPA, 1974), 91-
   94, 95, 96, 102, 119
Worth, D., 41
WPPA. *See* World Population Plan of Action (WPPA,
   1974)
Wulf, D., 211, 212, 213, 214
Wyon, J. B., 189

Yoruba people, 117-118, 152
Young, K., 128
Youssef, N. H., 153, 156

Zambia, *241*
Zeitlin, J., 10, 57, 183, 235-247
Zeitlin, M., 166
Zimbabwe, *144*, 197, 212, 220, *241*, 242
Zimmerman, M., 115, 118

Colophon
Book typeface: Adobe Garamond family.
Cover typeface: Adobe Utopia family.
Graphic design and production:
   Desktop Publishing & Design Co., Boston, MA.